PROGRESS IN CLINICAL AND BIOLOGICAL RESEARCH

RECENT TITLES

Please contact publisher for information about previous titles in this series.

EORTC Genitourinary Group Monograph 6

BCG IN SUPERFICIAL BLADDER CANCER

This symposium and publication have been made possible through a grant from Organon Teknika, n.v., Turnhout, Belgium.

ORGANON TEKNIKA

European Organization for Research on the Treatment of Cancer
Genitourinary Group Monograph Series

SERIES EDITORS

Louis Denis
Department of Urology
A.Z. Middelheim
Antwerp, Belgium

Fritz H. Schröder
Department of Urology
Erasmus University Rotterdam
Rotterdam, The Netherlands

EORTC Genitourinary Group Monograph 6

BCG IN SUPERFICIAL BLADDER CANCER

Proceedings of an EORTC Genitourinary Group Sponsored Meeting Held at Erenstein Castle Kerkrade, The Netherlands, on September 7–8, 1988

Organized by the Department of Urology, University of Nijmegen, The Netherlands

Editors

Frans M.J. Debruyne
Department of Urology
Radboud University Hospital
Nijmegen
The Netherlands

Louis Denis
Department of Urology
A.Z. Middelheim
Antwerp, Belgium

Ad P.M. van der Meijden
Department of Urology
Radboud University Hospital
Nijmegen
The Netherlands

ALAN R. LISS, INC. • NEW YORK

Library of Congress Cataloging-in-Publication Data

BCG in superficial bladder cancer : proceedings of the EORTC
  Genitourinary Group meeting, BCG-therapy in superficial bladder
  cancer, held at Erenstein Castle Kerkrade, the Netherlands,
  September 7th and 8th, 1988 / editors, Frans M.J. Debruyne, Louis
  Denis, Ad P.M. van der Meijden.
      p.   cm. -- (Progress in clinical and biological research ;.v.
  310) (EORTC Genitourinary Group monograph ; 6)
      "Proceedings of the First International Workshop on BCG in
  Superficial Bladder Cancer"--Foreword.
      Includes index.
      ISBN 0-8451-5160-6
      1. Bladder--Cancer--Immunotherapy--Congresses. 2. BCG
  vaccination--Congresses. I. Debruyne, F. M. J., 1941-   .
  II. Denis, L. III. Meijden, Ad P. M. van der. IV. European
  Organization for Research on Treatment of Cancer. Genito-Urinary
  Tract Cancer Cooperative Group. V. International Workshop on BCG in
  Superficial Bladder Cancer (1st : 1988 : Kerkrade, Netherlands)
  VI. Series: EORTC Genitourinary Group monograph ; 6. VII. Series:
  Genitourinary Group monograph series ; monograph 6.
      [DNLM: 1. BCG Vaccine--therapeutic use--congresses. 2. Bladder
  Neoplasms--therapy--congresses.   W1 PR668E v. 310 / WJ 504 B364
  1988]
  RC280.B5B38   1989
  616.99'46206--dc20
  DNLM/DLC
  for Library of Congress   89-8105
                                                       CIP

Contents

Contributors

Olof Alfthan, Urological Unit, Second Department of Surgery, Helsinki University, Helsinki, Finland **[271,335]**

Pierfrancesco Bassi, Department of Urology, University of Padova, Padova 35100, Italy **[81,253]**

Michael Belas, Department of Urology, Hôpital Cochin, Paris 75014, France **[153,161]**

B. Blumenstein, Department of Urology, West Virginia University, Morgantown, WV 26506 **[263]**

Laurent Boccon-Gibod, Department of Urology, Hôpital Bichat, Paris 75014, France **[153,161,325,335]**

Stanley A. Brosman, Department of Urology, Kaiser Permanente Medical Center, Los Angeles, CA 90027 **[171,193,311,335]**

P. Cárcamo, Service of Urology, La Paz Hospital, Universidad Autónoma, Madrid 28046, Spain **[237]**

G. Casanova, Department of Urology, University of Bern, Inselspital, 3010 Bern, Switzerland **[207]**

G.D. Chisholm, Department of Surgery/ Urology, Western General Hospital, Edinburgh EH4 2XU, Scotland **[93,335]**

E.D. Crawford, Department of Urology, West Virginia University, Morgantown, WV 26506 **[263]**

Ray Crispen, American International Hospital, Zion, IL 60099; and Northwestern University Medical School, Chicago, IL 60611 **[35]**

J. Crissmann, Department of Urology, West Virginia University, Morgantown, WV 26506 **[263]**

Bernard Debré, Department of Urology, Hôpital Cochin, 75014 Paris, France **[325]**

Frans M.J. Debruyne, Department of Urology, Radboud University Hospital and University Hospital Nijmegen, 6500 HB, Nijmegen, The Netherlands **[xv,11,67,285,311,335]**

Jean I. DeHaven, Department of Urology, West Virginia University, Morgantown, WV 26506 **[301]**

Wim H. de Jong, National Institute of Public Health and Environmental Protection, 6500 HB Bilthoven, The Netherlands **[11,67,285]**

The numbers in brackets are the opening page numbers of the Contributors'articles.

J.B. DeKernion, Division of Urology, UCLA Medical Center, Los Angeles, CA **[171]**

Louis Denis, Department of Urology, A.Z. Middelheim, Antwerp, Belgium **[xv]**

M. de Pauw, EORTC Data Center, B-1000 Brussels, Belgium **[125]**

Wim Doesburg, Department of Statistical Consultation, University of Nijmegen, 6500 HB Nijmegen, The Netherlands **[285]**

Hugh A.F. Fisher, Department of Urologic Oncology, Albany Medical College, Albany, NY 12208 **[275,335]**

L. Fiter, Service of Urology, La Paz Hospital, Universidad Autónoma, Madrid 28046, Spain **[237]**

Antonio Garbeglio, Department of Urology, University of Padova, Padova 35100, Italy **[253]**

M.J. García Matres, Service of Urology, La Paz Hospital, Universidad Autónoma, Madrid 28046, Spain **[237]**

H.B. Grossman, Department of Urology, West Virginia University, Morgantown, WV 26506 **[263]**

Stefano Guazzieri, Department of Urology, University of Padova, Padova 35100, Italy **[253]**

P. Guinan, Division of Urology, University of Illinois at Chicago, Chicago, IL 60612 **[171]**

M.G. Hanna, Jr., Organon Teknika, Bionetics Research Institute, Rockville, MD 20850 **[51,171,335]**

T.B. Hargreave, Department of Surgery/ Urology, Western General Hospital, Edinburgh EH4 2XU, Scotland **[93]**

J.M. Herve, Department of Urology, Hôpital Cochin, Paris 75014, France **[161]**

H.C. Hoover, Jr., Department of Surgical Oncology, Massachusetts General Hospital, Harvard Medical School, Boston, MA 02114 **[51]**

K. James, Department of Surgery, Western General Hospital, Edinburgh EH4 2XU, Scotland **[93]**

Gerhard Jaske, Urologische Klinik und Poliklinik, Klinikum rechts der Isar, Technische Universität, D-8000 Munich, Federal Republic of Germany **[187,335]**

Kari Jauhiainen, Department of Surgery, Mikkeli Central Hospital, Mikkeli, Finland **[271]**

Anne M. Jordan, Department of Pathology, Baptist Memorial Hospital, Memphis, TN 38146 **[215]**

O.P. Khanna, Department of Surgery, Hahnemann University, Philadelphia, PA 19102 **[171]**

R. Kraft, Institute of Pathology, Division of Diagnostic Cytology, University of Bern, 3010 Bern, Switzerland **[207]**

K.H. Kurth, Department of Urology, University of Amsterdam, 1105 AZ Amsterdam, The Netherlands **[125]**

D.L. Lamm, Department of Urology, West Virginia University School of Medicine, Morgantown, WV 26506 **[171,263,301,311,335]**

Christian Leleu, Department of Urology, Hôpital Cochin, Paris 75014, France **[153,161,325]**

J. Jimenez León, Service of Urology, La Paz Hospital, Universidad Autónoma, Madrid 28046, Spain **[237]**

J.A. Martinez-Pineiro, Service of Urology, La Paz Hospital, Universidad Autónoma, Madrid 28046, Spain **[237]**

L. Martinez-Pineiro, Jr., Service of Urology, La Paz Hospital, Universidad Autónoma, Madrid 28046, Spain **[237]**

Agostino Meneghini, Department of Urology, University of Padova, Padova 35100, Italy **[253]**

Claudio Milani, Department of Urology, University of Padova, Padova 35100, Italy **[81,253]**

J. Montie, Department of Urology, West Virginia University, Morgantown, WV 26506 **[263]**

Alvaro Morales, Department of Urology, Queen's University, Kingston General Hospital, Kingston K7L 2V7, Ontario, Canada **[3,335,361]**

J.A. Mosteiro, Service of Urology, La Paz Hospital, Universidad Autónoma, Madrid 28046, Spain **[237]**

William M. Murphy, Department of Pathology, Baptist Memorial Hospital, Memphis, TN 38146 **[215]**

J. Navarro, Service of Urology, La Paz Hospital, Universidad Autónoma, Madrid 28046, Spain **[237]**

J. Curtis Nickel, Department of Urology, Queen's University, Kingston K7L 2V7, Ontario, Canada **[361]**

Francesco Pagano, Department of Urology, University of Padova, Padova 35100, Italy **[81,253,335]**

Paolo Dalla Palma, Department of Urology, University of Padova, Padova 35100, Italy **[81]**

Anna Parenti, Department of Urology, University of Padova, Padova 35100, Italy **[81]**

Michele Pavone-Macaluso, Institute of Urology, University of Palermo, Palermo, 90127, Italy **[357]**

L.C. Peters, Organon Teknika, Bionetics Research Institute, Rockville, MD 20850 **[51]**

Alessandro Poletti, Department of Urology, University of Padova, Padova 35100, Italy **[81]**

S. Prescott, Department of Surgery/ Urology, Western General Hospital, Edinburgh EH4 2XU, Scotland **[93]**

Timothy L. Ratliff, Department of Surgery, Washington University School of Medicine and The Jewish Hospital of St. Louis, St. Louis, MO 63110 **[107]**

Anna Grazia Rebuffi, Department of Urology, University of Padova, Padova 35100, Italy **[81]**

D.J. Reitsma, Organon Teknika, Bionetics Research Institute, Rockville, MD 20850 **[171]**

Erkki Rintala, Urological Unit, Second Department of Surgery, Helsinki University, Helsinki, Finland **[271]**

Mell R.G. Robinson, Department of Urology, Pontefract General Infirmary, Friarwood, Pontefract WF7 7LP, England **[147]**

Joost E. Rultenberg, Department of Pathology, National Institute of Public Health and Environmental Protection, 6500 HB Bilthoven, The Netherlands **[xvii,67]**

Michael S. Sarosdy, Department of Surgery, Division of Urology, University of Texas Health Science Center, San Antonio, TX 78284 **[263,301]**

P. Scardino, Department of Urology, West Virginia University, Morgantown, WV 26506 **[263]**

Vincenzo Serrette, Interdepartment Center for Research in Clinical Oncology, University of Palermo, Palermo 91027, Italy **[357]**

Didier Sicard, Department of Medicine, Hôpital Cochin, 75014 Paris, France **[325]**

G. Simpson, Organon Teknika, Bionetics Research Institute, Rockville, MD 20850 **[171]**

J. Smith, Department of Urology, West Virginia University, Morgantown, WV 26506 **[263]**

J.F. Smyth, Imperial Cancer Research Fund, Medical Oncology Unit, University of Edinburgh, Western General Hospital, Edinburgh EH4 2XU, Scotland **[93]**

Mark S. Soloway, Department of Urology, University of Tennessee, Memphis, TN 38163 **[215]**

T. Stanisic, Department of Urology, West Virginia University, Morgantown, WV 26506 **[263]**

Peter A. Steerenberg, National Institute of Public Health and Environmental Protection, 6500 HB Bilthoven, The Netherlands **[11,67,285]**

Adolphe Steg, Department of Urology, Hôpital Cochin, Paris 75014, France **[153,161,325,335]**

U.E. Studer, Department of Urology, University of Bern, Inselspital, 3010 Bern, Switzerland **[207]**

J. Sullivan, Department of Urology, West Virginia University, Morgantown, WV 26506 **[263]**

R. Sylvester, EORTC Data Center, B-1000 Brussels, Belgium **[125]**

F. ten Kate, Department of Pathology, University of Rotterdam, 3015 GD Rotterdam, The Netherlands **[125]**

Giuseppe Tuccitto, Department of Urology, University of Padova, Padova 35100, Italy **[253]**

Ad P.M. van der Meijden, Department of Urology, University Hospital Nijmegen, 6500 HB, Nijmegen, The Netherlands **[xv,11,67,285,311,335]**

R.D. Williams, Department of Urology, University of Iowa Hospital and Clinic, Iowa City, IA 52242 **[171]**

E.J. Zingg, Department of Urology, University of Bern, 3010 Bern, Switzerland **[207]**

Foreword

This volume presents the proceedings of the First International Workshop on BCG in Superficial Bladder Cancer. The meeting was organized in Kerkrade, the Netherlands, September 7–8, 1988. Bacillus Calmette–Guérin (BCG) is now widely accepted as a highly effective therapy for carcinoma in situ of the urinary bladder. Its efficacy as an adjuvant therapy for superficial bladder cancer after complete or incomplete transurethral resection has also been proved. In the wake of these promising results, BCG is now promoted worldwide, after several decades during which intravesicular chemotherapeutic agents were used exclusively.

Despite increasing fundamental and clinical experience, the majority of questions raised ten years ago still have to be answered. The mechanisms that govern how BCG exerts its antitumor effect remain unclear. The preferred treatment schedule, the appropriate strain, and the optimal dose are unknown. The superiority of BCG over intravesicular chemotherapy has been demonstrated in several studies. Nevertheless, data from controlled prospective randomized trials are needed to determine the exact place of this form of nonspecific active immunotherapy. Since this adjuvant therapy seems to have more noticeable side effects than intravesicular chemotherapy, a careful risk–to–benefit analysis has to be made by urologists about whether BCG should be used in their patients. All these considerations led to the initiation of this first international workshop.

Outstanding researchers and clinicians from the United States and Europe, including nearly all the pioneers in this field, gathered to present their data, and above all to discuss controversial and unknown aspects of BCG. We are grateful for the support of the European Organisation for Research and Treatment of Cancer Genitourinary Group (EORTC–GU) and the Urological Research Foundation Nijmegen (STIWU) for helping to organize this meeting.

We thank Organon Teknika, Belgium, for generous financial support and the superb arrangements in Kerkrade,Mr. Grossblatt for revision of the contributions, and Mrs. D.M. Litjens–de–Heus for her editorial assistance and complete arrangement of all manuscripts.

Frans M.J. Debruyne
Louis Denis
Ad P.M. van der Meijden

Introduction

Bacillus Calmette–Guérin (BCG) and Immunotherapy

BCG immunotherapy in cancer has been a topic of experimental and clinical research for some time. The International Workshop on BCG in Superficial Bladder Cancer, held in Kerkrade, the Netherlands, offered a forum for discussion of several questions stemming from this research.

BCG, a bacterial adjuvant, has been used for immunostimulation since the late 1960s. It was found to have a profound effect on the immune system. The prophylactic and therapeutic antitumor activity of BCG was demonstrated in several animal tumor systems. However, clinical use of BCG immunotherapy in humans has been disappointing, with the exception of the success of treating superficial bladder cancer and carcinoma in situ. Although the mechanism by which BCG exerts its antitumor activity is still largely unknown, it has been suggested that local contact of BCG with tumor cells is needed. This contact may result in an immune reaction not only against BCG but also against the tumor cells themselves.

Laboratory studies have shown that BCG administration results in tumor-specific immunity in several animal systems. The effect of BCG depends on multiple factors like the BCG vaccine (strain of BCG, amount of dead material and additive present in the vaccine), the administered dose, the route of administration, and possibly the genetic background of the host. Immunologically, stimulation by BCG is partially mediated by the activation of T cells. General stimulation of the mononuclear phagocyte system and the induction of cytotoxic effector cells play a role as well. The result of BCG administration occurred apart from the induction of a granulomatous reaction concomitantly with the activation of the mononuclear phagocytic system. This result may be important for the eradication of residual disease or the prevention of recurrence.

BCG is certainly no panacea for clinical treatment of malignant disease. As in both experimental and spontaneous animal tumor models, so also in clincial tests, the most consistent results were obtained when BCG was used locally.

At this time, the use of BCG seems indicated for transitional bladder carcinoma. Several independent studies have demonstrated both the prophylactic effect of BCG in the prevention of recurrences and its efficacy for CIS. Further research is needed to examine whether the BCG effect in humans also depends on the induction of a specific immunity. Moreover, the possible role of BCG's immunopathological effects as a source of adverse reactions should be carefully monitored.

Urologists have a unique opportunity to study both the clinical and the immunological aspects of BCG therapy. Their work could provide a scientific foundation for the role of this form of cancer treatment. Such a foundation is urgently needed in the light of current renewed interest in biological response modifiers.

E.J. Ruitenberg

PART I. FUNDAMENTAL ASPECTS OF BCG-IMMUNOTHERAPY IN CANCER

EORTC Genitourinary Group Monograph 6:
BCG in Superficial Bladder Cancer, pages 3–10
© 1989 Alan R. Liss, Inc.

BCG IN THE TREATMENT OF BLADDER CANCER: STATE OF THE ART

Alvaro Morales

Department of Urology, Queen's University, Kingston,
Ontario, Canada

The organiszation of this workshop and the resulting collection, in one volume, of the experiences of groups in many countries is a welcomed event in urological oncology. The current status of BCG in the treatment of superficial bladder cancer is brought up to date by the reports of individuals working with a sense of purpose and a great deal of enthusiasm and dedication. New developments are occurring rapidly; therefore, there is a degree of urgency in communicating this information which can be of importance to the clinician and the researcher alike. Neither will be disappointed. Upon reaching the end of the book, the reader will have a clear view of what is known and what should be learned about the vaccine.

Much effort is being devoted to the understanding of superficial bladder cancer. Such an interest is justified since this tumor can be readily diagnosed and is, therefore, susceptible to local treatment which may spare the patient more extensive or disfiguring therapeutic modalities. The introduction of the Bacillus Calmette-Guérin (BCG) to the urological armamentarium has opened a new approach to the control of these neoplasms.

Since the development of the modified bacillus some 80 years ago, a large body of knowledge has emerged on its characteristics and biological effects both in animals and humans. In the specific area of genito-urinary neoplasms in general and bladder cancer in particular, we are just seeing the very early stages of its application.

Two areas in which particular interest has existed will be reviewed serving as an introduction to the new findings described in the various reports presented in the following chapters.

ANTITUMOR ACTIVITY AND MECHANISMS OF ACTION IN ANIMAL SYSTEMS

Clinical factors capable of inducing bladder cancer have been recognized for many years. This knowledge has facilitated the development of animal tumor systems with great similarity to their human counterparts. The availability of such models has permitted the elucidation of some aspects of the natural history of the disease and the assessment of anti-neoplastic agents employed in its treatment.

Perhaps the most valuable system is the MBT-2 tumor induced by formamide in C3H mice (Soloway, 1970). Studies with the MBT-2 tumor provided an explanation for the high incidence of recurrence observed in bladder cancer and possible avenues for the prevention of such recurrences (Soloway and Martino, 1976). Culture-adapted cells from this neoplasm were found to retain the capacity to induce progressive tumors in syngeneic mice. In amputation challenge experiments the MBT-2 tumor was found to be immunogenic and resistent to low doses of BCG (Morales et al., 1980; Soloway and Martino, 1976). However, larger doses of the vaccine were capable of preventing tumor takes and inducing tumor regression in animals with growing neoplasms (Pang and Morales, 1982a). Such findings provided a window to explain some of the mechanisms which may be operating not only in the malignant transformation of the urothelium but also in the regression of such tumors following non-specific active immunotherapy.

Animal systems have also provided a wealth of information in regard to the mechanisms of action of BCG. It is known that profound humoral and cellular immune changes occur as a consequence of BCG administration. This topic has been thoroughly reviewed by de Jong (de Jong et al., 1984). Suffice it to say that cell mediated responses appear to be fundamental in the appearence of antitumor effects, regardless of the solid tumor being investigated. Thus, T- and B-cells and macrophages as well as K- and

NK-cell activities are enhanced as a consequence of BCG treatment (Adams and Marino, 1981; Pang and Morales, 1982b; Ratliff et al, 1987). More recently, van der Meijden has demonstrated the presence of lymphokine-activated killer cell activity in the spleen and regional lymph nodes of guinea pigs one week after receiving the vaccine (van der Meijden et al., in press). Unfortunately, it is far from clear how the orchestration of these mechanisms result in tumor destruction. In fact, it has been postulated that the immunological alterations do not have a significant role in the elimination of superficial bladder tumors; the observed effects being simply the sloughing of the bladder mucosa as a result of the severe local inflammatory reaction. Although an inflammatory reaction may be of importance, such a simplistic view is not supported by the experimental evidence (Ratliff et al., 1987).

There is little doubt that animal studies will provide further insight into the unexplored areas of BCG activity in cancer therapy. After all, it should be remembered that the classical experiments of Coe and Feldman and the methodical studies of Zbar pointed the way to the human protocols leading to the application of BCG as an effective agent in the therapy of some solid tumors, including bladder cancer (Coe and Feldman, 1966; Zbar et al., 1972).

ANTITUMOR ACTIVITY AND MECHANISMS OF ACTION IN HUMANS

The introduction of BCG as an agent with activity against superficial bladder cancer was not the result of bladder cancer models but a logical deduction following the postulates of Coe and Feldman and Zbar (Coe and Feldman, 1966; Zbar et al., 1972). It is of interest that the results recorded in the very limited early pilot studies have been consistently borned out by larger controlled clinical investigation. Three distinct applications have been reported for intravesical administration of the vaccine in treating vesical mucosal malignancies.

Prophylaxis

This category has included patients with high incidence of recurrence (at least 3 new tumors in the preceding 24 months) but in whom all visible lesions have been surgically removed immediately prior to therapy. Unfortunately, the protocols have varied between investigators as to the source of the vaccine, the amount instilled and the frequency and duration of treatments. Nevertheless, the proportion of patients, with a previously unstable urothelium remaining disease-free after treatment ranges between 32% and 90% with an average amoung various reports being about 60% (Haaff et al., 1986; van der Meijden, 1988; Pinsky et al., 1982). It must be noted that, in addition to protocol discrepancies, the follow-up of patients has also been variable and may have a bearing on the interpretation of results.

Residual tumors

Included in this group are individuals in whom complete endoscopic elimination of superficial lesions was not accomplished. The results in these patients are also consistent and encouraging with complete responses in the vicinity of 60%, among the various investigators (van der Meijden, 1988).

Carcinoma in situ

Perhaps the most dramatic and consistent beneficial effects of BCG have been reported in the presence of carcinoma in situ. These tumors offer the advantage of a relatively prompt assessment of results and a more consistent definition of the tumor under treatment. The initial report about treating carcinoma in situ with BCG indicated a response rate of 71% (Herr et al., 1986; Lamm, 1985) which has been the recorded results in larger studies (Morales, 1980) but increasing to 94% with the modified protocol used by Brosman (Brosman, 1985).

Until a better definition of the most effective treatment is obtained, new protocols must take into consideration the recent report of Kavoussi in which the 6 week course of instillations has been found to be sub-optimal (Kavoussi et al., 1988), in the treatment categories mentioned above, and the outstanding results noted with an intensive, prolonged course of therapy (Brosman, 1985).

Comparative trials

The place of BCG among the various agents used for intravesical therapy is receiving increasing attention. Available controlled studies indicate that the vaccine is more effective than Thiotepa and Doxorubicin (Brosman, 1982; Lamm et al, 1987). The antitumor effect of Mitomycin has been found similar to that of BCG in the study of Debruyne (Debruyne et al., 1987). This topic has elicited a great deal of interest among co-operative organizations, thus, conclusive data may become available in the near future for the 3 therapy categories (prophylaxis, residual and CIS). Our experience with recombinant alpha-2B Interferon administered intravesically for the treatment of carcinoma in situ has been disappointing: no complete responses and only 1 partial response (positive cytology in the presence of negative biopsies) was noted in 8 patients. However, Torti has reported a complete response of 25% (4 of 16) in patients with papillary transitional cell carcinoma and of 32% (6 of 19) in patients with carcinoma in situ. In this study, as it was in our experience, the administration of Interferon was not accompanied by significant side effects.

The question of side effects secondary to BCG administration was recently addressed in a comprehensive study by Lamm (Lamm et al., 1986). The vast majority of unwanted symptoms is self-limiting and of a minor nature. Occasionally severe side effects are noted but they can be controlled with a short course of anti-tuberculous therapy. A complacent attitude is most unwise during administration of the vaccine. Bladder catheterization and intravesical delivery of a drug is a simple procedure. In inexperienced hands it may become a most dangerous weapon. An informed individual with the proper tools is the best warranty against complications. We have seen one near-fatal complication due to sepsis (presumably BCG-sepsis). In this as in all other cases, the underlying factor has been the presence of a traumatic catheterization. An awareness of this problem must be continuously emphasized. It is strongly recommended that if trauma during the catheterization occurs, the treatment be post-poned for one week. It is believed, albeit unproven, that a combination of trauma and forceful injection of the vaccine allows vascular entry and dissemination of the micro-organisms and the subsequent sepsis. An anaphylactic reaction may also explain part of the clincial picture; although it may present, it appears less likely.

Most of the available knowledge as to the mechanisms of action of the vaccine is derived from animal investigations. However, very early in our studies we documented the presence of a marked submucosal granulomatous reaction in humans receiving intravesical BCG (Morales, 1978). The presence of such vigorous reaction appeared to be of importance in the effectiveness of the treatment but the relevance of this finding has not been conclusively established (Torrence et al., 1988). Concerning immunological events, following BCG treatment, in humans, it is known that profound effects can be observed in the activity of different effector cell types including macrophages, B-, T-, K- and NK-cells as well as in humoral immunity (Morales and Ottenhof, 1983; Thatcher and Crowther, 1978). The individual and collective contribution of the local inflammatory effects and the systemic immune modulation to the antitumor activity, however, remains to be elucidated.

It is evident that BCG is now widely accepted as an effective addition to the urological armamentarium. Furthermore, as knowledge about the vaccine increases, the interest in its clincial application for other cancers has been rekindled with promising results (Hoover et al., 1985). This interest is perhaps most evident among the leading manufacturers of BCG. The initial development, remarkable come back and renewed applications of BCG in cancer therapy is a story of both human and scientific interest which does not seem to be completed yet.

REFERENCES

Adams DO, Marino PA (1981). Evidence for a multistep mechanism of cytolysis by BCG activated macrophages: the interrelationship between the capacity for cytolysis target binding and secretion of cytolytic factoc. J Immunol 126: 981.
Brosman SA (1982). Experience with BCG in patients with superficial bladder carcinoma. J Urol 128: 27.
Brosman SA (1985). The use of BCG in the therapy of bladder carcinoma in situ. J Urol 134: 36.
Coe JE, Feldman JD (1966). Extracutaneous delayed hypersensitivity, particularly in the guinea pig bladder. Immunology 10: 127.

Debruyne FMJ, van der Meijden APM (1987). BCG versus MMC intravesical therapy in patients with superficial bladder cancer. J Urol 137: 179A.

Haaff ED, Dresner SM, Ratliff TL, Catalona WJ. Two courses of intravesical BCG for transitional cell carcinoma of the bladder. J Urol 136: 820.

Herr HW. Pinsky CM, Whitmore Jr WF, Sogani PC, Oettgen HF, Melamed MR (1986). Long-term effect of intravesical BCG on flat carcinoma in situ of the bladder. J Urol 135: 265.

Hoover Jr HC, Surdijke MG, Dangel RB, Peters LC, Hanna Jr MG (1985). Prospective randomized trial of adjuvant active specific immunotherapy for human colorectal cancer. Cancer 55: 1236.

de Jong WH, Steerenberg PA, Kreeftenberg JG, Tiesjema RH, Kruizinga W, van Noorle Jansen LM, Ruitenberg EJ (1984). Experimental screening of BCG preparation produced for cancer immunotherapy: safety, immunostimulating and antitumor activity of four consecutively produced batches. Cancer Immunol Immunother 17: 18.

Kavoussi LR, Torrence RJ, Gillen DP, Hudson MA, Haaff EO, Dresner SM, Ratliff TL, Catalona WJ (1988). Results of 6 weekly intravesical Bacillus Calmette-Guérin instillations on treatment of superficial bladder tumors. J Urol 139: 935.

Lamm DL (1985). BCG immunotherapy for bladder cancer. J Urol 134: 40.

Lamm DL, Stogdill VD, Stogdill BJ, Crispen RG (1986). Complications of Bacillus Calmette-Guérin immunotherapy in 1278 patients with bladder cancer. J Urol 135: 272.

Lamm DL, Blumenstein B, Crawford ED, Montie JE, Scardino P, Stanisic IH, Grossman HB (1987). South-west Oncology Group comparison of Bacillus Calmette-Guérin and Doxorubicin in the treatment and prophylaxis of superficial bladder cancer. J Urol 137: 178A.

van der Meijden APM (1988). Aspects of non-specific immunotherapy with BCG in superficial bladder cancer: an overview. In "Non-specific immunotherapy with BCG -RIVM in superficial bladder cancer," Nijmegen: Thesis, Catholic University, pp 19.

van der Meijden APM, de Jong WH, de Boer EC, Steerenberg PA, Debruyne FMJ, Ruitenberg EJ (1988). Immunological aspects of intravesical administration of BCG in the guinea pig. Urol Res (in press).

Morales A (1978). Adjuvant immunotherapy in superficial blader cancer. In Bonney (ed): "Workshop on Genitourinary Cancer immunology," NCI Monograph 49, pp 315.

Morales A (1980). Treatment of carcinoma in situ of the bladder with BCG. Cancer Immunol Immunother 9: 69.

Morales A, Djeu J, Herberman RB (1980). Immunization by irradiated whole cells against an experimental bladder tumor. Invest Urol 17: 310.

Morales A, Ottenhof PC (1983). Clinical application of a whole blood assay for human NK-cell activity. Cancer 52: 667.

Pang ASD, Morales A (1982a). Immunoprophylaxis of a murine bladder cancer with high doses BCG immunizations. J Urol 127: 1006.

Pang ASD, Morales A (1982b). BCG induced murine peritoneal exudate cells: cytotoxic activity against a syngeneic bladder tumor cell line. J Urol. 127: 1225.

Pinsky CM, Camacho FJ, Kerr D, Braun Jr DW, Whitmore Jr WF, Oettgen HF (1982). Treatment of superficial bladder cancer with intravesical BCG immunotherapy of human cancer. In Terry WD, Rosenberg SA (Eds): "Excerpta Medica", New York: pp 309.

Ratliff TL, Gillen D, Catalona WJ (1987). Requirement of a thymus dependent immune response for BCG mediated antitumor activity. J Urol 137: 155.

Soloway MS (1970). Intravesical and systemic chemotherapy of murine bladder cancer. Cancer Res 30: 1309.

Soloway MS, Martino C (1976). Prophylaxis of bladder tumor implantation. Urology 7: 29.

Thatcher N and Crowther D. Changes in non-specific lymphoid (NK-, K- and T-cell) cytotoxicity following BCG immunizations in healthy subjects. Cancer Immunol Immunother 5: 105.

Torrence RJ, Kavoussi LR, Catalona W (1988). Prognostic factors in patients treated with intravesical BCG for superficial bladder cancer. J Urol 139: 941.

Torti FM, Shortliff LD, Williams RD (1988). Alpha-Interferon in superficial bladder cancer: A Northern California Oncology Group Study. J Clin Oncol 6: 476.

Zbar B, Bernstein ID, Bartlett GL, Hanna Jr MG, Rapp HJ (1972). Immunotherapy of cancer: regression of intradermal tumors and prevention of growth of lymph node metastases after intralesional injection of living Mycobacterium bovis. J Natl Cancer Inst 49: 119.

EORTC Genitourinary Group Monograph 6:
BCG in Superficial Bladder Cancer, pages 11–33
© 1989 Alan R. Liss, Inc.

ASPECTS OF NON-SPECIFIC IMMUNOTHERAPY WITH BCG IN SUPER-
FICIAL BLADDER CANCER: AN OVERVIEW

Ad P.M. van der Meijden, Frans M.J. Debruyne, Peter
A. Steerenberg, Wim H. de Jong
Department of Urology, University Hospital Nijmegen
(A.P.M.v.d.M., F.M.J.D.), National Institute of Public
Health and Environmental Protection, Bilthoven
(P.A.S., W.H.d.J.), The Netherlands.

INTRODUCTION

In 1908 Calmette and Guérin were working on the
development of an anti-tuberculosis vaccine. They observed,
while culturing a highly virulent strain of the tubercle
bacillus of bovine origin in a mixture of beef bile and
cooked potatoes, that the culture lost its characteristic
appearance (Guérin, 1980). After a transitory increase of
virulence, the tubercle bacillus was gradually losing its
noxious characteristics. Thirteen consecutive years and two
hundred and thirty one transplantings later the tubercle
bacillus had been tamed. It had become completely harmless
to animals but its antigenetic properties were unimpaired.
In 1921 the first human was vaccinated with the attenuated
bovine tubercle bacillus: Bacillus Calmette-Guérin (BCG).
Since then, more then 500 million vaccinations with BCG to
prevent tuberculosis were performed (Rosenthal, 1980). The
use of BCG for the prevention of tuberculosis was the most
important issue in the first half of this century, but
later on, the immunostimulating aspect of BCG became of
interest.

Pearl, in 1929, reported on the protective effect of
tuberculosis against cancer (Pearl, 1929). In an autopsy
study it was observed that a group of patients suffering
from tuberculosis significantly showed less malignant
tumors than a control group. Already during the last decade
of the nineteenth century Coley determined empirically a
therapeutic principle for the treatment of neoplasms
(Nauts et al., 1953). If different tumors were treated with

bacterial toxins, provoking an acute infection in or nearby the tumor site, tumor regression could be observed. Later, the working mechanism was interpreted as being a stimulation of the immune system causing tumor eradication. Rosenthal, in several studies in the mid thirty's, reported that, when the vaccin was administered to animals by various routes, not only a specific local response appeared, but also a generalized stimulation of the immune apparatus could be observed (Rosenthal, 1936; Rosenthal, 1938). Old and Clarke in the United States and Halpern in France demonstrated in 1959 that BCG was able to inhibit tumor growth in experimental tumors (Halpern et al., 1959; Old and Clarke, 1959).

In man immunotherapy with BCG was first used and reported by Mathé (Mathé et al., 1969). They used BCG as an adjuvant therapy in the treatment of acute lymphoblastic leukemia. Due to their promising results a number of trials were conducted in the U.S.A. and in Europe. However, the initial favorable results by Mathé could not be confirmed conclusively by other investigators.

Morton, in 1970, was the first to use BCG successfully by injecting the living bacilli intratumorally, in malignant melanoma (Morton et al., 1970). In 1976 a new approach to adjuvant therapy for superficial bladder cancer was developed by Morales et al. (Morales et al., 1976). They were the first to use Bacillus Calmette-Guérin as a nonspecific active immunotherapy. The preliminary results were very promising. In their study BCG was administered intravesically as well as intradermally. Morales started this new avenue for the treatment of superficial bladder cancer, making a linkage between the observations made by Coe and Feldman and the results of experiments performed by the research group of Zbar and Rapp (Coe and Feldman, 1966; Zbar at el., 1972).

In 1966, Coe and Feldman demonstrated that the bladder is a suitable organ for the development of delayed type hypersensitivity reactions. In immunized guinea pigs, exposed to an antigenic challenge, strong delayed type hypersensitivity reactions were observed in the skin and in the bladder. Responses, observed in the kidney, testis or muscle, were particularly weaker or absent. So, the induction of antigen specific responses in the guinea pig can be demonstrated by eliciting a delayed type hypersensitivity reaction not only in the skin, but also in the bladder wall.

The research group of Zbar and Rapp, in a number of experiments, investigated the basic principles for successful non-specific active immunotherapy in a guinea pig tumor system (Zbar et al., 1972). In inbred strain 2 guinea pigs, the line 10 hepatocarcinoma, a chemically induced tumor, could be completely cured by intratumoral injection of Bacillus Calmette-Guérin. Not only the primary tumor, but also micrometastases in the regional lymph nodes, present at the time of treatment, were eradicated. Furthermore, the existence of tumor immunity could be demonstrated as BCG-cured animals rejected a second tumor cell challenge. Optimum results in antitumor activity were obtained if certain basic principles were fulfilled:
1. Tumor burden must be small.
2. Direct contact between tumorcells and BCG is essential.
3. The dose of immunizing agent must be adequate.
4. Tumors respond better, when confined to the parent organ or, in case of metastases, when spread is limited to the regional lymph nodes.

It was remarkable, however, that important information for the development of immunotherapy with BCG in bladder cancer in man was obtained without the use of experimental bladder tumors. Bloomberg et al. observed a marked inflammatory reaction in the bladder of healthy dogs after intravesical instillation of BCG. Cellular infiltrates built up from histiocytes and macrophages were present in the bladder wall (Bloomberg et al., 1975). This observation, together with the results of studies by Coe and Feldman and by Zbar and Rapp provided the basis for immunotherapy protocols in bladder cancer (Coe and Feldman, 1966; Zbar et al., 1972). Now, a decade has past and the effectiveness of BCG in superficial transitional cell carcinoma has been determined conclusively. However, a number of issues on this therapy are still questionable or remain unclear.

About the optimal route of administration consensus has been reached during recent years. However, no consensus has been reached about the optimal treatment schedule, optimal dose, and appropriate strain.

Some of these problems, which are controversial or indistinct will be discussed below.

THE ROUTE OF ADMINISTRATION

Five different routes of BCG-administration for the treatment of superficial bladder cancer have been used sofar:
- percutaneous administration
- intralesional injection
- oral administration
- intravesical instillation combined with percutaneous administration
- intravesical instillation alone.

Percutaneous administration of BCG in superficial bladder cancer was investigated by Martinez-Pineiro and Muntanola (Martinez-Pineiro and Muntanola, 1977; Martinez-Pineiro, 1984). Per week ten scarifications measuring 5 cm in length were administered. At each treatment a 0.5 ml dose of lyophilized Pasteur BCG vaccin, containing 300 mg/ml was used. Only 7 patients were treated and many variable factors (different periods of treatment, patients with or without residual bladder tumors) made it impossible to estimate the value of this intensive therapy, but anti-tumor effect was observed.

Intralesional administration was performed by the same authors in two patients by injection 37.5 mg of BCG into their bladder tumor. One patient developed a serious hyper-sensitivity reaction, resulting in an allergic shock. Thereafter this way of administration was abolished.

The antitumor effect of oral administration of BCG was studied by several investigators (Lamm, 1987 and 1988; Netto and Lemos, 1984). Netto and Lemos treated 10 patients with muscle invasive bladder cancer using fresh BCG of the Moreau strain in high doses. A complete response was obtained in 7 patients. Lamm used oral administration of the Tice BCG-strain in muscle invasive bladder cancer in patients, who could not be treated by radiation or cyst-ectomy. Although tumor regression was observed the results were less impressive compared with those from Netto and Lemos (Lamm, 1987 and 1988).

Lamm also investigated the effect of oral administered BCG (200 mg Tice-BCG, three times per week) in superficial bladder tumors (Lamm et al. 1986). No measurable antitumor effect, however, was observed in patients treated that way.

The most thoroughly investigated route of administration is the intravesical instillation, initially combined with percutaneous administration. Morales developed an empirically based therapeutic scheme which remained the treatment modality in superficial bladder cancer for many years (Morales et al., 1976). He instilled BCG in a watery solution in the bladder once weekly, for 6 consecutive weeks.

At the same time BCG was administered percutaneously at the anterior surface of the thigh by a multiple puncture apparatus. After 10 years of experience, reviewing his results, Morales reported a complete response in 50% of the patients using BCG as a prophylactive therapy. In 58% of patients with residual disease and in 77% of patients with carcinoma in situ complete response was achieved (Morales and Nickel, 1986). Two prospective randomized clinical trials, using the Morales treatment schedule, were conducted in the U.S.A. (Camacho et al., 1980; Lamm et al., 1981). Responses were in the same range as obtained by Morales. Herr used intravesical and percutaneous BCG for the treatment of carcinoma in situ. A complete response was noted in 65% of the patients (Herr et al., 1983; Herr et al., 1986).

Excellent results of intravesical BCG instillation without percutaneous administration were reported by Brosman (Brosman, 1982). In a randomized study patients were treated either with Thiotepa instillations or with BCG instillations. BCG was administered intravesically weekly for 12 consecutive weeks, followed by instillations every 2 weeks for 3 months and thereafter every month until a recurrent tumor developed or the patient had been treated for a total period of 2 years.

No recurrences have been observed in the BCG-treated group, while 40 per cent in the Thiotepa group suffered from recurrences.

Treating carcinoma in situ, 94 per cent of the patients were rendered free of tumor (Brosman, 1985). Brosman stated that patients do not require pre-sensitization or continued intradermal inocculations of BCG as he observed that all his patients, when treated with intravesical instillations alone converted from a negative PPD skin reaction to a positive one, after 9 instillations. A problem in these studies was the increasing toxicity of the prolonged instillation therapy.

At the moment percutaneous supportive inocculation has been abandoned by most investigators. It is considered as not essential for the antitumor effect of BCG immunotherapy in superficial bladder cancer (Lamm, 1987 and 1988). At the moment intravesical administration of BCG alone is accepted in most centres to be the best route of administration in treating patients with superficial transitional cell carcinoma of the urinary bladder.

The PPD skin test conversion, which indicates a systemically induced immunisation against BCG, seems to show a correlation to treatment results (Kelley et al., 1985). Most investigators noted that patients, whose PPD skin test converted from negative to positive after BCG treatment, were the best responders to the therapy (Catalona et al., 1987; Haaff et al., 1986; Kelley et al., 1985). Badalament, however, observed that patients with a reactive tuberculin test before and after 6 weeks BCG had significantly less tumor recurrences than patients with different PPD skin test results (Badalament et al., 1987).

TREATMENT SCHEDULE

Till 1985 the overall complete response rate for BCG therapy of papillary carcinoma and carcinoma in situ tumors obtained from all published reports is approximately 67 per cent (Haaff et al., 1985).

The cumulative experience with BCG as a non-specific immunotherapy for superficial bladder cancer is depicted in Table 1. The response rate for prophylaxis after TUR, for residual disease after TUR and for carcinoma in situ is presented separately. It must be strained that remarkable differences exist in duration of follow-up, used strain, therapeutic regime and route of administration.

It was clearly demonstrated that BCG therapy is superior to standard endoscopic resection alone (Lamm et al., 1981; Morales et al., 1976) to adjuvant intravesical chemotherapy with Thiotepa (Camacho, 1980) or Doxorubicin (Lamm et al., 1987). Although the response rate to BCG appears to be superior to other forms of intravesical therapy, a considerable number of patients fail when only the initially proposed 6 weeks BCG-regimen is used (Kavoussi, 1988).

TABLE 1. Cumulative BCG experience in superficial bladder tumors

INVESTIGATOR	NO. OF PATIENTS	WITHOUT RECURRENCE
PROPHYLAXIS:		
Morales et al., 1986	46	50%
Lamm et al., 1987	53	72%
Pinsky et al., 1982	25	32%
Brosman et al., 1984	53	88%
deKernion et al., 1984	22	64%
Haaff et al., 1986	29	90%
RESIDUAL:		
Douville et al., 1978	6	67%
Morales et al., 1986	24	58%
Martinez-Pineiro et al., 1977	5	0%
Brosman et al., 1984	27	63%
deKernion et al., 1984	22	36%
Schellhammer et al., 1986	24	71%
Haaff et al., 1986	13	69%
CIS:		
Morales et al., 1986	26	77%
Lamm et al., 1987	77	75%
Brosman et al., 1984	33	94%
Herr et al., 1986	47	68%
deKernion et al., 1984	19	68%
Haaff et al., 1986	19	68%

An appropriate adjuvant therapy for those patients failing one course of 6 weeks BCG has not been determined yet. At the moment two fundamental treatment schedules have become of interest and both schedules have presented favorable tumor responses compared with an instillation scheme of 6 weeks only (Brosman, 1982; 1985; Catalona et al., 1987; Haaff et al. 1986; Kavoussi, 1988).

The first schedule is the so called maintenance therapy, first advocated by Brosman (Brosman, 1982). This treatment regimen consisted of intravesical instillations once per week for 6 weeks, biweekly for 3 months and monthly until recurrence or the completion of a 2-year course. The response rate was far more favorable than ever previously reported. In a randomized trial patients with superficial bladder tumors were treated with Thiotepa or BCG intravesically. Twentyseven patients were allocated to the BCG group and 12 additional patients were treated after they had failed previous Thiotepa therapy. These 39 patients showed no recurrences. In treating 33 patients with carcinoma in situ, 31 patients (94 per cent) were rendered free of tumor (mean follow-up 5.2 years). However, the local and systemic toxicity of this prolonged therapy was severe and significantly worse than in other protocols (Lamm et al., 1986). Regarding the increased toxicity, the maintenance therapy as used by Brosman, can be considered in a number of patients as an unnecessary over-treatment. On the other hand this therapy may be suitable for patients with strongly recurrent tumors, resistant to any previous treatment.

The second treatment schedule has become of interest during the last 2 years. It was reported that adding a second 6-week course of BCG therapy for those patients failing the first course, could improve the response rate from approximately 60% after a single 6-week course up to approximately 80% following the second 6-week course (Catalona et al., 1987; Haaff et al., 1986). This overall response rate approaches that reported by Brosman. Moreover, the 2-course treatment could spare unnecessary toxicity for those patients who respond rapidly to BCG therapy and appears to provide adequate therapy for those patients needing more extensive treatment.

Another point that must be emphasized concerning multiple BCG treatments is the inability to identify patients who will not respond to BCG and who are at risk for invasive bladder cancer while being treated with maintenance BCG therapy or multiple courses of BCG.

Catalona conducted a risk-to-benifit analysis of repeated courses of intravesical BCG therapy (Catalona et al., 1987). Their results suggest that many patients who failed 1 course of therapy respond to a second course of 6 weeks. On the other hand the risk of developing invasive cancer or metastases in patients who have failed 2 courses exceed the prospects of eradicating the superficial cancer with further BCG treatment. In 100 consecutive patients treated with repeated 6-week courses of BCG they observed a 30 per cent risk of developing invasive cancer and a 50 per cent risk of metastatic disease in those patients who relapsed after 2 courses of BCG. In other words to treat patients with more than 2 courses may be dangerous with regard to development of invasive disease. However, it remains unclear whether or not patients developing invasive cancer after 2 courses of BCG should have done so, if they were treated with maintenance therapy from the start.

Although most investigators are convinced that a single 6-week course of intravesical BCG is a suboptimal therapy, Badalament, however, in a prospective randomized study comparing maintenance versus non-maintenance therapy, could not demonstrate a significant difference between the two groups. Patients receiving maintenance therapy had similar recurrence and progression rates as those who were treated with a single 6-week course (Badalament et al., 1987). It must be stated, however, that patients starting with maintenance therapy did so, 5 to 8 weeks after completing the initial 6-week course, thus lacking intra-vesical instillation up to two months between the end of the initial 6-week course and the start of the maintenance scheme.

Prognostic factors in each individual patient should be considered in order to decide which treatment schedule should be used from the start. Summarizing it can be stated that more prospective randomized studies are needed to establish the optimal treatment regimen.

VIABILITY, DOSE AND APPROPRIATE STRAIN

Comparative studies of different strains of BCG in a murine model revealed that the immunogenicity of a BCG-preparation was related directly to the viability of the vaccin (Mackaness et al., 1984). Shapiro, in a murine bladder tumor model observed variations in the viability and efficacy of different lots of BCG (Shapiro et al., 1983).

The immunizing efficacy of a BCG vaccin depends on at least 2 factors: the number of bacilli and the ability of the organisms to multiply in vivo, that is the viability (Dubos and Pierce, 1956). Kelley investigated the effect of BCG viability on treatment results in human superficial bladder cancer (Kelley et al., 1985). They noted differences in the number of colony-forming units between different lots of BCG of the same strain and among different strains. In the Pasteur strain (Institute Armand Frappier, Quebec, Canada) the number of colony-forming units differed from $6x10^6$ till $1x10^{12}$ per ampule and in the Tice strain (Institution Tuberculosis Research, Chicago, U.S.A.) from $3x10^7$ till $4.6x10^{11}$ per ampule. In general one or two ampules are used for intravesical instillation. Treatment failures occurred more frequently among patients who received a preparation with low viability. Patients treated with $6x10^6$ c.p. per ampule had recurrent tumors in 71 per cent, while those patients treated with $3x10^{11}$ c.p. per ampule showed recurrences in 25 per cent.

The dose of BCG in the two BCG strains mostly used for intravesical instillation (Pasteur, Quebec and Tice, Chicago) is 120 mg per instillation. The BCG preparations are lyophilized and dissolved in 50 ml of saline. The amount of culturable particles per vial seems to be more important than the dry weight or biomass in the preparation. It was demonstrated in an experimental model that the antitumor activity increased with the dose, but after an optimal dose has been reached, further augmentation results in decreasing antitumor effect (Lamm, 1987 and 1988).

A dose of $5x10^8$ till $5x10^9$ c.p. is considered to be the optimal dose, but again no conclusive evidence has been reached on this subject.

Sofar the results of 6 strains used for immunotherapy in superficial bladder cancer have been published. These preparations are Pasteur (Quebec, Canada), Tice (Chicago, USA), Connaught (Toronto, Canada), Pasteur (Paris, France), Glaxo (Greenford, England) and Moreau (Sao Paulo, Brasil).

Originally, most of these preparations were derived from the Pasteur strain in Paris. The Pasteur (Quebec) and the Tice strain have been investigated most thoroughly in superficial bladder cancer. Few reports have been published on results obtained by the preparations of Glaxo and

Moreau. The Moreau strain was administered in fresh form orally in few patients and the Glaxo strain turned out to be of weak immunogenicity, probably due to a moderate biomass and viability in the vials used initially (Morales and Nickel, 1986; Netto and Lemos, 1984). It seems that the efficacy of Pasteur (Quebec), Tice and Connaught BCG is comparable, but no prospective randomized clinical trials have been conducted sofar to determine which strain is the most appropriate one.

From 1985 onwards, a Dutch BCG-preparation produced at the Rijksinstituut voor Volksgezondheid en Milieuhygiène (RIVM), the National Institute of Public Health and Environmental Protection has been used for the treatment of superficial bladder cancer in the Netherlands. This strain has been derived from a seed lot of the French Pasteur strain in 1964.

In culturing BCG-bacilli the mycobacteria usually are grown as a pellicle on the surface of a liquid medium. At harvesting the pellicle is ground in a ball mill to a paste. This results in a preparation not containing live BCG bacilli only, but also dead micro organisms and abundant subcellular debris. However, another method of culture, used at the RIVM, the Netherlands, is to grow the BCG-bacteria in a homogeneously stirred deep culture system. Higher viability per mg dry weight can be obtained if a detergent is added to the culture medium. This culture method ensures a relatively high ratio of viable organisms and a small quantity of subcellular debris and dead bacilli. After both methods of culture, the vaccines are harvested and can be lyophilized. Although differences in immunostimulating activity and antitumor activity have been observed, BCG-preparations cultured by these different methods show similar antitumor activity (Ruitenberg et al., 1981). The antitumor potency of BCG-RIVM conclusively was established in different animal tumor systems e.g. murine fibrosarcoma (Ruitenberg et al., 1981), line 10 hepatocellular carcinoma in the guinea pig (de Jong et al., 1984), bovine ocular squamous cell carcinoma (Klein et al., 1982) and equine sarcoid (Klein et al., 1986).

TOXICITY

Local and systemic toxicity may occur after BCG

immunotherapy. Important factors for these side effects are the route of administration, the dose of BCG and the number of repeated administrations. In superficial bladder cancer BCG has been administered orally, percutaneously and intravesically, of which the latter has proved to be the most important route. Only few patients have been treated orally (Lamm, 1987 and 1988; Netto and Lemos, 1984). No complications or side effects were reported, if the oral route was used.

The local side effects of percutaneous BCG application are well known from the extensive experience with BCG vaccination for the prevention of tuberculosis (Sparks, 1976). More than 500 million vaccinations have been performed all over the world (Rosenthal, 1980). The post-vaccination reaction normally consists of erythema, in most cases followed by the formation of a crusted nodule, which may show ulceration. Moderate swelling of the regional lymph nodes is regarded as a normal reaction. As local complications of intradermal application are considered persistent ulceration, localized abcess, granuloma formation and regional lymphadenitis (Sparks, 1976).

Systemic complications after intradermal application caused by generalized BCG infection have rarely been observed (Sparks, 1976) and if they are present, patients often suffered from immunodeficiency syndroms. Hypersensitivity reactions, arthritis, granulomatous hepatitis and pneumonitis have been reported (de Jong et al., 1987).

The toxicity of intravesical instillation of BCG is of major importance in the treatment of superficial bladder cancer. The complications of intravesical BCG in 1278 patients were reviewed by Lamm (Lamm et al., 1986). This author compiled the data of 195 patients treated by himself and from 1083 patients reported by 13 different investigators in the USA and Europe. These patients were treated with 5 different strains of BCG. No difference in the incidence or severity of side effects were observed in patients treated with Pasteur (Armand Frappier), Tice and Connaught preparations. Local side effects, restricted to the bladder were seen frequently. More than 90 per cent of the patients suffered from cystitis with frequency and dysuria. Hematuria was seen in 43 per cent, sometimes in severe form (0.5%) requiring catherization. The histological substrate of the cystitis consists, on biopsy, of acute and chronic inflammation with granuloma formation in the stroma of the bladder wall. Patients generally have symptoms of cystitis for a short period and find relief with non-steroidal anti-inflammatory agents. The bladder irritability usually begins after 2 or 3 instillations and may persist for about 2 days. The vesical symptoms however increase with the frequency and duration of BCG administration.

During maintenance therapy (monthly BCG) it is sometimes necessary to reduce dose and to treat patients with anti-tuberculosis drugs for these severe local side effects.

Moderate systemic side effects were observed as well consisting of fever till 39°C (28 per cent), malaise (24 per cent) and nausea (8 per cent) (Lamm et al., 1986). These side effects generally will subside spontaneously. Severe local and systemic side effects, regarded as complications, were encountered in about 5% of all patients (see Table 2).

TABLE 2. Complications of intravesical BCG-instillation in 1278 patients with superficial bladder cancer
(Reproduced from Lamm et al., 1986 J Urol 135:146A with permission of William and Wilkins, Inc. Baltimore.)

Fever more than 39°C	3.9%
Granulomatous prostalitis	1.3%
BCG pneumonitis/hepatitis	0.9%
Arthritis/arthralgia	0.5%
Skin rash	0.4%
Ureteral obstruction	0.3%
Epididymo-orchitis	0.2%
Hypotension	0.1%
Cytopenia	0.1%
Contracted bladder	0.2%

If local or systemic complications, as described before, are encountered patients must be treated with anti-tuberculous drugs.

In case of severe or prolonged irritative vesical symptoms, fever, chills, or malaise it is recommended to lower the dose of BCG till half the normal dose and to treat the patients with Isoniazid (I.N.H.) 300 mg per day starting one day before instillation and continuing for 3 days or until symptoms resolve. If severe systemic complications are present BCG administration must be withholded and a combination anti-tuberculous therapy is started. This therapy consists of Isoniazid 300 mg per day and Rifampicin 600 mg per day for 3 months. Fatal reactions to BCG in general can occur. In vaccination programs for tuberculosis one death per 50 million patients was observed (Lotte et al., 1984). A higher mortality rate (1 death per 12,500 patients) occurred when BCG was administered as an immunotherapy for cancer. Almost all patients, however, had pre-existing defects in cellular immunity. In the literature, until recently, no fatalities have been reported in patients with bladder tumors treated with intravesical BCG. However, Rawls and Lamm have reported recently one death after intravesical BCG administration (Rawls et al., 1988).

The same authors and also Steg have reported six cases of severe life threatening systemic complications of BCG intravesical therapy (Rawls et al., 1988; Steg et al. 1988). In almost all cases traumatic catheterisation was noted before the onset of disseminated BCG sepsis. This means that no BCG instillations should be performed within 24 hours after traumatic catheterisation nor immediately after TUR or biopsy of bladder tumors. If a life-threatening BCG infection or anaphylaxis should occur patients must be treated with 500 mg cycloserine twice daily for 3 days in addition to the combination anti-tuberculous therapy because rapid action of this drug may be life saving.

In summary, it can be concluded that intravesical BCG administration for superficial bladder cancer generally is well tolerated and has produced no serious complications in more than 95 per cent of the patients treated. However, significant morbidity can occur and therefore urologists should be familiar with anti-tuberculous therapy.

EFFECTOR MECHANISM(S) OF BCG IN CANCER

Of all issues concerning BCG-immunotherapy the most intriguing problem remains the unclarified mechanism(s) by which BCG exerts its antitumor activity. Although second and third generation of immunotherapeutics (recombinant DNA products) are available nowadays, BCG probably remains the most important Biologic Response Modifier for bladder cancer. It has the potential to act as a non-specific immunopotentiator most likely, not by a single mechanism, but by a variety of actions involving a range of cells of the immune system including T- and B- lymphocytes, macrophages, K-(killer), and NK- (natural killer) cells. Three different effector mechanisms have been proposed (Merguerian et al., 1987).

1) Live BCG provokes immediately an inflammatory response in which macrophages, being the effector cells, may be activated directly by BCG without the participation of T-cells.

2) A delayed type hypersensitivity reaction in which macrophages ingest BCG and additionally stimulate BCG-sensitized T-cells to produce lymphokines, which results in a further cascade of activation of parts of the immune system.

3) The induction of tumor-specific immunity in which BCG stimulated proliferating T-cells may interact with macrophages that have ingested both BCG and cellular debris of tumor cells.

An overview of the different possibilities of BCG to interact with the immune system is presented in Fig. 1 (according to de Jong et al., 1987). What the eventual result of BCG administration will be, stimulation or suppression of the immune system, depends on multiple factors such as the genetic background, strain of BCG, administered dose and the route of administration. However, all interactions of BCG with the immune system depicted in Fig. 1, may occur.

The enhancing effect of BCG on antibody synthesis was frequently demonstrated. It can be the result of a direct effect on B-cells or indirectly via helper T-cells (Brown et al., 1979). When BCG is administered intravenously or subcutaneously the concentration ("trapping") of lymphocytes in lymph nodes is increased (Zatz, 1976). This trapping phenomenon is T-cell dependent.

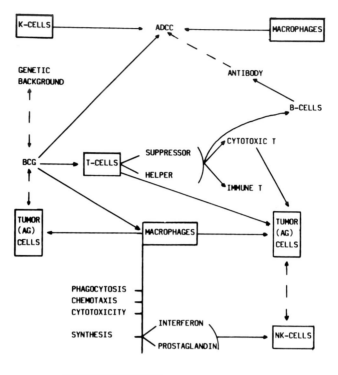

Figure 1. Possible interactions of BCG with the immune system (Reproduced from de Jong et al., 1987 Res Monogr Immunol 11:283-307 with permission of Elsevier Publishers.)

Cell mediated immunity to thymus dependent antigens is enhanced by BCG (Florintin et al., 1976) and furthermore BCG appears to be mitogenic for T-cells (Mitchel et al., 1975). BCG may induce enhancement of the immune system, but also suppression can occur. Part of the suppression may be the effect of induction of T-suppressor cells (Collins and Watson, 1979). It was demonstrated that BCG increases metabolic activity, resulting in release of extracellular enzymes, migration and pinocytosis of macrophages (Poplack et al., 1976).

BCG-activated macrophages can attack tumor cells directly or by mediating cytotoxic T-cell precursors (Adams and Marino, 1981; Mitchel et al., 1973). Spleen macrophages, activated by BCG, produce enhanced lymphocyte activating factor (L.A.F.) so called interleukin 1.

Besides macrophages, BCG enhances the activity of non T, non B lymphoid cells which show non-specific cytotoxic activity against tumor cells, the so called natural killer cells (NK-cells) (de Jong et al., 1983; Wolfe et al., 1976).

Finally, antibody dependend cellular cytotoxicity (ADCC) was enhanced, after injection of BCG, in two kinds of spleen cell populations, probably macrophages and K-cells (Pollack et al., 1977).

The mentioned activities and interactions by which BCG may exert its antitumor effect, are extremely complicated and not fully understood yet.

In experimental and spontaneously arising animal tumors, BCG has conclusively proved to have the potency to inhibit tumor growth and even to eradicate tumors completely. The local presence of BCG and the induction of a granulomatous reaction, together with activation of the mononuclear phagocytic system is regarded to be important. The conditions considered necessary for optimal BCG immunotherapy as advocated by Zbar and Rapp are present in superficial bladder tumors (Zbar et al., 1972).

At this moment, the clinical use of BCG for non-specific immunotherapy appears to be indicated only in superficial bladder cancer. In other tumors, like carcinoma of the head and neck region (Bier et al., 1981) and melanoma (Morton et al., 1970) promising preliminary results were obtained, but the efficacy of BCG-therapy was not conclusively determined.

However, recent data show that treatment of colon carcinoma with a mixture of BCG and autologous tumor cells may be successful (Hoover et al., 1984; Hoover et al., 1985).

For superficial bladder cancer the next decade has to give an answer how to use BCG successfully. More controlled clinical trials are needed to obtain knowledge about optimal treatment of superficial bladder tumors with Bacillus Calmette-Guérin.

REFERENCES

Adams DO, Marino PA (1981). Evidence for a multistep mechanism of cytolysis by BCG activated macrophages: the interrelationship between the capacity for cytolysis, target binding and secretion of cytolytic factor. J Immunol 126: 981.

Badalament RA, Herr HW, Wong GY, Gnecco G, Pinsky CM, Whitmore Jr WF, Fair WR, Oettgen HF (1987). A prospective randomized trial of maintenance versus non-maintenance intravesical Bacillus Calmette-Guérin therapy of super-ficial bladder cancer. J Clin Oncol 5: 441.

Bier J, Rapp HJ, Borsos T, Zbar B, Kleinschuster S, Wagner H, Rollinghof M (1981). Randomized clinical study on intratumoral BCG-cell wall preparation (C.W.P.) therapy in patients with squamous cell carcinoma in the head and neck region. Cancer Immunol Immunother 12: 71.

Bloomberg SD, Brosman SA, Haasman MS, Cohen A, Battenberg JD (1975). The effects of BCG on the dog bladder. Invest Urol 12: 423.

Brosman SA (1982). Experience with Bacillus Calmette-Guérin in patients with superficial bladder carcinoma. J Urol 128: 27.

Brosman SA (1984). BCG in the management of superficial bladder cancer. Urology (suppl. to April): S2.

Brosman SA (1985). The use of Bacillus Calmette-Guérin in the therapy of bladder carcinoma in situ. J Urol 134: 36.

Brown CA, Brown IN, Sljivic VS (1979). Suppressed or enhanced antibody responses in vitro after BCG treatment of mice: importance of BCG viability. Immunology 38: 481.

Camacho FJ, Pinsky CM, Kerr D, Whitmore Jr WF, Oettgen HF (1980). Treatment of superficial bladder cancer with intravesical BCG. Proc Amer Ass Cancer Res and Amer Soc Clin Oncol 21: 359.

Catalona WJ, Hudson, M'Liss A, Gillen DP, Andriole GL, Ratliff TL (1987). Risk and benefits of repeated courses of intravesical Bacillus Calmette-Guérin therapy for superficial bladder cancer. J Urol 137: 220.

Coe JE, Feldman JD (1966). Extracutaneous delayed hyper-sensitivity, particularly in the guinea pig bladder. Immunology 10: 127.

Collins FM, Watson SR (1979). Suppressor T-cells in BCG-infected mice. Infect Immun 25: 491.

Dubos RJ, Pierce CH (1956). Differential characteristics in vitro and in vivo of several substrains of BCG IV. Immunizing effectiveness. Amer Rev Tuberc 74: 699.

Douville Y, Pelouze G, Roy R, Charrois R, Kibrite A, Martin M, Dionne L, Coulonval L, Robinson J (1978). Recurrent bladder papillomata treated with Bacillus Calmette-Guérin: a preliminary report (phase I trial). Cancer Treat Rep 62: 551.

Florentin I, Huchet R, Bruley-Rosset M, Halle-Pannenko O, Mathé G (1976). Studies on the mechanism of action of BCG. Cancer Immunol Immunother 1: 31.

Guérin C (1980). The history of BCG. In Rosenthal SR (Ed): "BCG vaccine: tuberculosis-cancer," Littleton, Massachusetts: P.S.G. Publishing Company Inc., p. 37.

Haaff EO, Dresner SM, Kelley DR, Ratliff TL, Shapiro A, Catalona WJ (1985). Role of immunotherapy in the prevention of recurrence and invasion of urothelial bladder tumors: a review. World J Urol 3: 76.

Haaff EO, Dresner SM, Ratliff TL, Catalona WJ (1986). Two courses of intravesical Bacillus Calmette-Guérin for transitional cell carcinoma of the bladder. J Urol 136: 820.

Halpern B, Biozzi G, Stiffel C, Morton D (1959). Effet de la stimulation du système réticulo endothélial par l'inoculation du bacille de Calmette-Guérin sur le dévelopement de l'épitheliome atypique T-S Guérin chez le rat. G.R. Biol (Paris) 153: 919.

Herr HW, Pinsky CM, Whitmore Jr WF, Oettgen HF, Malamed MR (1983). Effect of intravesical BCG on carcinoma in situ of the bladder. Cancer 51: 1323.

Herr HW, Pinsky CM, Whitmore Jr WF, Sogani PC, Oettgen HF, Melamed MR (1986). Long-term effect of intravesical Bacillus Calmette-Guérin on flat carcinoma in situ of the bladder. J Urol 135: 265.

Hoover HC Jr, Surdijke MG, Dangel RB, Peters LC, Hanna MG Jr (1984). Delayed cutaneous hypersensitivity to autologous tumor cells in colorectal cancer patients immunized with an autologous tumor cell: Bacillus Calmette-Guérin vaccine. Cancer Res 44: 1671.

Hoover Jr HC, Surdijke MG, Dangel RB, Peters LC, Hanna Jr MG (1985). Prospective randomized trial of adjuvant active-specific immunotherapy for human colorectal cancer. Cancer 55: 1236.

de Jong WH, Ursen PS, Kruizinga W, Osterhaus ADME, Ruitenberg EJ (1983). Effect of Bacillus Calmett-Guérin on natural killer cell activity in random bred rats. In Crispen RG (ed): "Cancer: Etiology and Prevention," New York: Elsevier Biomedical, pp 213.

de Jong WH, Steerenberg PA, Kreeftenberg JG, Tiesjema RH,

Kruizinga W, van Noorle Jansen LM, Ruitenberg EJ: Experimental screening of BCG preparations produced for cancer immunotherapy: safety, immunostimulating and antitumor activity of four consecutively produced batches. Cancer Immun. Immunoth. 17: 18, 1984.

de Jong WH, Steerenberg PA, Ruitenberg EJ. Bacillus Calmette-Guérin (BCG) and its use for cancer immunotherapy (1987). In Otter W den, Ruitenberg EJ (eds): "Tumor Immunology - Mechanisms, Diagnosis, Therapy", Amsterdam: Elsevier, pp.

Kavoussi LR, Torrence RJ, Gillen DP, Hudson MA, Haaff EO, Dresner SM, Ratliff TL, Catalona WJ (1988). Results of 6 weekly intravesical Bacillus Calmette-Guérin instillations on treatment of superficial bladder tumors. J Urol 139: 935.

Kelley DR, Ratliff TL, Catalona WJ, Shapiro A, Lage JM, Bauer WC, Haaff EO, Dresner SM (1985). Intravesical Bacillus Calmette-Guérin therapy for superficial bladder cancer: effect of Bacillus Calmette-Guérin viability on treatment results. J Urol 134: 4.

deKernion JB, Huang M, Lindner A, Smith RB, Keufman JJ (1984). Management of superficial bladder tumors and urothelial atypia with intravesical Bacillus Calmette-Guérin (BCG). J Urol 133: 139A.

Klein WR, Ruitenberg EJ, Steerenberg PA, de Jong WH, Kruizinga W, Misdorp W, Bier J, Tiesjema RH, Kreeftenberg JG, Teppema JS, Rapp HJ (1982). Immunotherapy by intravesical injection of BCG cell walls or live BCG in bovine ocular squamous cell carcinoma: a preliminary report. J Natl Cancer Inst 69: 1095.

Klein WR, Bras GE, Misdorp W, Steerenberg PA, de Jong WH, Tiesjema RH, Kersjes AW, Ruitenberg EJ (1986). Equine sarcoid: BCG immunotherapy compared to cryosurgery in a prospective randomized clinical trial. Cancer Imm Immunoth 21: 133.

Lamm DL, Thor DE, Harris SL, Reyna JA, Stogdill VD, Radwin HM (1980). Bacillus Calmette-Guérin immunotherapy of superficial bladder cancer. J Urol 124: 38.

Lamm DL, Thor DE, Winters WD, Stogdill VD, Radwin HM (1981). BCG immunotherapy of bladder cancer: inhibition of tumor recurrence and associated immune responses. Cancer 48: 82.

Lamm DL, Stogdill VD, Stogdill BJ, Crispen RG (1986). Complications of Bacillus Calmette-Guérin immunotherapy in 1278 patients with bladder cancer. J Urol 135: 272.

Lamm DL, Pilot S, Sardosi MF (1986). Oral Bacillus

Calmette-Guérin versus intravesical plus percutaneous Bacillus Calmette-Guérin in superficial transitional cell carcinoma. J Urol 135: 186A.

Lamm DL, Blumenstein B, Crawford ED, Montie JE, Scardino P, Stanisic TH, Grossman HB (1987). South-west Oncology Group comparison of Bacillus Calmette-Guérin and doxorubicin in the treatment and prophylaxis of superficial bladder cancer. J Urol 137: 178A.

Lamm DL (1987 and 1988). Personal communication.

Lotte A, Wasz-Höckert O, Poisson N, Dumitrescu N, Verron M, Couvet E (1984). BCG complications. Estimates of the risks among vaccinated subjects and statistical analysis of their main characteristics. Adv Tuberc Res 21: 107.

Mackaness GB, Auclair DJ, Langrange PH (1973). Immunopotentiation with BCG. Immune response to different strains and preparations. J Natl Cancer Inst 51: 1655.

Martinez-Pineiro JA, Muntanola P (1977). Non-specific immunotherapy with BCG vaccine in bladder tumors. A Preliminary report. Eur Urol 3: 11.

Martinez-Pineiro JA (1984). BCG vaccine in superficial bladder tumors: eight years later. Eur Urol 10: 93.

Mathé G, Amiel J, Schwartzenberg L, Schneider M, Catton A, Schlumberger J, Hayat M, De Vassal F (1969). Aucte immunotherapy for acute lymphoblastic leukemia. Lancet 1: 697.

Merguerian PA, Donahue L, Cockett ATK (1987). Intraluminal interleukin 2 and Bacillus Calmette-Guérin for treatment of bladder cancer: a preliminary report. J Urol 136: 216.

Mitchel MS, Kirkpatrick P, Mokyr MB, Gery I (1973). On the mode of action of BCG. Nature, New Biol 243: 216.

Mitchel MS, Mokyr MB, Kahane I (1975). Effect of fractions of BCG on lymhoid cells in vitro. J Natl Cancer Inst 55: 1337.

Morales A, Eidinger D, Bruce AW (1976). Intracavitary Bacillus Calmette-Guérin in the treatment of superficial bladder tumors. J Urol 116: 18.

Morales A, Nickel JG (1906). Immunotherapy of superficial bladder cancer with BCG. World J Urol. 3: 209.

Morton DL, Eilber FR, Malmgren RA (1970). Immunologic factors which influence response to immunotherapy in malignant melanoma. Surgery 68: 158.

Nauts HC, Fowler GA, Bogatka F (1953). A review of the influence of bacterial infection and of bacterial products (Coley's toxins) on malignant tumors in man. Acta Med Scand 276: 5.

Netto Jr NR, Lemos GC (1984). Bacillus Calmette-Guérin

immunotherapy of infiltrating bladder cancer. J Urol 132: 675.

Old L, Clarke D (1959). Effect of Bacillus Calmette-Guérin infection on transplanted tumors in the mouse. Nature 184: 291.

Pearl R (1929). Cancer and tuberculosis. Am J Hyg 9:97.

Pinsky CM, Camacho FJ, Kerr D, Braun Jr DW, Whitmore Jr WF, Oettgen HF (1982). Treatment of superficial bladder cancer with intravesical BCG immunotherapy of human cancer. In Terry WD, Rosenberg SA (Eds): "Excerpta Medica", New York: pp 309.

Pollack SB (1977). Effector cells for antibody-dependent cell mediated cytotoxicity. I. Increased cytotoxicity after priming with BCG-SS. Cell Immunol 29: 373.

Poplack DG, Sher NA, Chaparas SD, Blaese RM (1976). the effect of Mycobacterium bovis (Bacillus Calmette-Guérin) on macrophage random migration, chemotaxis and pinocytosis. Cancer Res 36: 1233.

Rawls WH, Lamm DL, Eyolfson MF (1988). Septic complications in the use of Bacillus Calmette-Guérin for non-invasive transitional cell carcinoma. J Urol 139: 300A.

Rosenthal SR (1936). Focal and general tissue responses to an avirulent tubercle bacillus (BCG) intracardiac route. Arch Pathol 22: 348.

Rosenthal SR (1938). The general tissue and humoral response to an avirulent tubercle bacillus. In University of Illinois Press (ed): "Illinois Medical and Dental monographs", Urbana Ilinois

Rosenthal SR (1980). BCG vaccine: tuberculosis - cancer. P.S.G. Publishing Company Inc., Littleton, Massachusetts, foreword.

Ruitenberg EJ, de Jong WH, Kreeftenberg JG, Steerenberg PA, Kruizinga W, van Noorle Jansen LM (1981). BCG preparations, cultured homogeneously dispersed or as a surface pellicle, elicit different immunopotentiating effects but have similar antitumor activity in a murine fibrosarcoma. Cancer Immunol Immunoth 11: 45.

Schellhammer PF, Warden SS, Ladaga LE (1986). Bacillus Calmette-Guérin (BCG) in the treatment of transitional cell carcinoma (TCC) of the bladder. J Urol 135: 261.

Shapiro A, Ratliff TL, Oakley DM, Catalona WJ (1983). Reduction of bladder tumor growth in mice treated with intravesical Bacillus Calmette-Guérin and its correlation with Bacillus Calmette-Guérin viability and natural killer cell activity. Cancer Res 43: 1611.

Sparks FC (1976). Hazards and complications of BCG immunotherapy. Med Clin North Am 60: 499.

Steg A, Leleu C, Debre B, Boccon-Gibod L (1988). Systemic Bacillus Calmette-Guérin infection in patients treated by intravesical Bacillus Calmette-Guérin therapy for bladder cancer. J Urol 139: 300A.

Wolfe SA, Tracey DE, Henney CS (1976). Induction of natural killer cells by BCG. Nature 262: 584.

Zatz MM (1976) Effects of BCG on lymphocyte trapping. J Immunol 116: 1587.

Zbar B, Bernstein ID, Bartlett GL, Hanna Jr MG, Rapp HJ (1972). Immunotherapy of cancer: regression of intradermal tumors and prevention of growth of lymph node metastases after intralesional injection of living Mycobacterium bovis. J Natl Cancer Inst 49: 119.

EORTC Genitourinary Group Monograph 6:
BCG in Superficial Bladder Cancer, pages 35–50
© 1989 Alan R. Liss, Inc.

HISTORY OF BCG AND ITS SUBSTRAINS

Ray Crispen

American Intl Hospital, Northwestern University, Zion,
Chicago, Illinois, USA

At the turn of the century there was widespread
activity to develop vaccines from attenuated microorganisms
following Pasteur's succesful result using such an approach
with a chicken cholera vaccine. Many medical investigators
throughout the world were examining mycobacteria in the
laboratory from various sources to attunuate the virulence
in order to create a safe but effective vaccine. At that
time most of the adult population was or had been infected
with the tuberculosis bacillus and with a mortality rate of
about 25% tuberculosis was a major public health problem.
It was in the midst of this intense race that Calmette and
Guérin began their work. Calmette had established a branch
of the Pasteur Institue in Lille, France in 1894 and with
the help of Guérin he explored the possibility of
developing the successful vaccine. The initial strain of
mycobacteria that was to become the Bacillus Calmette and
Guérin (BCG) was isolated from a young cow with tuberculous
mastitis by A Nocard in 1904 (Guérin, 1957). This was a
highly virulent strain and was being used routinely in
their laboratory for virulent challenge of animals. One of
the major problems in mycobacteria laboratories was that
because of the clumping of the bacteria to make a
suspension for injections the mass of culture had to be
ground with a mortar and pestle. The addition of beef bile
during this procedure allowed a homogeneous suspension to
be made suitable for innoculation onto culture media or
into animals. A major step was taken in 1908 when Calmette
and Guérin decided to add the beef bile as an ingredient to
the culture medium in expectation that this would result in
changes in the bacteria. After initially increasing in

virulence, the culture became increasingly attenuated and over the next several years the virulence for animals gradually decreased and by 1920 the culture was considered avirulent. It took 231 transfers and over 13 years to accomplish this result (Guérin, 1957). This special strain of MYCOBACTERIUM BOVIS was called the Bacillus of Calmette and Guérin (BCG) in honor of the two discoverers.

DISPERSION OF B.C.G. CULTURES

1921	Pasteur Institute, FRANCE
1924	USSR
	BULGARIA (1958)
1924	BRAZIL
1924	NETHERLANDS
1925	JAPAN
1926	ROUMANIA
1926	SWEDEN
	EQUADOR (1954)
	NORWAY (1966)
1930	BELGIUM
1931	DENMARK (State Secum Institute)
	CZECHOSLOVAKIA (1947)
	EGYPT (1954)
	UNITED KINGDOM (1952)
	SWITZERLAND (1959)
	JAPAN (1965)
	INDIA (1967)
1934	U.S.A. (Chicago)
1937	CANADA (Quebec)
	CANADA (Toronto) (1949)
1948	U.S.A. (New York)
	AUSTRALIA(1951)
1957	TUNISIA
1963	SENEGAL
1965	NETHERLANDS
1965	CHINA
1966	KOREA

Figure 1.

In July 1921 the culture was first given by Weill-Halle to a newborn of a tuberculous mother with a grand-mother also with tuberculosis residing in the same house-hold. The child suffered no ill effects from the vaccina-tion and subsequently grew to adulthood without developing tuberculosis. At the last report the child had reached the age of 33 and was living in the United States (Guérin, 1957). Following this early succes further vaccinations were given, and soon BCG was being given in many countries.

At this time BCG vaccination was by means of freshly prepared cultures. The ability to store the vaccine was limited extending only for a few days or weeks even with refrigeration. This precluded shipping the vaccine through-out the world using the BCG culture developed by Calmette and Guérin. The time line of this dispersion is outlined in Figure 1 (Perkins, 1971; Trudeau, 1970).

TIME THAT DIFFERENT BCG LABORATORIES IN VARIOUS COUNTRIES RECEIVED BCG CULTURES FROM THE PASTEUR INSTITUTE AND THE OTHER COUNTRIES TO WHICH SUBSEQUENTLY WERE PASSED THE CULTURES AND THE DATES OF PASSAGE

Some of the laboratories received subcultures of BCG directly from the Pasteur Institute while others obtained theirs as secondary cultures from these laboratories. Many of the laboratories continue to use the original subculture received while others use newer lots or a number of sub-strains. The results of this random and nearly uncontrolled dispersion were many. The manner of propagation the cultures at that time were such that it was possible for a mixture of genotypes to be continually transferred. In 1927 Petroff and Steenken (Petroff et al., 1929) demonstrated what appeared to be two distinct subcultures from the BCG vaccine: the R-varient and the S-varient. Other labora-tories substantiated this finding for a short time but sub-sequently this differentiation disappeared. It was during this discovery that the Lubeck Disaster happened in 1930. Of 251 newborns vaccinated orally with BCG, 72 died of tuberculosis, 135 showed symptoms of tuberculosis and 44 became positive reactors to the skin test. None of the 161 children born at the same time but not vaccinated were affected and none died of tuberculosis within the next three years. A thorough investigation of the episode by German authorities established that the vaccine had been prepared accidently from a mixture of BCG and a virulent strain of Mycobacterium tuberculosis. Recurring episodes of different culture forms being dissociated on culture are still appearing with some differences also appearing in animal testing (Portelance et al., 1976; Mokyr et al., 1980; Osborn, 1971 and 1986). With the different culture conditions and ingredients of the media being used through the world the slow evaluation of the dispersed daughter strains of BCG have become evident. The genetic drift of BCG can be stabilized by the use of the seed lot system for BCG being established by each laboratory as recommended by the World Health Organization (Guld, 1971). As a result, the reproducibility of production lots is now more reliable, but the differences of the various daughter strains can still be demonstrated by laboratory comparison (Mokyr at al., 1980). Even within the individual substrains, there still exists subtle differences as reported from some laboratories even though the propagation procedures remain the same (Bennet et al., 1983). Each laboratory has established the preferred means of producing the culture and the resulting methodology gives rise to differences in substrains. Pellicle growth on the surface of the medium or subsurface growth in deep culture are obvious differences of preparation that are likely to result in differing characteristics (Ruitenberg at al., 1981).

Although all current vaccines used in anti-tuberculosis programs appear to have maintained their ability to stimulate immunity to tuberculosis, albeit to different degrees, the use of these BCG substrains and other substrains developed in various laboratories for cancer research and therapy, has resulted in a redefinition of variations in the BCG strains (Crispen, 1976). A review of much of this early work published in 1972 set the stage for further research on the potential of BCG immunotherapy mechanisms of immune activation by BCG (Crispen, 1972; Crispen, 1974; Davies, 1982).

In the early 1970's I began to experiment with the Tice substrain to determine whether it was suitable for use as an antitumor agent. Experiments in mice and rats (Crispen, 1972) established that it was effective in tumor models (El-Domeiria et al., 1978a) and several clinical trials were begun to study its effectiveness in humans. Results in lung cancer (Crispen et al., 1977; Warren et al., 1978), melanoma (El-Domeiria et al. 1978b), prostate (Guinan et al. 1979), and bladder cancer (Brosman, 1982; Crispen, 1984) have proven the efficacy of this new substrain of the original Tice daughter strain. During the 1970's further work in my laboratory resulted in increasing effectiveness evolving in the new substrain through the IL 74 intermediate seed until the seed strain 105 was finally developed (Crispen, 1978). Laboratory and clinical tests demonstrated the IL 74 surpassed the original Tice sub-strain (9-8S) and that the new seed lot 105 was superior to IL 74 (Bennet et al., 1983). This was proven to be the most effective of the BCG strains used in bladder cancer (Guinan et al., 1987); Khanna et al., 1988). Similar research is continuing in many other laboratories (De Jong et al., 1984).

The use of BCG to treat cancer in humans was first reported by Holmgren in Sweden (Holmgren, 1935). He reported some successes with 185 injections in 28 patients without serious side effects. This report was not followed-up for several years until in 1963 Vilasor in the Philli-pines reported the use of BCG with some success in 43 patients with various types of cancer (Vilasor, 1965). The modern use of BCG in cancer therapy was begun with the report of controlled clincial trials such as the ones by Mathe in 1969 with the dramatic decrease of acute leukemia in children (Mathe et al., 1969) and Hadsiev in Bulgaria of the use of BCG in bronchial carcinoma that showed increased survival of 71 patients (Hadsiev and Kavaklieve-Dimitrova, 1969), and the additional report from the United States by Morton of the successful use of direct injection of BCG into melanoma nodulcs (Morton et al., 1970). These reports clearly established BCG as an important cancer treatment. These results gave rise to many clinical studies, but the inability to reproduce the results of the early trials lcd to the reduced use of BCG. At the same time the advances of other forms of therapy resulted in the reduction of the apparant advantage of BCG immunotherapy.

The major exception was in the use of BCG in the treatment of bladder cancer. This use of BCG was begun by Morales and associates in the 1970's (Morales et al., 1976). BCG is now widely used through the world as the preferred treatment for the superficial stagcs of bladder cancer. Recently thc American Medical Association in a report of a panel of 23 medical experts on the Diagnostic and Therapeutic Technology Accessment (DATTA), determined that BCG immunotherapy was both safe and effective for such use (DATTA, 1988). A recent report by Lamm on the use in 1,278 patients has been instrumental in establishing the basis of the expected range of treatment effects and side effects with recommendations for control of untoward effects (Lamm et al., 1986). Guiman reviewed the experience of several trials of BCG immunotherapy (Guiman et al., 1987). Many other publications have appeared from the laboratories and clinics of the speakers of this meeting.

Reports from throughout the world in such use of BCG daughter strains have been uniformly positive with two exceptions. Flamm reported that the use of BCG from Connaught Laboratories (Toronto) was ineffective (Flamm and Grof, 1981), although many others have found this substrain to be effective. Robinson reported that the Glaxo substrain yielded poor results (Robinson et al., 1980). It is likely that these reported failures were the result of inadequate doses. Kaisary in a comparison of Glaxo and Pasteur substrains found that similarily good results for both could be obtained if the dosage was adjusted to adequate levels (Kaisary, 1987).

The major requirement for the successful use of BCG in bladder cancer therapy is that the dosage be high enough and that the preparation contains a high proportion of viable mycobacteria (Kelley et al., 1985). Non-viable preparations do not have antitumor activity (Mackaness et al., 1973). With the repeated administration of BCG on a weekly basis for several weeks the cumulative dosage (in conjunction with the multiplication of the mycobacteria) is sufficient to make all the BCG substrains useful (adequate) for the treatment of bladder cancer.

The differences in the various substrains of BCG in laboratory and animal tests is well established, although clinical trials may not reveal these differences. The tests for viability are sufficiently complex that inter-laboratory comparisons cannot be done effectively even though the tests are done in laboratories producing BCG and experienced in doing BCG viability tests. In the usual clinical laboratories the results of such viability tests are even more difficult to interpret (Kelley et al., 1985). The USA Food and Drug Administration has mandated the method for viability tests for BCG vaccine licensed in the USA using the semi-solid agar tube method (Federal Registration, 1979). The major problem of determining viability of BCG preparations is the fact that it is reported in Colony Forming Units (CFU). Each CFU, while theoretically is a single live organism, is in reality probably also a clump of organisms. The high lipid content of the outer wall structure of mycobacteria (up to 60% of the dry weight) makes it difficult to separate the mycobacteria sufficiently to result in single cell counts. Even the dispersed deep culture growth using wetting agents results in small clumps averaging three bacilli while the pellicle growth with subsequent homogenization results in clumps of 10-1,000 cells. The resulting mixtures of live and dead cells comprise the innoculum. Although the live cells are essential to the proper immunostimulation, the portion of the dosage that contains killed cells and cell debris also contributes to the response and may even be responsible for much of the less desirable side effects (Mackaness et al., 1973). Figure 2 is an electron micrograph of mycobacteria showing the coating that causes the bacteria to clump (Crispen, 1967).

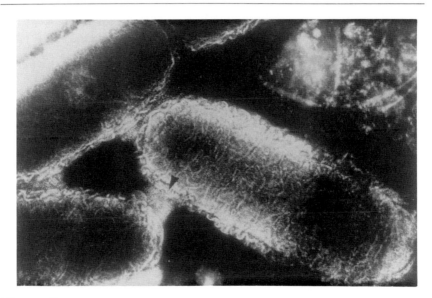

Figure 2.

THE THICK OUTER WALL OF THE MYCOBACTERIA IS SHOWN AND THE ADHERENCE OF THE CELLS CAN BE SEEN. CELL FRAGMENTS ARE ALSO PRESENT. MAGNIFICATION 40,000x.

The patient's immunological status is important in adjusting the route and dosage of BCG to obtain the maximum benefit without serious side effects. The immune response has a finite capacity and from animal studies it is known that the dosage necessary to trigger the immune response is different in sensitized versus non-sensitive hosts. There is a limit to the immune response even in normal individuals, although, it varies with the genetic make-up and state of health. BCG affects a wide spectrum of specific and non-specific immune phenomena such as antibody responses (Miller et al., 1973; Florentin et al., 1976), non-specific anti-bacterial immunity (Blanden et al., 1969), allograph rejection (Sparks and Breeding, 1974), as well as tumor rejection. These responses are due to the effect of BCG on different cell types including T-cells, B-cells, macrophages, killer (K) cells, and natural killer (NK) cells. Figure 3 is a diagram of the different branches of the immune system that are involved in actions against a tumor.

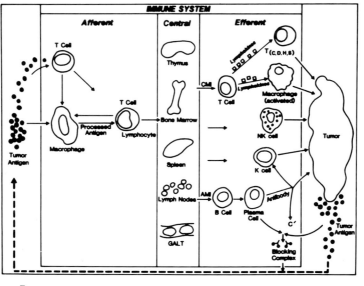

Figure 3.

DIAGRAM OF THE THREE BRANCHES OF THE IMMUNE SYSTEM

The afferent branch is the recognition stage; BCG is able to preactivate this branch either by the fact that it shares common antigens with some tumors or develops more sensitive cells by non-specific means. The central arm is the reservoir whereby new cells can be generated and/or potential (stem) cells can be activated. BCG causes both hyperactivity and hyperplasia resulting in a vigorous response (Bansal and Sjogren, 1973). The effector branch is the action branch that is able to exert cytotoxic or cytostatic effects on the tumor. This is accomplished by several means: the activation of cytotoxic T-cells, the modification of macrophages to the activated stage, and the production of specific antibodies by plasma cells against the tumor. BCG has been shown to have the ability to activate each of these branches and phases within the branches. The different substrains affect these activations to differing degrees, but if the dosages are sufficient, full activation is reached by all the present substrains. BCG acts by activating macrophages by means of T-lympho- cytes, presumably CD 4 helper cells, which are specifically reacting with the antigenic determinants of the microbes. These may share antigens between some tumor systems and BCG as reported by different laboratories (Minden, 1976). A repeated exposure of the resulting clone of CD 4 helper cells eventually generates the necessary numbers and quality of signals to convert macrophages into cells with the capacity to kill tumor cells as well as the inciting organisms (Mitchell et al., 1973). Ruco reported that in animal experiments for the full activation of macrophages to be tumoricidal, a sequence of signals is required (Ruco and Melther, 1977). The macrophage activation factor (MAF) plus a second signal of bacterial antigen caused the macrophages to develop their tumoricidal potential to the fullest. This is in agreement with the "arming/activation" sequence proposed earlier. (Evans and Alexander, 1972). Other investigators found that the macrophages could be activated by either of the signals but that there was a synergistic effect if both signals were present (Sone and Fidler, 1981). As a result of these and other experiments it has been shown in animals that the use of BCG and lymphokines can have more effect than either alone. BCG stimulates the production of lymphokines, but the use of BCG with exogenous lymphokines can be even more effective. Early experiments along this line in humans with bladder cancer have shown promising results in which the use of IL 2 with BCG allows the dose of BCG to be reduced by one half (Merguerian et al., 1987).

Numerous mechanisms are proposed for the effects of BCG on tumors (Crispen, 1974). These mechanisms include lymphoid cells becoming sensitized against tumor antigens and specifically attacking the tumor, macrophages being activated by a number of stimuli resulting in cytolysis or inhibition of the tumor, K-cells developing cytotoxic activity against the tumor after the tumor has been sensitized by specific antibody, and increased NK-cell activity against tumors which is antibody dependent. Within this range BCG has the ability to insure tumor regression by both specific and non-specific mechanisms. The specific mechanism includes the typical delayed type hypersensitivity after intralesional injection of BCG where the tumor cells are attacked non-specifically as "bystanders", and the increase of tumor specific immunity as the result of prior sensitization by the tumor (Florentin et al., 1976). The non-specific mechanism includes the generalized stimulation of the entire phagocytic monocyte system causing hyperplasia and hyperreactivity of its cellular components. BCG affects the distribution of lymphoid cells through the body, possibly by means of a T-cell subpopulation-mediated mechanism (Zatz and Gershon, 1974) and lymphocyte trapping (Zatz, 1976). Florintin reported that BCG adjuvant effect was not dependent on lymphocyte trapping but on a modification of the localization of normal lymphoid cells by depressed migration (Florintin et al., 1976). The homing pattern of thoracic duct lymphocytes could be altered by BCG to direct more lymphocytes to the thymus reducing those to the bone marrow (Sutherland et al., 1979), thereby increasing the number of recirculating lymphocytes together with increased lymphocyte-mediated cytotoxicity (Bansal and Sjogren, 1973). BCG, thereby, plays a multiple role in the activation of T-cells. Much of this work has been reviewed recently (Davies, 1982; de Jong 1985).

It may be a result of the concentration of the finite immune response of the host that has been responsible for the high degree of success of BCG immunotherapy against bladder cancer. Such a concentration of the limited resources of the immune system thus may pre-empt immune responses against other new primary tumors. Such an effect could explain the presence of unrestricted growth of such tumors in successfully treated patients as reported recently (Hardeman et al., 1988; Khanna et al., 1988). This result can be expected and explained by the rational given previously for the mechanisms of BCG antitumor actions. The immune system has a finite response capacity. If this capacity has been maximally stimulated by BCG and focused on the initial tumor, i.e. bladder cancer, then by the various migration inhibiting factors and trapping activities of the

BCG stimulation there would be insufficient reserves to react against the second tumor, especially if the second tumor lacks the anti-genicity to stimulate the immune response. It has been conclusively demonstrated in the Strain 2 guinea pig model that the successful immunization to the line 10 tumor does not result in any immunity to the distinctly different line 1 tumor (De Jong et al., 1985). Surgery remains a primary treatment for cancer but due to the fact that many tumors have metastasized before surgery this form of treatment has only limited potential for permanent cure and then only for early cancer. Chemotherapy and radiation therapy, although increasing in effectiveness with the newer drugs and treatment protocols, use first order kinetics in killing a decreasing portion of tumor cells with each successive treatment and resistant tumor cells frequently allow the tumor to regrow. Immunotherapy, as with BCG, follows zero order kinetics and can potentially destroy the last tumor cells but is dependent, however, on the amount of response that the host can generate and is limited in the number of tumor cells that response can destroy.

Other biological agents have been prepared to replace BCG but none have been adequate - other mycobacterial strains, killed cell vaccines, extracts of BCG and other bacteria and viruses (Zatz and Gershon, 1974; Scott and Bomford, 1976) have been tried but have not surpassed the effectiveness of BCG and most are not as effective. The unique advantage of BCG remains its viability and the ability to stimulate the immune system over long periods of time. The viability results in the self leveling dosage when the host's response acts to reduce the BCG cells by natural means. The addition safety factor of the ability to use the anti-tuberculosis drugs is an added feature that none of the other agents possess.

The use of a combination of modalities of treatment and a combination of agents can be additive in effect. The recent availability of lymphokines and their usefulness with the various substrains of BCG has opened a new era of BCG immunotherapy. Just what is the best substrain to use with each lymphokine and for what indication is yet unknown. Experiments have begun in cloning the DNA of BCG which adds a further dimension to our research (Thole et al., 1985). It is certain that the search for the definitive BCG substrain begun by Calmette and Guérin will continue and be strengthened by the clear demonstration of the effectiveness of BCG treatment of bladder cancer as defined by this meeting.

The history of BCG and its substrains continues.

REFERENCES

Additional Standards For Bacterial Products. Part 620: BCG Vaccine: Final Rule (1979). Federal Register 44: 14541-14548.

Bansal S, Sjogren H (1973). Effects of BCG on various facets of the immune response against polyoma tumors in rats. Int J Cancer 11: 162-171.

Bennett J, Gruff H, Mc Kneally M, Zelterman D, Crispen R (1983). Differences in biological activity among batches of lypholized Tice BCG and their association with clinical course in Stage 1 lung cancer. Cancer Res 43: 4183-4290.

Blanden R, Lefford M, Mackaness G (1969). The host response to BCG infection in mice. J Exp Med 129: 1079-1107.

Brosman SA (1982). Experience with BCG in patients with superficial bladder carcinoma. J Urol 128: 27-34.

Crispen R (1967). Laboratory data, Northwestern University, Chicago.

Crispen R (1972). Laboratory data, Department of Micro-biology University of Illinois.

Crispen R (1974). BCG in perspective. Semm Oncology 1: 311-317.

Crispen R (1976). Actions of immuntherapy agents. In Crispen R (ed): "Neoplasma Immunity: Mechanisms," Chicago, ITR Pub, pp.

Crispen R, Warren S, Nika B (1977). Immunotherapy for advanced lung cancer. In Salmon S, Jones S (eds): "Adjuvant Therapy of Cancer," Amsterdam: North-Holland Pub, pp 251-256.

Crispen R (1978). Tice Laboratory and Tice Clinic data, ITR, Univesity of Illinois.

Crispen R (1984). RE Experience with Bacillus Calmette-Guérin in patients with superficial bladder carcinoma (letter). J Urol 131: 558.

Davies M (1982). BCG as an antitumor agent: The interaction with the cells of the mammalian immune system. Biochem Biophisic Acta 651: 143-174.

Diagnostic and Therapeutic Technology Assessment (DATTA)

(1988). BCG immunotherapy in bladder cancer: A reassessment. J Amer Med Assoc 259: 2153-2155.

El-Domeiria A, Crispen R, DasGupta T, Trippon M, Simo C, Sabat T (1978a). Immunization against methylcolanthrene induced sarcoma in A/J mice. J Reticuloendothelial Soc 24: ab 4716.

El-Domeiria A, DasGupta T, Trippon M, Simo C, Sabet T, Crispen R (1978b). Adjuvant chemotherapy and immunotherapy in high risk patients with melanoma. Surg Gynecol Obstet 146: 230-232.

Evans R, Alexander P (1972). Mechanism of immunologically specific killing of tumor cells by macrophages. Nature 236: 168-170.

Florentin I, Hucket R, Bruley-Rosset M, Halle-Pannenko O, Mathe G (1976). Studies on the mechanisms of action of BCG. Can Immun Immunother 1: 31-39.

Flamm J, Grof F (1981). Adjuvante lokale Immunotherapy mit BCG in der Behandlung des Urothelkarzinoms der Harnblase. Wien Med Wochenschr 131: 501-506.

Guérin C (1957). Early history of BCG. In Rosenthal SR (ed): "BCG Vaccination Against Tuberculosis," Boston: Little Brown, pp 48-53.

Guinan P, Crispen R, Baumgartner G, Rao R, Totchi E, Ablin R (1979). Adjuvant immunotherapy with Bacillus Calmette-Guérin in prostatic cancer. Urology 14: 561-565.

Guinan P, Crispen R, Rubenstein M (1987). BCG in management of superficial bladder cancer. Urology 30: 515-519.

Guld J (1971). Use of the seed lot system. Symp Series Immunobiol Stand 17: 143-146.

Hadziev S, Kavaklieve-Dimitrova J (1969). Application du BCG dans le cancer chez l'homme. Folia Med Neerl 11: 8-14.

Hardeman S, Perry A, Soloway M (1988). Transitional cell carcinoma of the prostate following intravesical therapy for transitional cell carcinoma of the bladder. J Urol 140: 289-292.

Holmgren I (1935) La tuberculine et le BCG chez les cancereuz. Schwiez Med Wochenschr 65: 1203-1206.

de Jong W, Steerenberg P, Kreeftenberg J, Tiesjema R, Kruizinga W, van Noorle Jansen L, Ruitenberg E (1984). Experimental screening of BCG preparations produced for cancer immunotherapy: safety, immunostimulating and anti-tumor activity of four consecutive produced batches. Can. Imm Immunother 17: 18-27.

de Jong W, van der Plas M, Steerenberg P, Kruizinga W, Ruitenberg E (1985). Selective localization of tumor immune spleen cells at the tumor challenge site adoptive transfer of line 10 tumor immunity in strain 2 guinea pigs. J Immunol 134: 163-187.

de Jong W (1985). Thesis, University of Utrecht, the Netherlands.

Kaisary A (1987). Intravesical BACG therapy in the management of multiple superficial bladder cancer: A comparison between Glaxo and Pasteur strains. Br J Urol 59: 554-558.

Kelley D, Ratliff T, Catalona W, Shapiro A, Lage J, Bauer W, Haaff E, Dresner S (1985). Intravesical BCG therapy for superficial bladder cancer: Effect of BCG viability on treatment results. J Urol 134: 48-53.

Khanna O, Chou R, Son D, Mazer H, Read J, Nugent D, Cottone R, Heeg M, Viek N, Uhlman R, Freidmann M (1988). Does BCG immunotherapy accelerate growth and cause metastatic spread of secondary primary malignancy? Urology 31: 459-468.

Khanna O, Son D, Mazer H, Read J, Nugent D, Cottone R, Heeg M, Rezvan M, Viek N, Uhlman R, Freidmann M (1988). Superficial bladder cancer treated with intravesical BCG or adriamycin: Follow-up report. Urology 31: 287-293.

Lamm DL, Stogdill V, Stogdill B, Crispen R (1986). Complications of Bacillus Calmette-Guérin immunotherapy in 1,278 patients with bladder cancer. J Urol 135: 272-274.

Mackaness G, Auclair D, Lagrange P (1973). Immunopotentiation with BCG: Immune response to different strains and preparation. J Nat Can Inst 5: 1655-1658.

Mathe G, Amiel J. Schwarzenberg L, Schneider M, Catton A, Schlumberger J, Hayat M, Vassal F de (1969). Acute immunotherapy for acute lymphoblastic leukemia. Lancet 1: 679-699.

Merguerian P, Donahue L, Cockett A (1987). Intraluminal interleukin 2 and BCG for treatment of bladder cancer: A preliminary report. J Urol 137: 216-219.

Miller T, Mackaness G, Lagrange P (1973). Immunopotentiation with BCG: II Modulation of the response to sheep red blood cells. J Natl Can Inst 51: 1669-1676.

Minden P (1976). Shared antigens between animal and human tumors and microorganisms. In Lamourreux F, Portelance V, Turcotte R (eds): "BCG in cancer immunotherapy," New York: Grune and Stratton, pp 73-76.

Mitchell M, Kirkpatrick D, Mokyr M, Gery I (1973). On the mode of action of BCG. Nature 243: 216-217.

Mokyr M, Bennett J, Hengst J, Mitchell M, Dray S (1980). Opposite effects of different strains or batches of the same strain of BCG on in vitro generation of syngeneic and allogeneic antitumor cytotixicity. J Nat Can Inst 64: 339-344.

Morales A, Eidinger D, Bruce A (1976). Intracavitary Bacillus Calmette-Guérin in the treatment of superficial bladder tumors. J Urol 116: 180-183.

Morton DL, Eilber F, Malmgren R, Wood W (1970). Immunological factors with influence response to immunotherapy in malignant melanoma. Surgery 68: 158-164.

Osborn T (1971). Studies "in vitro" of BCG daugther strains. Symp Series Immunobiol Stand 17: 125-132.

Osborn T (1986). Some effects of nutritional components on the morphology of BCG colonies. Dev Biol Stand 58: 79-94.

Perkins F (1971). Analysis of the replies to a questionaire. Symp Series Immunobiol Stand 17: 5-40.

Petroff SA, Branch A, Steenken W (1929). Study of Bacillus Calmette and Guérin (BCG): biological characteristics, culture "dissociation" and animal experiments. Amer Review Tuber 19: 9-49.

Portelance V, Boulanger RP, Duranleau-Dragon D (1976). Comparative virulence and antitumor activity of BCG substrains. In Lamoureux G, Turcotte R, Portelance V (eds): "BCG in Cancer Immunotherapy," New York: Grune and Stratton, pp.

Robinson M, Richard B, Adib R, Akdas A, Rigby C, Pugh R (1980). Intravesical BCG in the management of T1 Nx Mx transitional cell tumors of the bladder: a toxicity study. In Pavone-Macaluso M, Smith P, Edsmyr F (eds): "Bladder tumors and other topics in urological oncology," New York: Plenum Press, pp 171-174.

Ruco L, Melther M (1977). Macrophage activation for tumor cytotoxicty; induction of tumoricidal macrophages by supernatants of PPD stimulated BCG immune spleen cells and cultures. J Immunol 119: 889-896.

Ruitenberg E, de Jong W, Kreeftenberg J, Steerenberg P, Kruizinga W, van Noorle Jansen L (1981). BCG preparations, cultured homogeneous dispersed or as a surface pellicle, elicit different immunopotentiation effects but have similar antitumor activity in a murine fibrosarcoma. Can Immun Immunother 11: 45-51.

Scott M, Bomford R (1976). Comparison of the potentiation of specific tumor immunity in mice by Corynebacterium parvum or BCG. J Nat Can Inst 57: 555-559.

Sone S, Fidler I (1981). In vitro activation of tumoricidal properties in rat alveolar macrophages by synthetic muramyl dipeptide encapsulated in liposomes. Cell Immunol 57: 42-50.

Sparks F, Breeding J (1974). Tumor regression and enhancement resulting from immunotherapy with BCG and neuraminidase. Cancer Res 34: 3262-3269.

Sutherland R, Spardaro-Antonelle M, Lawrence V, Quagliata F
(1979). Immunosupressive activity of BCG; effects of
adjuvant disease, lymphocyte subpopulations and homing of
thoracic duct cells in rats. Infect Immun 25: 310-319.

Thole J, Dauwerese H, Das P, Groothuis D, Schouls L, van
Embden J (1985). Cloning of Mycobacterium bovis (BCG) DNA
and expression of antigens in Escherichia coli. Infect
Immun 50: 800-806.

Trudeau Mycobacterial Catalogue (1970).

Villasor RP (1965). The clinical use of BCG vaccine in
stimulating host resistance to cancer. II immunotherapy
in advanced cancer. J. Philippine Med Assoc 41: 619-632.

Warren S, Crispen R, Nika B (1978). Survival of patients
with bronchogenic carcinoma modified by BCG immunotherapy. Am Surgery 44: 428-431.

Zatz M, Gershon R (1974). Thymus dependence of lymphocyte
trapping. J Immunol 112: 101-106.

Zatz M (1976). Effects of BCG on lymphocyte trapping. J
Immol 116: 1587-1591.

EORTC Genitourinary Group Monograph 6:
BCG in Superficial Bladder Cancer, pages 51–65
© 1989 Alan R. Liss, Inc.

FUNDAMENTALS OF ACTIVE SPECIFIC IMMUNOTHERAPY OF CANCER USING BCG-TUMOR CELL VACCINES

M.G. Hanna Jr., L.C. Peters and H.C. Hoover Jr.

Organon Teknika, Bionetics Research Institute, Rockville, and Massachusetts General Hospital, Harvard Medical School, Boston, USA

INTRODUCTION

The success of immunotherapy both in experimental animals and in man depends upon the stage of the tumor at the time of treatment. The major potential for immunotherapy is its use as an adjunct to chemotherapy or surgery of the primary tumor when there is only minimal regional lymph node metastasis and micrometastatic disease in the visceral organs. Non-specific immunomodulation with the aim to enhance immune reactivity against disseminated minimal residual malignancy has been attempted clinically with such microbial vaccines as Mycobacterium bovis strain Bacillus Calmette-Guérin (BCG), Corynebacterium parvum, several polynucleotides, levamisole, and lately Interferon. The unsuccessful or equivocal results of these problematic, albeit feasible, clinical protocols may be partly attributable to the low degree of antigenicity of human tumors, while the successful animal models for non-specific immunotherapy involved relatively antigenic transplantable murine tumors. Although immunopotentiators can enhance immune responses in general, the complicated host-tumor interrelationship indicates that in the immunocompetent host the immune response has a finite capacity to counteract any given antigen. Thus, it is unlikely that generalized immunopotentiation will result in a sufficiently elevated immunological capacity that would significantly alter the growth of a weakly antigenic tumor or affect micrometastases.

There has also been a substantial effort to actively immunize autochthonous or syngeneic hosts with irradiated or chemically modified tumor cells in an attempt to achieve active specific immunotherapy. Inherent in this approach is the assumption that tumor cells express tumor-specific transplantation antigens. Treatment of tumor cells with a variety of unrelated agents such as radiation, Mitomycin-C, lipophiloc agents, neuraminidase, viruses, or admixture of the cells with bacterial adjuvants has yielded non-tumorigenic tumor cell preparations that are immunogenic upon injection into syngeneic hosts (Bartlett and Zbar, 1972; Bekesi et al., 1971; Martin et al, 1971; Prager and Baechtel, 1973; Ray et al., 1975). Basically, these results support the concept that antigens not found in normal adult tissues are frequently found in tumors and that the immunogenicity of these tumor cells can be expressed and even enhanced in normal and tumor-bearing hosts. These experimental results have validated the rationale of active specific immunotherapy of neoplasia.

Beginning with the pioneering studies of Mathé, who treated acute lymphocytic leukemia with BCG (Mathé et al., 1973), killed leukemic blasts, or both, similar protocols for treatment of acute or chronic granulocytic leukemia (Powles et al., 1973; Sokal et al., 1973), malignant melanoma (Morton et al., 1976), and lung tumor (Hollingshead, 1978) have produced encouraging results by prolonging disease-free intervals. However, as of now, none of the treatments have significantly increased patient survival. Not all immunotherapy trials have been successful, even with respect to maintenance of disease-free intervals, as shown by recent studies of stage IIB malignant melanoma in which allogeneic or autochthonous tumor cells were used (Hedley et al., 1978). The approach of active specific immunotherapy, although recognized as biologically sound, has been burdened by technical limitations that must be overcome before being practical in the laboratory or clinic (Prager, 1978).

The weakly immunogenic L10 hepatocarcinoma of strain 2 guinea pigs has proven to be a useful experimental model for examining certain aspects of active specific immunotherapy and has provided a system to evaluate a potent immunostimulant, Mycobacterium bovis (BCG). Intratumoral injection of viable BCG produced regression of established tumors of limited size growing in the skin and the elimination of regional lymph node metastases (Hanna et al., 1972; Zbar and Tanaka, 1971); it also conferred immunity to a second intradermal (i.d.) challenge with L10 tumor cells (Hanna et al., 1973; Zbar et al., 1972). More recently, it has been demonstrated that vaccines composed of viable BCG organisms admixed with metabolically active but non-tumor-igenic L10 cells were effective in eliminating established visceral micrometastases (Hanna and Peters, 1978a,b). These observations imply that mixing the BCG with tumor cells may provide an effective immune stimulus despite the weak anti-genicity of the tumor cells. In this guinea pig model the resultant tumor-specific immune response can eliminate established micrometastases. It is important to note that common to both the elimination of localized tumor by BCG alone and the induction of tumor-specific immunity by BCG-tumor cell vaccination is the development of a chronic inflammatory reaction resulting in epithelioid granuloma formation (Hanna and Bucana, 1979). The relationship between the chronic BCG-induced granulomatous inflammation (Adams, 1976; Boros, 1978) and the induction of systemic, tumor-specific immunity in this experimental guinea pig model is unclear.

Of the two therapeutic approaches, intratumoral BCG or BCG plus tumor cell immunization, the latter would appear to be more generally applicable in cancer treatment. Recent investigations have focused on various parameters of the vaccine preparation and administration. The two variables of BCG dose and tumor cell viability were found to pro-foundly influence the efficacy of the vaccine in the guinea pig immunotherapy model (Hanna et al., 1979; Peters et al., 1979). Significant protection against disseminated tumor required a minimum of two vaccinations administered 1 week apart with the initial immunization containing at least 10^7 viable BCG organisms admixed with 10^7 or more tumor cells. Tumor cell viability above 85% in the final vaccine prepa-ration was critical. Thus, any manipulation of the tumor cells such as disaggregation from a solid tumor, cryobio-logic preservation, or X-irradiation would have to be accomplished while maintaining the prerequisite of cell viability. As well, no protection was achieved when another syngeneic, but antigenically distinct, hepatocarcinoma was used in the vaccine, thus suggesting that this was active specific immunotherapy.

An important feature of the model is its adaptability

to studies of active specific immunotherapy as an adjunct to surgery (Hanna and Peters, 1978a). This allows the translation of information from this model to cases in which specific immunotherapy is used to treat micrometastasis after surgical excision of the primary tumor.

EXPERIMENTAL STUDIES OF ACTIVE SPECIFIC IMMUNOTHERAPY IN THE GUINEA PIG TUMOR MODEL SYSTEM

A major contribution to understanding the principles of active specific immunotherapy has been the development and biological characterization of an adequate experimental model that fulfills the requirements for studying effective immunotherapy of established tumors.

A BCG-L10 tumor cell vaccine was developed that successfully stimulated systemic tumor immunity in strain 2 guinea pigs. A series of studies (Hanna et al., 1972, 1973, 1979; Peters et al., 1979) demonstrated that BCG admixed with tumor cells could induce a degree of systemic tumor immunity that could eliminate a small disseminated tumor burden (Table 1) when the vaccine was carefully controlled for such variables as the number of viable, but non-tumorigenic tumor cells (10^7 optimal), the ratio of viable BCG organisms to tumor cells (1:1), and the vaccine regimen (3 vaccines, 1 week apart) is carefully administered (Table 2). Most prior clinical trials of tumor vaccines have used either non-viable (metabolically inactive) autologous tumor cells or allogenic tumor cells, both found to be totally ineffective in the guinea pig.

TABLE 1. Survival of guinea pigs after immunotherapy of established metastases

Vaccination schedule (days after tumor injection)	Survival rate %	Size of pulmonary metastases (day measured)
No vaccinations	0	
1,7,14	70	<5 cells (day 1)
4,11,18	65	5-10 cells (day 4)
7,14,21	40	0.1-0.2 mm (days 7-10)
10,17,24	20	0.35-0.5 mm (days 21-24)

Inbred strain 2 guinea pigs were injected i.v. with 10^6 syngeneic line-10 hepatocarcinoma cells. Each animal subsequently received two intradermal injections of 10^7 BCG admixed with viable but nontumorigenic line-10 cells which had been exposed to X-rays (20,000 rads), and one injection of irradiated line-10 cells alone. The data are pooled from three experiments (a total of 45 guinea pigs per group).

TABLE 2. Vaccines for active specific immunotherapy

Adjuvant

a) BCG (Phipps, Tice, Connaught): lyophilized, frozen
    (dose-dependence $>10^6 = 10^7 - 10^8$)
b) C. Parvum (Wellcome Labs)
    (dose-dependence >7 μg $= 70$ μg <700 μg)

Tumor Cells

a) Enzymatic dissociation
    1) Collagenase type I (1.5-2.0 U/ml HBSS)
    2) DNase (450 K.U./ml HBSS)
    3) 37°C with stirring
b) Cryopreservation
    1) Controlled-rate freezing (-1°C/min) (7.5% DMSO,
        5% FBS, HBSS)
    2) Viability $\geq 80\%$
c) X-irradiation
    1) Rendered nontumorigenic at 12,000-20,000 R.

Components and Administration[a]

a) Ratio of adjuvant to tumor cells--10:1-1:1 (optimum)
b) 10^7 tumor cells (optimum)
c) 2-3 I.D. vaccinations at weekly intervals (third vaccination
    contains tumor cells only)

---

[a]INH chemoprophylaxis of BCG infection optional.

A most dramatic influence on vaccine efficacy was demonstrated when low tumor cell viability ($<50\%$) was compared to high tumor cell viability ($>70\%$). The latter was best achieved with proper dissociation procedures and optimal cryopreservation (Peters et al., 1980). Another important factor in vaccine efficacy was dose of adjuvant (Figure 1). Variation in dose of either C. Parvum or BCG, with constant tumor cell dose (10^7) had a marked influence in percentage survival of vaccinated guinea pigs injected with line 10 cells. In general, low adjuvant mixture was ineffective and more adjuvant (>70 μg CP or 10^7 BCG) was not necessarily beneficial.

In our studies, as well as other investigator's (G.B. Mackaness, personal communications) there were salient observations in the properties of various BCG preparations, which may be relevant to the success of application of BCG to tumor cell vaccines. All commercially produced, freeze-dried BCG vaccines are poorly disperged. Of the pellicle-grown vaccines, the Pasteur product is the least and Tice the most highly dispersed of those examined. Even the Glaxo vaccine, which is grown as a submerged culture, is strongly aggregated. This fact results in mis-represented colony counts since a single colony may result from an aggregate of 10 or more bacteria. On the other hand, the fresh-frozen cultures, (not freeze-dried) are inherently less aggregated, and based on our experience the cell density may vary by a factor of 3 versus 10 or more in the freeze-dried vaccine. This variable is of importance in maintaining constant non-toxic doses of BCG for administration to either guinea pigs or man. In keeping with differences in the state of dispersion, reconstituted vaccine shows heavy deposits of varying bulk when centrifuged. Moreover, the supernatant after centrifugation showed varying degrees of opacity which reflected the content of subcellular particles resulting form dispersion of pellicle-grown vaccines. Since we do not know how these factors of aggregation and subcellular particles may influence the immune response and in an attempt to control BCG dose within a limited range in these studies, we used fresh-frozen Tice BCG at a dose of 10^7 organisms per tumor cell vaccine.

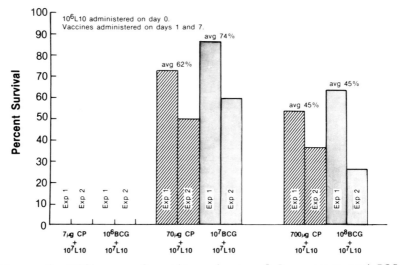

Figure 1. Efficacy of various doses of <u>C. parvum</u> and BCG as adjuvants in L10 tumor cell vaccines.

MECHANISMS OF ACTION OF BCG-TUMOR CELL VACCINES IN THE GENERATION OF SYSTEMIC TUMOR IMMUNITY

The effect of surgical excision of the dermal immunization site and regional lymph node

The granulomatous inflammation produced by BCG-tumor cell vaccines administered i.d. is associated with potent tumor-specific immunity. Mycobacteria and tumor cells injected at separate sites are ineffectual immunostimulants, suggesting that granulomagenesis, and immune induction are synergistically interrelated. In orde to identify those stages of immunization that are requisite for systemic tumor, we examined the effect of interrupting granulomagenesis on the induction of immunity. The vaccination site (groups A-F) or both the vaccination site and regional SDA lymph nodes (groups G-L) were surgically excised at various times (i.e., 1, 4, 7, 11, 15, and 22 days) after vaccination with 10^8 BCG organisms admixed with 10^7 X-irradiated L10 cells (Table 3).

TABLE 3. Effect of surgical excision of vaccination site and superficial distal axillary lymph nodes on the development of systemic tumor immunity after BCG tumor cell vaccination

Treatment group	Vaccinate 10^8 BCG, 10^7 L10 i.d. / Surgery (days)	Tumor challenge 10^6 L10 i.d.	Progressors/total	%
	Excise vaccination site			
A	+ +	+	8/16	50
B	+ +	+	1/16	6
C	+ +	+	0/16	0
D	+ +	+	0/16	0
E	+ +	+	0/16	0
F	+ +	+	2/16	13
	Excise vaccination site + SDA nodes			
G	+ +	+	5/5	100
H	+ +	+	6/6	100
I	+ +	+	5/6	83
J	+ +	+	4/6	67
K	+ +	+	2/6	33
L	+ +	+	2/5	40
	No surgery			
M	+	+	3/16	19
N		+	15/15	100

[a] Numbers indicate days after vacinnation with 10^8 BCG organisms admixed with 10^7 X-irradiated L10 cells.

An i.d. challenge of 10^6 viable L10 cells was consistently fatal to unvaccinated animals, whereas vaccinated, but surgically untreated, animals (group M) were almost completely protected when challenged 37 days after vaccination (100% and 19% mortality, respectively). Excision of vaccination sites at 4-22 days after immunization had no discernible effect on the induction of tumor immunity, since the incidence of progressive tumor growth did not differ from that of animals not subjected to surgery (M), as determined by the Fisher exact probability test ($p > 0.05$). Though it may appear that excision of immunization sites 1 day after vaccination blocked the development of immunity in group B (50% progressors) as opposed to the untreated controls (19%), this difference was not statistically significant.

Excision of the vaccination site and the regional lymph nodes, however, resulted in a severe impairment in the generation of systemic antitumor immunity. Progressive tumor growth occured in 100% of animals surgically treated 1 and 4 days after vaccination (G and H); only partial protection was conferred to animals surgically treated 7 or more days after vaccination (I-L).

The length of time that the vaccination sites and regional lymph nodes remained intact was critical to the development of antitumor immunity. The incidence of progressive tumor growth steadily declined as the time increased between vaccination and surgical excision. For groups A-G and H-L, this trend was highly significant, using the Cochran-Armitage test for analysis of trends (one-tailed test, $p < 0.005$ and < 0.001, respectively). The data suggest that early stages of the inflammatory response prior to granulomagenesis are associated with maximal induction of antitumor immunity and that the involvement of the vaccination site at the regional lymph nodes is minimal after 4 and 15 days, respectively.

CLINICAL STUDIES OF ACTIVE SPECIFIC IMMUNOTHERAPY

Over the past 5 years, we have translated the results of our experiments with the guinea pig model of active specific immunotherapy into a prospectively randomized, controlled clincial trial of therapy for colorectal cancer in humans (Hoover et al., 1984, 1985). Two questions were asked: (1) Can the delayed cutaneous hypersensitivity (DCH) to autologous tumor cells be boosted by immunotherapy, and (2) can active specific immunotherapy improve the disease-free interval and/or survival when used as an adjuvant to surgery? Primary tumors were removed by standard surgical techniques and were enzymatically dissociated and cryo-preserved by techniques which maintain cell viability. Adjacent normal colon mucosa was processed similarly. Patients with transmural extension of tumor or nodal metastases were randomized into groups receiving immunotherapy. Skin testing with irradiated, autologous tumor cells and mucosa cells was done 3 weeks postoperatively before immunotherapy began. Immunized patients received one intra-dermal vaccination weekly for 2 weeks of 10^7 irradiated, autologous tumor cells and 10^7 BCG and one vaccination of 10^7 irradiated, autologous tumor cells alone in the third week. Skin tests were repeated at 6 weeks, 6 months, and 1 year post-vaccination. To date, 74 patients have parti-cipated in the trial. Immunized patients demonstrated a significant boost in the DCH response to their autologous tumor cells (Figure 2). Control patients did not react significantly to tumor or mucosa cells at any test period. Reactivity to tumor cells diminished at 6 months and 1 year but continued to be significantly elevated over control values. Histologic analysis of positive skin-test sites revealed marked perivascular infiltrates suggestive of cell-mediated hypersensitivity.

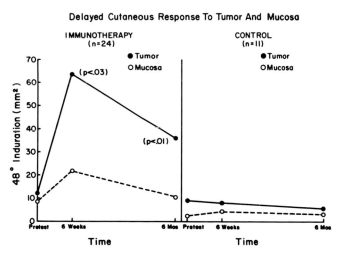

Figure 2. DCH response to tumor and mucosa cell prepara-
(legend continued on page 60.)

CLINICAL OUTCOME

We considered two outcomes: time to recurrence and time to death. Among the 44 colon cancer patients, 23 received active specific immunotherapy (ASI); in this group there were 8 deaths and 10 recurrences. Twenty-one were in the control group (12 deaths and 15 recurrences). Among the 30 rectal cancer patients, 14 recieved ASI (6 deaths and 7 recurrences). One patient from each group died of causes unrelated to cancer. Because of wide variation in follow-up for individual patients, estimates of the distribution of time-to-event are the only statistical bases for comparing the groups. Comparing treatment groups among all patients, there is a significant difference in the distributions of time-to-recurrence by the Mantel-Haenszel test (p-value is 0.037) and a significant difference in the distributions of time-to-death (p-value 0.031). Both comparisons favor the ASI group. Most of the differences was due to the subgroup with colon cancer. Perhaps because of small sample sizes and insufficient statistical power, less clear conclusions emerge from the separate examination of colon and rectal patients. Colon patients obtain a moderately significant benefit (p=0.041) from ASI in delaying recurrences but not for time-to-death (p=0.085). It should be noted, however, that three control patients with colon cancer remain alive with extensive resectable metastases, whereas only one patient in the treated group has no disease. One treated patient is clinically free of disease after resection of a mesenteric recurrence. Therefore, the number of deaths in the control group is likely to increase substantially in the near future. No significant treatment differences are seen among the 30 rectal cancer patients despite a 7-1 ratio of recurrence rates between 9 and 15 months in favor of ASI. But, as noted above, upon combining these patients with the colon cancer patients, stronger conclusions emerge than from either group alone.

That colon cancer patients would benefit more than rectal cancer patients is not suprising, and, in fact, could have been predicted from our animal model. In the

---

tions in autologous tumor cell-immunized and non-immunized patients. The differences between 48-hr induration of tumor and mucosa were statistically significant at 6 weeks (p < 0.03) and 6 months (p < 0.01) in the treated patients.

guinea pig model, the draining lymph nodes are imperative to the efficacy of the vaccine for 21 days following immunization. Rectal cancer patients start pelvic radiation, including the draining lymph nodes, within a few days to 1 week after completing immunization. Theroretically, the lymph nodes that have been stimulated by immunotherapy were destroyed by the 5020 rad X-irradiation before they could impact fully upon the immunologic response. Our plan is to obviate this problem in future protocols by immunizing via lymph node basins, such as the axillary nodes, that are not within the radiation field.

The Cox model estimate of the ratio of the instantaneous risk of death in the control group to the risk in the ASI group (hazard ratio) is 2.46. A two-sided 95% confidence interval for this ratio is (0.96, 6.32), and a one-sided lower 90% confidence limit is 1.18 regarding recurrence. The Cox model estimate of the hazard ratio (control to ASI) is 2.14; a two-sided 95% confidence interval is (0.95, 4.84), and a one-sided lower 90% confidence limit is 1.08. The credibility of these results, which suggest a substantial but not yet significant benefit for ASI, is enhanced by the agreement between the actuarial and Cox model estimates.

We now have three lines of evidence that ASI has immunologic impact in patients with colorectal cancer: (1) we have previously reported a significant boost in reactivity to autochthonous tumor cells in vaccinated patients (Hoover et al., 1984); (2) we have reported the peripheral blood lymphocytes from these immunized patients as sources for the development of stable clones of human B-lymphocytes that produce colon tumor-specific monoclonal antibodies (Haspel et al., 1984) in which lymphocytes harvested from unimmunized patients appear to be less effective in producing tumor-specific monoclonal antibodies; and (3) the sustained differences in clinical outcome between immunized and non-immunized groups of patients in our study are encouraging even with the small numbers.

We must ask whether this is another small trial showing a benefit from an innovated approach that will be negated in larger and better controlled trials. The literature is replete with the failures of others who have tried to develop effective immunization procedures against human malignancies. How can we explain our modest success in the

face of so many past failures of attempts to control malignant disease by immune manipulations? A repraisal of the
past failures in the light of current studies in experimental animal models may clarify the reasons for the failures
and suggest other new immunologic aproaches. Our clinical
protocol was borne out of nearly 8 years of intensive
investigation and the many lessons learned in the animal
model, using the syngeneic line-10 hepatocarcinoma in
inbred strain 2 guinea pigs.

CONCLUSION

To address the problem of disseminated and locally in-
accessible human tumors, we modified the guinea pig hepatocarcinoma model to make it more relevant to the clinical
situation. The ability to achieve systemic tumor immunity
by means of an intradermal BCG/autochthonous tumor cell
vaccine was a major advance in the guinea pig immunotherapy
model. A series of studies has demonstrated that BCG mixed
with tumor cells is effective in inducing a degree of
systemic immunity capable of eliminating a limited disseminated tumor burden only when BCG and tumor cells were carefully controlled for variables, such as the number of tumor
cells (10^7 optimal), the ratio and source of BCG organisms
to tumor cells (1:1), maintenance of metabolically viable
tumor cells, and vaccination regimen (three vaccines, 1
week apart). Further studies in the guinea pig model demonstrated the feasibility of preparing tumor cells suspen-
sions from enzymatically dissociated solid tumors without
loss of immunogenicity, a requirement for the preparation
of human tumor vaccines. Furthermore, the regional lymph
nodes draining the intradermal vaccination site were found
to be critical. If the nodes were removed before 21 days
after vaccination, the effectiveness was lost. It was
possible in this model to demonstrate that neither allogeneic cells, dead cells, or cell components (antigeneic
extracts) were effective. It was also demonstrated that BCG
components were not effective substitutes for whole viable
BCG cells. Autochthonous tumor cells alone or BCG alone
were ineffective.

While the therapeutic effectiveness of ASI as learned
from the guinea pig model as an adjunct to surgical
resection of colorectal cancer is suggested by our clinical
data, it is presumed that the optimal vaccination and

treatment protocols have not yet been achieved. If we are to optimize all aspects of treatment, further experimental and clinical investigations are required. To date, efforts to develop therapeutic vaccines have concentrated primarily on vaccine preparation and administration. Another equally important aspect of immunization is the capacity of the host to respond adequately to potentially immunogenic vaccines. Still another clinical strategy to improve host response with ASI may be through addition of other biologic agents, such as IL-2. Studies are under way to look at the potential immune-enhancing effects of IL-2 combined with ASI. With the suggestion of clinical efficacy of immunotherapy identified by our data, it also becomes increasingly important that methods of immune monitoring other than the DCH be developed. Efforts to this end are ongoing in our laboratory.

REFERENCES

Adams DO (1976). The granulomatous inflammatory response. A review, Am J Pathol 84: 164-191.

Bartlett GL, Zbar B (1972). Tumor-specific vaccine containing Mycobacterium bovis and tumor cells: safety and efficacy. J Natl Cancer Inst 49: 1709-1726.

Bekesi JG, St. Arneault G, Holland JF (1971). Increase of leukemia L1210 immunogenicity by Vibrio cholerae neuraminidase treatment. Cancer Res 31: 2130-2132.

Boros DL (1978). Granulomatous inflammations. Progr Allergy 24: 183-267.

Hanna Jr MG (1972). Histopathology of tumor regression and intralesional injection of Mycobacterium bovis. I. Tumor growth and metastasis. J Natl Cancer Inst 48: 1441-1455.

Hanna Jr MG, Snodgrass MJ, Zbar B, Rapp HJ (1973). Histopathology of tumor regression after intralesional injection of Mycobacterium bovis. IV. Development of immunity to tumor cells and BCG. J Natl Cancer Inst 51: 1897-1908.

Hanna Jr MG, Peters LC (1978a). Specific immunotherapy of established visceral micrometastases by BCG tumor cell vaccine alone or as an adjunct to surgery. Cancer 42: 2613-2625.

Hanna Jr MG, Peters LC (1978b). Immunotherapy of established micrometastases with Bacillus Calmette-Guérin tumor cell vaccine. Cancer Res 38: 204-209.

Hanna Jr MG, Bucana C (1979). Active specific immunotherapy of residual micrometastasis: the acute and chronic inflammatory response in induction of tumor immunity by BCG tumor cell imunization. J Reticuloendothel Soc 26: 439-452.

Hanna Jr MG, Brandhorst JS, Peters LC (1979). Active specific immunotherapy of residual micrometastasis: an evaluation of sources, doses, and ratios of BCG with tumor cells. Cancer Immunol Immunother 7: 165-173.

Haspel MV, McCabe RP, Pomato N, Janesch NJ, Knowlton JV, Peters LC, Hoover Jr HC, Hanna Jr MG (1985). Generation of tumor cell reactive human monoclonal antibodies using peripheral blood lymphocytes from actively immunized colorectal carcinoma patients. Cancer Res 45: 3951-3961.

Hedley DW, McElwain TJ, Currie GA (1978). Specific active immunotherapy does not prolong survival in surgically treated patients with stage IIB malignant melanoma and may promote early recurrence. Br J Cancer 37: 491-496.

Hollingshead AC (1978). Active-specific immunotherapy. In Hersh E (ed): "Immunotherapy of human cancer," New York: Raven Press, pp 213-233.

Hoover Jr HC, Surdyke M, Dangel RB, Peters LC, Hanna Jr MG (1984). Delayed cutaneous hypersensitivity to autologous tumor cells in colorectal cancer patients immunized with an autologous tumor cell Bacillus Calmette-Guérin vaccine. Cancer Res 44: 1671-1676.

Hoover Jr HC, Surdyke M, Dangel RB, Peters LC, Hanna Jr MG (1985). Prospectively randomized trial of adjuvant active specific immunotherapy for human colorectal cancer. Cancer 55: 1236-1243.

Martin WJ, Wunderlich JR, Fletcher F, Inman JK (1971). Enhanced immunogenicity of chemically-coated syngeneic tumor cells. Proc Natl Acad Sci USA 68: 469-472.

Mathé G, Weiner R, Pouillart P, Schwarzenberg L, Jasmin C, Schneider M, Hrynt M, Amiel JL, DeVassal F, Rosenfeld C (1973). BCG in cancer immunotherapy. I. Experimental and clinical trials of its use in the treatment of leukemia and/or residual disease. Natl Cancer Inst Monogr 39: 165-175.

Morton DL, Eilber FR, Holmes EC, Sparks FC, Ramming KP (1976). Present status of BCG immunotherapy of malignant melanoma. Cancer Immunol Immunother 1: 93-98.

Peters LC, Brandhorst JS, Hanna Jr MG (1979). Preparation of immunotherapeutic autologous tumor cell vaccines from solid tumors. Cancer Res 39: 1353-1360.

Powles RL, Crowther C, Bateman CJT, Beard MEJ, McElwain TJ, Russel J, Lister TA, Whitehouse JMA, Wrigley PFM, Pike M, Alexander P, Fairly GH (1973). Immunotherapy for acute myelogenous leukemia. Br J Cancer 28: 365-376.

Prager MD, Baechtel FS (1973). Methods for modification of cancer cells to enhance their antigenicity. In Bush H (ed): "Methods in cancer reseach," vol 9, New York: Academic press, pp 339-400.

Prager MD (1978). Specific cancer immunotherapy. Cancer Immunol Immunother 3: 157-161.

Ray PK, Tahkur VS, Sundaram K (1975). Antitumor immunity. I. Differential response of neuraminidase-treated and X-irradiated tumor vaccine. Eur J Cancer 11: 1-8.

Sokal JE, Aungst CW, Grace Jr JT (1973). Immunotherapy of chronic myelocytic leukemia. Natl Cancer Inst Monogr 39: 195-198.

Zbar B, Tanaka T (1971). Immunotherapy of cancer: regression of tumors after intralesional injection of living Mycobacterium bovis. Science 172: 271-273.

Zbar B, Bernstein ID, Bartlett GL, Hanna Jr MG, Rapp HJ (1972). Immunotherapy of cancer: regression of intradermal tumors and prevention of growth of lymph node metastases after intralesional injection of living Bacillus Calmette-Guérin. J Natl Cancer Inst 49: 119-130.

EORTC Genitourinary Group Monograph 6:
BCG in Superficial Bladder Cancer, pages 67–79
© 1989 Alan R. Liss, Inc.

INTRAVESICAL BCG ADMINISTRATION IN THE GUINEA PIG.
HISTOMORPHOLOGICAL ASPECTS

Ad P.M. van der Meijden, Wim H. de Jong, Peter A.
Steerenberg, Frans M.J. Debruyne, Joost E. Ruitenberg
Department of Urology, University Hospital Nijmegen
(A.P.M.v.d.M., F.M.J.D.), National Institute of Public
Health and Environmental Protection, Bilthoven
(W.H.d.J., P.A.S., J.E.R.), The Netherlands.

INTRODUCTION

Bacillus Calmette-Guérin (BCG) has received much
attention for its important role in the prophylaxis and
treatment of superficial bladder carcinoma and primary
carcinoma in situ of the urinary bladder in man. After the
initial study of Morales et al. in 1976, several investigators published favorable results obtained with BCG
(Badalament et al., 1987; Brosmann, 1982; Haaff et al.,
1985; Herr et al., 1983; Lamm et al., 1980).

Relatively few descriptions of the morphological
changes induced by BCG in the bladder are reported. Granulomatous inflammatory reactions and mononuclear cell infiltration in the subepithelial layer of the bladder have been
described in man (Lage et al. 1986). These inflammatory
reactions were frequently accompanied by epithelial ulceration. In dogs, minor inflammatory reaction resembling early
granulomas, were present after combined intravesical and
intradermal BCG administration (van der Meijden et al.,
1986). Intravesical instillation only, induced minimal
changes into the dog bladder, whereas extensive inflammation was present after injection of BCG into the bladder
wall (Bloomberg et al., 1975). In a study in rats, part of
mononuclear infiltrate present after repeated BCG instillations, could be identified as T-cells (Guinan et al.,
1986). The granulomatous reactions were non-caseating.

We used guinea pigs as a model to study the histopathological changes induced in the bladder, the regional

iliac lymph nodes, the spleen, liver and lungs after intravesical administration of different doses of BCG. The
guinea pig was chosen because this animal is known to be
very susceptible to mycobacteria (Rosenthal, 1980).
Furthermore, the guinea pig also shows delayed type hypersensitivity reactions inside the bladder wall after a
second intravesical antigen challenge (Coe and Feldman,
1966). It is not known whether BCG-bacilli are capable of
penetrating the intact bladder wall and of dissemination.
Therefore, in addition we investigated whether BCG-bacilli
or parts of it were present in the bladder wall, in the
regional retroperitoneal (iliac) lymph nodes and spleen
after a course of six weekly bladder instillations.

MATERIAL AND METHODS

Animals

Thirty random bred female albino and inbred female
Sewall-Wright strain 2 guinea pigs, age 4-6 months, weigh-
ing 400-600 g were used for the experiments.

Bacillus Calmette-Guérin (BCG)

The BCG used for intravesical administration was
produced at the RIVM, the Dutch Institute of Public Health
and Environmental Protection. BCG-RIVM has shown antitumor
activity both in laboratory animal tumor systems (de Jong
et al., 1984) and in spontaneously occurring bovine ocular
squamous cell carcinoma (Klein et al., 1982; Misdorp et
al., 1985) and equine sarcoid tumor of the skin (Klein et
al., 1986). BCG-RIVM, originally obtained as a seed lot
from the Institute Pasteur (Paris, France) is cultured in a
homogeneous deep culture suspension under continuous stir-
ring, and is freeze dried after harvesting.

Experimental design

The BCG was administered intravesically in a volume of
1.0 ml in an empty bladder, and kept in the bladder for 0.5
or 1 hour by leaving the closed sheath in the bladder. In
pilot experiments the normal bladder capacity was found to

be 3 to 5 ml. Thereafter, the bladders were emptied by gentle compression at the suprapubic region. The procedure was repeated weekly for six consecutive weeks. After the instillation procedure, no signs of tissue damage, such as blood present on the catheter, were observed. Control animals were instilled intravesically with a placebo preparation. At week 7 animals were sacrificed.

RESULTS

Detection of mycobacteria

After twelve weeks of incubation at 36°C, no bacterial colonies were detected in Löwenstein-Jensen cultures from the (iliac) lymph nodes draining the bladder and from the spleen. In tissue sections stained by the Ziehl-Neelsen method, no BCG bacilli, recognisable as slightly curved acid fast rods, were found at the surface or in the epithelial or muscle layer of the bladder, nor in the iliac lymph nodes.

Histopathology after intravesical BCG administration

Bladder. The microscopical anatomy of the guinea pig bladder is shown in Fig. 1. The mucosal covering consists of 4 to 5 layers of transitional epithelial cells and so-called 'umbrella' cells are present. The basement membrane is well established and intact. Underlying the epithelium is the submucosa or lamina propria, containing blood vessels. Underlying the submucosa is the muscular wall consisting of smooth muscle tissue arranged in criss-cross bundels. the outside of the bladder is covered by a serosal layer. Perivesical fatty tissue is present locally in the subserosal area.

Intravesical instillation of BCG-RIVM induced an inflammatory reaction in the bladder wall of the guinea pig. This imflammatory response consisted of a mononuclear infiltrate varying from small accumulation of lymphoid cells to larger, more distinct areas (Fig. 2) composed of mononuclear cells with both lymphoid and histiocytic characteristics. Occasionally lymphoid follicles were observed in the larger inflammatory lesions. In approximately 50% of the

animals, epithelioid cells, forming non-caseating granulomas, were present (Fig. 3). Occasionally, multinucleated
giant cells were observed in the larger granulomatous reactions. Generally, the mucosal layer covering the inflammatory reactions, remained intact.

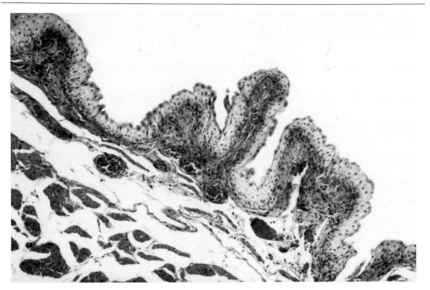

Figure 1. Microscopical anatomy of guinea pig bladder
showing transitional epithelial cells lamina propria and
muscular wall. HE staining x80.

There seemed to be a correlation between the dose of
BCG administered intravesically, and the composition and
extent of the inflammatory reactions. In the bladder wall
of animals treated with 10^5 c.p. of BCG or less, no pathological lesions were observed. When 10^6 c.p. BCG were
administered, mild reactions in the submucosal connective
tissue were present, consisting of small accumulations of
lymphocytes, without epithelioid cells. When the intravesical dose of BCG was increased to 10^7 c.p., the same
morphological changes were present in the lamina propria,
but were more frequent. Moreover, after treatment with
$1x10^7$ or $5x10^7$ c.p. BCG, epithelioid cell clusters and
well-developed non-caseating granulomas were observed. In
bladders from animals treated with the highest dose ($5x10^7$
c.p.) the most severe inflammatory reactions were present.

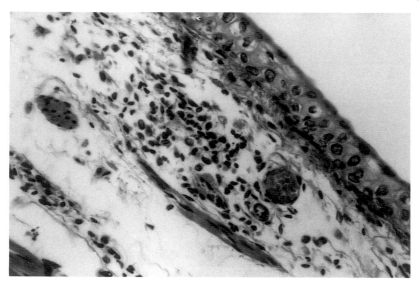

Figure 2. Mild inflammatory reaction in the bladder after intravesical BCG (5x10^7 c.p.) administration (once a week for six consecutive weeks). HE Staining x320.

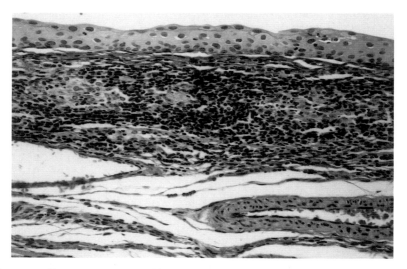

Figure 3. Severe inflammatory reaction in the lamina propria of the bladder after intravesical BCG (1x10^7 c.p.) administration (once a week for six consecutive weeks). Note cluster of epithelioid cells indicating a granulomatous type of reaction. HE staining x200.

Regional (iliac) lymph nodes. In animals receiving intravesically 10^6 c.p. BCG or more, the primary iliac lymph nodes draining the bladder were enlarged to at least twice the normal size. No enlargement was noticed in the iliac lymph nodes of animals which were treated with 10^7 c.p. BCG intradermally and in animals treated with 0.9% saline intravesically. Histologically, the iliac lymph nodes in animals treated with 10^6 BCG showed besides regions of normal lymph node architecture, clusters of epithelioid cells and small granulomas located predominantly in the paracortex. Lymph nodes from the axillary and para-aortal region showed no histological changes.

Using higher doses of BCG (1×10^7 and 5×10^7 c.p.), epithelioid cells were clearly present varying from small clusters to large typical granulomatous lesions (Fig. 4). These granulomatous reactions showed the same histological pattern as those present in the bladder wall. The histiocytes in a granuloma contained a pale nucleus and an large amount of cytoplasm. Langhans-type giant cells were sometimes present within the lesions. Occasionally, in the larger granulomas central necrosis (caseation) was noticed (Fig. 4a). Neutrophilic leukocytes were not encountered.

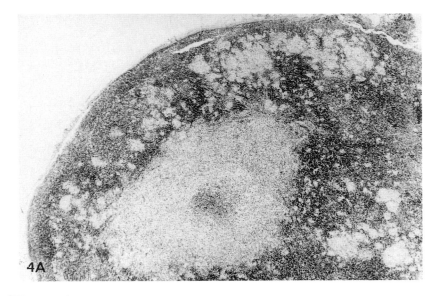

4A

(Figure 4A. Legend on facing page.)

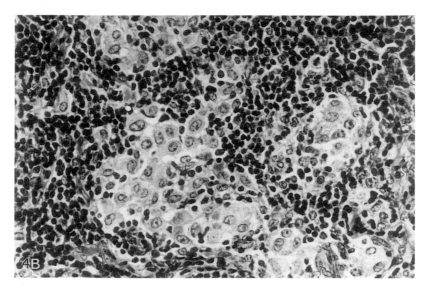

Figure 4. Granulomatous reaction in the primary draining iliac lymph node of the bladder after intravesical BCG (1×10^7 c.p.) administration (once a week for six consecutive weeks). **A:** Note the presence of granulomas varying in size from small epithelioid cell clusters to large granulomas with central necrosis. **B:** Detail of epithelioid cell cluster. HE Staining A x32, B x320.

Other organs. At autopsy no gross pathologic changes were observed. In addition to the bladder and regional lymph nodes, liver, lung and spleen were examined histologically. The liver of 5 from the 18 BCG treated animals showed infiltrates. These infiltrates contained epithelioid cells indicating a granulomatous type of reaction (Fig. 5).

In the lungs of 3 from the 29 BCG (5×10^7 c.p.) -treated animals, granulomatous lesions were observed, as indicated by the presence of epithelioid and occasional giant cells. The BCG lesions showed more or less rounded configurations which were composed of epithelioid cells with a large pale nucleus and abundant cytoplasm, accompanied by lymphocytes.

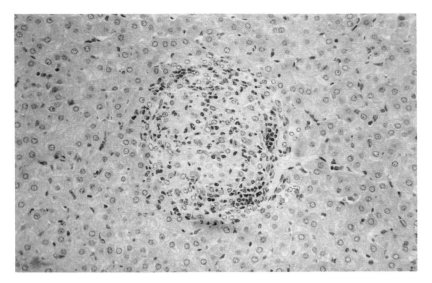

Figure 5. Granulomatous hepatitis after intravesical BCG
(5x10^7 c.p.) administration (once a week for six
consecutive weeks). Note the presence of epithelioid cells
surrounded by lymphoid infiltrate, and the rounded
configuration of the lesion.
HE staining x320.

In 16 BCG (5x10^7) -treated animals, the spleen was
examined histologically (data not shown). In two of the BCG
treated animals the spleens showed a granulomatous
reaction, with epithelioid cells and Langhans multinuclear
giant cells. These BCG granulomas were found mainly in the
red pulp and occasionally in the white pulp of the spleen.
These two animals also showed granulomatous lesions in
liver and lungs. Furthermore, in the same animals
granulomas were found in distant (axillary) lymph nodes.

It appeared that these animals were suffering from a
generalized inflammatory reaction to BCG.

DISCUSSION

During the last decade, intravesical BCG administration has attained an important role as a non specific adjuvant immunotherapy for the treatment of recurrent superficial bladder cancer (Shapiro et al. 1982, Morales 1984, Haaff et al. 1985, Morales and Nickel 1986). Although it is generally thought that BCG exerts its antitumor activity by stimulation of the immune system, the precise mechanism is still unknown. Generally, the toxicity of BCG is limited to the site of administration and the primary draining lymph nodes. Disseminated infection is extremely uncommon (Sparks 1976, Pitlik et al. 1984).

When BCG is administered intravesically, a relatively large mucosal surface is exposed. However, most of the inflammatory foci observed in our study, were scattered throughout the submucosa underlying the epithelium. Even when a severe lymphocytic inflammation was present in a large submucosal area, no disruption of the epithelium was present. Our observations in guinea pigs are similar to observations in dogs, in which BCG instillation also provoked a submucosal reaction (Bloomberg et al. 1975, Van der Meijden et al. 1986). With regard to the intensity of the inflammation in the bladder, the guinea pigs showed a more extensive reaction compared with the dogs. In patients with superficial bladder cancer treated with intravesical BCG, subepithelial granulomas, accompanied by erosion of the covering epithelial layer, were observed (Lage et al. 1986). Several factors may enhance BCG attachment and thereby increase the local BCG effect inside the bladder wall. In particular, endoscopic resection of bladder tumors probably results in enhanced adherence of BCG to the bladder wall. It has been demonstrated that BCG adheres minimally to undamaged murine bladders, but the adherence is increased more than 100-fold in bladders damaged by electrocautery (Ratliff et al. 1987). In particular the extracellular matrix protein fibronectin was found to mediate BCG adherence. Fribronectin is a major constituent of healing wounds (Grinnel et al. 1980). Intravesical wounds, causing fibrin-clot formation, are induced by transurethral resection and electrocautery of bladder tumors.

It was suggested by Ratliff, that fibronectin acts as an attachment matrix to mediate BCG retention, thus allowing induction of the immune response Ratliff et al., 1987). Although in our studies, it cannot be excluded completely that the instillation procedure caused epithelial lesions in the bladder mucosa, in none of the animals investigated (both BCG and placebo treated) were there, indications for epithelial damage on histological examination. Thus, our observations strongly suggest that a local and regional immune reaction can occur through an intact bladder epithelium. This is indicated by the induction of a lymphocytic inflammation in the submucosa underlying an intact epithelium and by the granulomatous reaction in the primary draining lymph nodes. In addition, guinea pigs treated intravesically with BCG (once a week for six consecutive weeks) developed a delayed type hypersensitivity (DTH) skin reaction to purified protein derivative (PPD) of Mycobacterium tuberculosis (Van der Meijden et al., 1988). This DTH reaction is the result of antigen-specific priming of T cells, which occurs only after a proper immunization procedure. Thus, the contact of BCG with an (apparently) intact bladder wall results in a systemic immunological reaction. We conclude that a damaged bladder wall is not required in order to provoke a BCG mediated immune reaction to BCG itself. Whether a damaged bladder is needed for the expression of the antitumor activity of BCG remains to be established.

Besides a local granulomatous reaction in the primary draining lymph nodes, occasionally granulomatous lesions were also observed in the liver and the lungs. The reactions in liver and lungs may be considered as unwanted side effects. In cancer patients, granulomatous hepatitis has been reported after intralesional and intradermal BCG administration. These reactions appeared to be allergic in nature since viable organisms could not be recovered from these lesions (Hunt et al. 1973, Bodurtha et al. 1974). It is likely that the development of hepatic granulomas represents a hypersensitivity reaction to the BCG antigens. In addition, another source of antigen exposure may be the BCG processing by phagocytizing mononuclear cells. We were not able to find viable mycobacteria in the draining (retroperitoneal) lymph nodes of the bladder or in the spleen and it is probably that these reactions were also allergic in nature. In man, after intravesical BCG administration, serious side effects are encountered in approximately 2% of patients. Generally, the side effects are limited to the bladder, although BCG pneumonitis and hepatitis have been described occasionally (Lamm et al. 1986). Serious side effects, however, can be treated effectively by anti-tuberculous therapy.

Although the intensity of the inflammatory reaction in the bladder wall was occasionally very severe, the presence of the specific mycobacterial granulomatous component in the inflammation was limited. In contrast the primary draining (iliac) lymph nodes showed a more consistent reaction. Mycobacteria invoke a granulomatous inflammation including epithelioid cells and T-cells (MGregor 1975). After intravesical BCG administration in the rat, the mononuclear cellular infiltrate contained particularly T-cells (Guinan et al. 1986). This suggests a T-cell-mediated immune response. The occurence of such an immune response was demonstrated by the development of a positive PPD skin reaction in the guinea pigs treated only intravesically with BCG. These results will be reported elsewhere. Whether this BCG-specific antigen response is accompanied by an antitumor response of antigen specific or non-specific nature, is still unknown. Further studies are required to elucidate the mechanism by which BCG exerts its antitumor activity.

REFERENCES

Badalament RA, Herr HW, Wong SY, Gnecco C, Pinsky CM, Whitmore WF, Fair WR, Oettgen HF (1987). A prospective randomized trial of maintenance versus non maintenance intravesical Bacillus Calmette-Guérin therapy of superficial bladder cancer. J Clin Oncol 5: 441-449.

Bloomberg SD, Brosman SA, Hausman MS, Chohen A, Battenberg JD (1975). The effects of BCG on the dog Bladder. Invest Urol 12: 423-427.

Bodurtha A, Kim YH, Laucius JF, Donato RA, Mastrangelo MJ (1974) Hepatic granulomas and other hepatic lesions associated with BCG immunotherapy for cancer. Am J Clin Pathol 61: 747-752.

Brosman SA (1982) Experience with Bacillus Calmette-Guérin in patients with superficial bladder carcinoma. J Urol 128: 27-30.

Coe JE, Feldman JD (1966) Extracutaneous delayed hypersensitivity, particularly in the guinea pig bladder. Immunology 10: 127-136.

Grinnel F, Billingham RE, Burgess L (1980). Distribution of fibronectin during wound healing in vivo. J Invest Dermat 76: 181-189.

Guinan P, Shaw M, Ray V (1986). Histology of BCG and Thiotepa treated bladders. Urol Res 14: 211-215.

Haaff EO, Dresner SM, Kelley Dr, Ratliff TL, Shapiro A, Catalona WJ (1985). Role of immunotherapy in the prevention of recurrence and invasion of urothelial bladder tumors: a review. World J Urol 3: 76-85.

Herr HW, Pinksy CM, Whitmore Jr WF., Oetggen HF, Melamed MR (1983). Effect of intravesical Bacillus Calmette-Guérin (BCG) on carcinoma in situ of the bladder. Cancer 51: 1323-1326.

Hunt JS, Silverstein MJ, Sparks FC, Haskell CM, Pilch YH, Morton DL (1973). Granulomatous hepatitis: a complication of BCG immunotherapy. Lancet 2: 820-821.

de Jong WH, Steerenberg PA, Kreeftenberg JG, Tiesjema RH, Kruizinga W, van Noorle Jansen LM, Ruitenberg EJ (1984). Experimental screening of BCG preparations produced for cancer immunotherapy: safety and immunostimulating and antitumor activity of four consecutively produced batches. Cancer Immunol Immunother 17: 18-27.

Klein WR, Ruitenberg EJ, Steerenberg PA, de Jong WH, Kruizinga WH, Misdorp W, Bier J, Tiesjema RH, Kreeftenberg JG, Teppema JS, Rapp HJ (1982). Immunotherapy by intralesional injections of BCG cell walls or live BCG in bovine ocular squamous cell carcinoma: a preliminary report JNCI 69: 1095-1103.

Klein WR, Brass GE, Misdorp W, Steerenberg PA, de Jong WH, Tiesjema RH, Kersjes AW, Ruitenberg EJ (1986). Equine sarcoid: BCG immunotherapy compared to cryosurgery in a prospective randomised clinical trial. Cancer immunol immunother 21: 133-140.

Lage JM, Bauer WC, Kelley DR, Ratliff TL, Catalona WJ (1986). Histological parameters and pitfalls in the interpretation of bladder biopsies in Bacillus Calmette-Guérin treatment of superficial bladder cancer. J Urol 135: 916-919.

Lamm DL, Thor DE, Harris SC, Reyna JA, Stogdill VD, Radwim HM (1980). Bacillus Calmette-Guérin immunotherapy of superficial bladder cancer. J Urol 124: 38-43.

Lamm DL, Stogdill VD, Stogdill BJ, Crispen RG (1986). Complications of Bacillus Calmette-Guérin immunotherapy in 1,278 patients with bladder cancer. J Urol 135: 272-274.

McGregor DD (1975). Cytokinetics and fate of sensitized

lymphocytes. J Reticuloendoth Soc 17: 126-132.

van der Meijden APM, Steerenberg PA, De Jong WH, Bogman MJJT, Feitz WFJ, Hendriks BT, Debruyne FMJ, Ruitenberg EJ (1986). The efeects of intravesical and intradermal application of a new BCG on the dog bladder. Urol Res 14: 207-210.

van der Meijden APM (1988). Non-specific immunotherapy with BCG-RIVM in superficial bladder cancer. Histological, immunological and therapeutic aspects. Thesis, Nijmegen, The Netherlands.

Morales A. Eindinger D, Bruce AW (1976). Intracavitary Bacillus Calmette-Guérin in the treatment of superficial bladder tumors. J Urol 116: 180-183.

Morales A (1984). Long-term results and complications of intracavitary Bacillus Calmette-Guérin therapy for bladder cancer. J Urol 132: 457-459.

Morales A, Nickel JC (1986). Immunotherapy of superficial bladder cancer with BCG. World J Urol 3: 209-214.

Misdorp W, Klein WR, Ruitenberg EJ, Hart G, De Jong WH, Steerenberg PA (1985). Clinico-pathological aspects of immunotherapy by intralesional injection of BCG cell walls or live BCG in bovine ocular squamous cell carcinoma. Cancer Immunol Immunother 20: 223-230.

Pillik SD, Fainstein V, Hopfer RL, Bodey SP (1984). Isolations of Bacille Calmette-Guérin after immunotherapy for cancer. J Inf Dis 149: 476.

Ratliff TL, Palmer JO, McCarr JA, Brown E (1987). Intravesical Bacillus Calmette-Guérin therapy for murine bladder tumors: initiation of the response by fibronectin mediated attachment of Bacillus Calmette-Guérin. Cancer Res 47: 1762-1766.

Rosenthal SR (1980). BCG vaccine: tuberculosis-cancer. PSG Publishing Company, Inc., Littleton, Ma, USA.

Shapiro A, Kadmon D, Catalona WJ, Ratliff TL (1982). Immunotherapy of superficial bladder cancer. J Urol 128: 891-894.

Sparks FC (1976). Hazards and complications of BCG immunotherapy. Med clin North Am 60: 499-509.

EORTC Genitourinary Group Monograph 6:
BCG in Superficial Bladder Cancer, pages 81–91
© 1989 Alan R. Liss, Inc.

PATHOLOGIC AND STRUCTURAL CHANGES IN THE BLADDER AFTER BCG
INTRAVESICAL THERAPY IN MEN

Francesco Pagano, Pierfrancesco Bassi, Claudio Milani,
Paolo Dalla Palma, Anna Grazia Rebuffi, Alessandro
Poletti, Anna Parenti
Departments of Urology, Pathology, and Cytology,
University of Padova, Padova, Italy

INTRODUCTION

Since the first publication of Morales (Morales et
al., 1976), numerous controlled clinical trials with intravesical Bacillus Calmette-Guérin (BCG) have confirmed its
value in reducing the rate of tumor recurrence and progression in patients with superficial transitional cell carcinoma (TCC) of the bladder (Brosman, 1985; Herr et al.,
1986; Lamm, 1985). Over 10 years later, there are still
many efforts to identify the mechanism of action and the
most appropriate treatment schedule (Lamm, 1987). Better
understanding of the morphologic findings after treatment
is also needed and a pathomorphologic method that can be
used in the diagnosis and monitoring of BCG-treated
patients is being sought.

We have reviewed our experience with 98 patients
treated since February 1986 and analysed the value of the
common pathologic methods of characterizing the structural
changes observed after BCG treatment. We emphasized routine
histopathology, cytology, and electron microscopy, rather
than immunopathology.

MATERIALS AND METHODS

BCG immunotherapy for superficial bladder cancer was
used to prevent recurrences after transurethral resection
(TUR) (prophylaxis) and to treat carcinoma in situ (therapy).

Patients

Since February 1986, a total of 98 patients were treated with intravesical BCG. Of these, 58 patients had multiple (more than three) papillary superficial bladder tumors (stage Ta, T1a, and T1b) and 40 patients had carcinoma in situ with or without concurrent papillary tumors. Follow-up of 60 patients (33 in the papillary-tumors group and 27 in the carcinoma-in-situ group) has been 12 months or more. Of these 98 patients, 29 -- 17 in the papillary-tumor group and 12 in the carcinoma-in-situ group -- had been previously treated unsuccessfully with intravesical chemotherapy (Mitomycin and Adriamycin). All visible papillary lesions were removed by transurethral resection; washing cytology and multiple biopsies in abnormal- and normal-looking bladder mucosa were performed as a routine procedure in all patients.

BCG therapy

The induction course consisted of 75 mg (5×10^8 CFU) of BCG-Pasteur (Institute Pasteur-Paris, France) administered in 50 cc of saline solution intravesically and kept in the bladder for 2 hours. Treatment was initiated within 3 weeks after endoscopy. BCG was administered weekly for 6 consecutive weeks. No intradermal inoculations of vaccine were given. When tumors were not demonstrated after the induction course, maintenance therapy was started and given monthly by instillation for a year and quarterly for a second year. Patients who did not respond to induction therapy -- that is, tumors recurred or persisted without progression -- were given and additional 6-week course. Serial endoscopic evaluations with bladder-washing cytology and multiple biopsies were performed in all patients after treatment. All post-treatment evaluations were done 30-40 days after the last BCG instillation. A PPD skin test was not performed. No further course of therapy was given to the patients who did not respond to the second course.

Response criteria

Clinical results were classified as complete response or no response; partial responses were not considered. A complete response in prophylaxis and therapy groups was

defined as no tumor recurrence and negative cytologic
results. Evidence of tumors histologically proved or consisting of positive cytologic results alone, was considered
as no response. Tumor recurrence or progression after an
initial complete response was defined as a relapse.

Histology

We examined 892 non-neoplastic histologic specimens
from 98 patients -- both complete responders and non-
responders to an induction course of BCG therapy. For routine histology, bladder tissue was fixed and stained with
hematoxylin and eosin, PAS (periodic acid-schiff stain)
with or without diastase digestion. Biopsy specimens were
examined by the same pathologist. The histologic changes in
urothelium, deep subepithelial connective tissue, muscular
wall of the bladder, and prostatic urethra were evaluated.
Particular attention was paid to mucosal changes --
sloughing, severe denudation, inflammatory changes, severe
dysplasia, hyperplasia and granuloma. Dysplasia was defined
as low-grade cytohistologic alterations that were distinct
from reactive-reparative epithelial response on the one
hand and from carcinoma on the other (Dean and Murphy,
1987). Staging was according to UICC tumor classification
modified to distinguish between stage T1a (tumor invading
only the fibrovascular core) and stage T1b (tumor invading
the lamina propria of the bladder wall); tumors were graded
according to WHO classification.

Cytology

We examined 391 bladder washing specimens from 98 patients.
Bladder washing (with 80 ml of sterile saline solution) was
performed for cytologic evaluation before every cysto-endo-
scopy. The centrifuged sediment was smeared on four glass
slides and stained according to the standard Papanicolaou
procedure. The examination was done by the same experienced
cytopathologist without reference to endoscopic or histologic findings. According to established criteria, specimens were considered negative, suspicious, or positive.
When multiple cytologic specimens were available, the one
with the most ominous interpretation was accepted.

Electron microscopy

We evaluated 55 serial specimens (at least two per patient) from 24 patients (16 complete response, 5 no response, and 3 relapse), with a follow-up of at least 12 months, with reference to the presence of the most established electron microscopic markers of neoplasia -- presence of pleomorphic microvilli, loss of asymmetric unitary membrane, thinckening of basal membrane, and loosening of tight intercellular junctions (Jacobs et al., 1981). Small specimens were fixed in 4% glutaraldehyde and then in osmium tetroxide; ultrafine sections were evaluated with transmission electron microscopy.

Clinical correlation

The clinical course of 60 BCG-treated patients with a follow-up of at least 12 months was correlated with dysplasia, granuloma, severe denudation, and cytologic features. Inflammatory changes and sloughing were not considered for clincial correlation, because they appeared in most of the patients. We also evaluated the agreement of bladder-washing cytology and routine histology in the detection of tumors.

RESULTS

The clinical results of BCG therapy appeared substantially similar to those already reported (Brosman, 1985; Herr et al., 1986; Lamm, 1985), however, with a significant reduction in toxicity. These data will be reported elsewhere in this volume.

Histology

Thirty to forty days after the induction course of BCG, foci of sloughing (98%), severe dysplasia (38%), severe denudation (23%), and hyperplasia (4%) of the mucosa were evident in non-neoplastic specimens. All patients had intense inflammatory cell infiltration with lymphocytes, plasma cells, histiocytes, and polymorphonuclear leukocytes; capillary proliferation and interstitial edema were also seen in deep subepithelial connective tissue and in the subjacent muscular wall. In 24% of cases, we observed a characteristic granuloma composed of epithelioid cells with multinucleate Langhans's cells in the deep subepithelial connective tissue. Acid-fast baccilli identified with Ziehl-Neelsen stain were never detected.

TABLE 1. Relative incidence of bladder histologic findings in non-neoplastic areas 30-40 days after induction therapy (overall, CR, NR), and after 1 year

| | After induction therapy | | | After 1 year of monthly |
	Overall N=98 No. %	CR N=59 No. %	NR N=39 No. %	maintenance N=60 No. %
Inflammation	98 100	59 100	39 100	41 68
Sloughing	96 98	58 98	38 97	13 22
Severe dysplasia	37 38	14 24	23 59	9 15
Severe denudation	23 23	16 27	7 18	8 13
Granuloma	24 24	13 22	11 28	2 3
Hyperplasia	4 4	2 3	2 5	17 28

The histologic findings were the same after 1 year of monthly maintenance; however, the incidence of every finding considered, except hyperplasia, was decreased. Hyperplasia was more frequent (28%) than immediately after induction (4%).

Correlation of histologic findings and clinical course

The most evident correlation between histologic findings and clinical course (Table 1) was found for dysplasia, which was more frequent in non-responders (59%) than in responders (24%). The outcome of dysplasia in complete responders after induction therapy was considered. After 6 months, 37 of the 98 evaluable patients had persistent dysplasia and 14 were tumorfree. After 12 months, 12 patients were evaluable; all were tumorfree, but seven had dysplasia. After 18 months, only seven patients were evaluable; three patients were tumorfree and had no dysplasia, one had severe dysplasia, and three patients had tumors (relaps).

Severe denudation was evident after the induction course in 16 (27%) of the 59 complete responders. No relapse was reported in the 10 patients (four with papillary tumors and six with carcinoma in situ) evaluable at 12 months. At 18 months, only seven patients were evaluable, and one of them experienced relapse.

Granulomas were found in 24 patients (24%) after the induction course. Comparison of clinical response with the relative distribution of the granuloma in the long-term follow-up patients (eigth with papillary tumors and seven with carcioma in situ) failed to show significant prevalence in non-responders (11 of 39, or 28%) or in responders (13 of 59, or 22%).

Tumor progression and radical surgery

Of our 98 patients seven (three with multiple papillary tumors and four with carcinoma in situ) underwent radical cystectomy because of tumor progression, and three because of non-response without progression. In six of the seven with tumor progression, glandular metaplasia (in one patient with papillary tumor and one with carcinoma in situ) or squamous metaplasia (in one patient with papillary tumor and three with carcinoma in situ) was evident from the first observation on. However, squamous or glandular metaplasia were more frequent in carcinoma is situ (three patients) than in papillary tumor (one). It must be emphasized that no tumor with glandular or squamous metaplasia responded to BCG therapy.

Cytology

No significant differences in accuracy of bladder-washing cytology were observed between BCG-treated and control patients. Cytologic tests only rarely revealed structural alterations specifically related to BCG immunotherapy. An increase in number of lymphocytes and macrophages was evident after treatment in 22% of the cases. Epithelioid Langhans's cells were observed in one patient.

Transitional cells showed slight, non-specific inflammatory features.

Correlation of histologic findings and washing cytologic findings

Of the 58 patients with papillary tumors, cytologic findings were negative in six cases: all six patients had low-grade tumors (Table 2). In two patients, dysplasia was associated with positive cytologic findings.

TABLE 2. Correlations between histologic and washing cytologic findings in 58 patients with papillary tumors after induction therapy

Cytologic findings	Histologic findings, no. patients		
	Positive	Dysplasia	Negative
Positive	10	2	0
Suspicious	2	13	2
Negative	6	0	33

Of the 40 patients with carcinoma in situ, cytologic findings were positive in three patients with negative histologic findings and in five with evidence of dysplasia (Table 3)

TABLE 3. Correlation between histologic and washing cytologic findings in 40 patients with carcinoma in situ after induction therapy

Cytologic findings	Histologic findings, no. patients		
	Positive	Dysplasia	Negative
Positive	9	5	3
Suspicious	1	2	3
Negative	1	1	15

All our patients with positive cytologic findings were
considered as non-responders and were treated with an
additional course of therapy, to which eight responded.

Electron microscopy

The presence of pleomorphic microvilli was the only
significant structural tumor marker at electron microscopic
examination. It appeared related to the clinical course of
the patients; pleomorphic microvilli were present in four
of five non-responders, in two of three patients who
relapsed, and in none of the complete responders. Other
structural markers (loss of the asymmetric unitary membrane, thickening of basal membrane, loosening of tight
intercellular junctions, and modifications of Golgi apparatus) were distributed in all groups of patients without
significant prevalence. However, pleomorphic microvilli
disappeared after initially successful therapy but later,
they appeared again when there was clinical and histologic
evidence of relapse.

DISCUSSION

Cytology and histology

The common histologic finding in bladders of BCG-
treated patients was non-specific inflammatory changes.
When granulomas are present, it is the only specific
feature. Inflammatory changes and sloughing are diffuse and
constant. All those features abate, however, in most
patients within 6 months after the end of treatment, as
reported by Lage (Lage et al., 1986). The cytologic pattern
is substantially non-specific in most patients. Only rarely
does the evidence of multinucleate giant cells characterize
previous BCG treatment. The inflammatory pattern evoked by
BCG is an inherent aspect of the antitumor effect, as
suggested by Lamm (Lamm, 1987). Stimulated either directly
or indirectly by mycobacterial antigens, lymphocytes and
macrophages kill or inhibit tumor growth by direct contact
or through the release of tumoricidal factors. Therefore,
the local inflammatory response seems critical for the
continuous destruction of neoplastic cells.

In our series, urothelial hyperplasia increased with the long-term administration of BCG. This effect can be interpreted as the expression of a chronic inflammation. The evidence of severe urothelial dysplasia must be carefully considered (Dean and Murphy, 1987; Hofstädter et al., 1986), because it could indicate persistent neoplastic activity. Three of seven patients with 18-months follow-up who experienced tumor relapse had persistent dysplasia. It is not known whether that is due to the progression of the dysplasia preceeding a recurrent tumor or to the persistence of a tumor that was undetected after induction therapy. Conditions were different for patients previously treated with endovesical chemotherapy or radiation, because of the presence of dysplasia induced by the previous treatment (Murphy et al., 1981). When these patients are given BCG immunotherapy, interpretation can be difficult.

Previous trials reported a high percentage of granulomas in BCG-treated patients (Lamm, 1987). It was suggested that the granulomatous response is correlated with the clinical response. However, it has not been demonstrated that granuloma formation provides an accurate predictive index of therapeutic response, even when the patient population was divided into patients treated for carcinoma in situ and patients treated for papillary tumors. We observed microscopic granulomas in only 24% of patients after induction therapy. In our series, no statistical correlations between presence of granuloma and response to treatment were possible. None of our patients with squamous or glandular metaplasia responded to BCG therapy, and all experienced early tumor progression. If confirmed in a larger series of patients, that observation could constitute a useful indicator of poor prognosis and suggest early alternative therapeutic choices.

Histologic and washing cytologic findings did not correlate perfectly in BCG-treated patients. Washing cytology appeared unreliable in low-grade tumors, but detected 10 tumors (two papillary tumors, and eight carcinomas in situ) not proved histologically. The high incidence of histologic error could be attributed to the wellknown limitations of random biopsies, to the elusivity of endoscopic appearances, and to mucosal denudation. In fact, the denudation evident in bladder biopsies of 23% of BCG-treated patients reduces the diagnostic value of histologic examination Severe denudation also must be clearly distinguished from so called "denuding cystitis" (Eliot et al., 1973).

Electron microscopy

The presence of pleomorphic microvilli seems to be a useful diagnostic pathomorphological marker of neoplasia in normal-looking epithelium of BCG-treated patients. (It is interesting to note its disappearance after successful BCG therapy.) Other markers in our limited series of patients seem less useful. In our experience, electron microscopy did not yield early detection of patients who later experienced tumor progression or recurrence. The presence of severe denudation in urothelium after BCG therapy reduces the number of pathologic specimens evaluable and thus does not seem useful for diagnostic application in BCG-treated patients.

CONCLUSIONS

1. After BCG therapy, cytologic and histologic findings are often non-specific, particularly cytologic findings.

2. Granuloma formation is a BCG-related feature, but probably not a reliable prognostic factor, because of its low incidence.

3. Severe denudation is non-specific and cannot be correlated with clinical course.

4. Dysplasia is a relatively frequent finding (24% in responders; its persistence in responders makes the search for persistent tumor activity mandatory even in patients previously given chemotherapy.

5. Washing cytology improves diagnostic accuracy, particularly in the presence of dysplasia.

6. Electron microscopy failed to help in early detection of tumors in patients who later had relaps of tumor. The presence of pleomorphic microvilli after BCG therapy appears to be correlated with clinical course.

ACKNOWLEDGMENT

We thank Marina Calore for her editorial assistance in the preparation of this manuscript.

REFERENCES

Brosman SA (1985). The use of Bacillus Calmette-Guérin in the therapy of bladder carcinoma in situ. J Urol 134: 36.

Dean PJ, Murphy WM (1987). Carcinoma in situ and dysplasia of the bladder urothelium. World J Urol 5: 103.

Elliot GB, Molonei PS, Anderson GH (1973). Denuding cystitis and in situ urothelial carcinoma. Arch Pathol 96: 91.

Herr HW, Pinsky CM, Whitmore Jr WF, Sogani PC, Oettgen HF, Melamed MR (1986). Long-term effect of intravesical Bacillus Calmette-Guérin on flat carcinoma in situ of the bladder. J Urol 135: 265.

Hofstädter F, Delgado R, Jakse G (1986). Urothelial dysplasia and carcinoma in situ of the bladder. Cancer 57: 356.

Jacobs JB, Cohen SM, Farrow GM, Friedell GH (1981). Scanning electron microscopy features of human urinary bladder cancer. Cancer 48: 1399.

Lage JM, Bauer WC, Kelley DR, Ratliff TL, Catalona WJ (1986). Histological parameters and pitfalls in the interpretation of bladder biopsies in Bacillus Calmette-Guérin treatment of superficial bladder cancer. J Urol 135: 916-919.

Lamm DL (1985) Bacillus Calmette-Guérin immunotherapy for bladder cancer. J Urol 134: 40.

Lamm DL (1987). BCG immunotherapy for superficial bladder cancer. In Ratliff TL, Catalona WJ (eds): "Genitourinary cancer," Boston: Martinus Nijhoff Publishers, pp 205-224.

Morales A, Eidinger D, Bruce AW (1976). Intracavitary Bacillus Calmette-Guérin in the treatment of superficial bladder tumors. J Urol 116: 18.

Murphy WM, Soloway MS, Finebaum PJ (1981). Pathological changes associated with topical chemotherapy for superficial bladder cancer. J Urol 126: 461.

EORTC Genitourinary Group Monograph 6:
BCG in Superficial Bladder Cancer, pages 93–105
© 1989 Alan R. Liss, Inc.

IMMUNOPATHOLOGICAL EFFECTS OF INTRAVESICAL BCG THERAPY

S. Prescott, K. James, T.B. Hargreave, G.D. Chisholm,
J.F. Smyth
Department of Surgery/Urology and Imperial Cancer
Research Fund Medical Oncology Unit, department of
Oncology Western General Hospital, Edinburgh, Scotland

INTRODUCTION

Bacillus Calmette-Guérin (BCG) was the first immuno-adjuvant found to have antitumor activity and was therefore widely used via the percutaneous or intralesional routes for a variety of tumors including leukaemia, malignant melanoma and lung cancer (Bast et al., 1974). The disappointing results of treatment lead to abandonment of the use of BCG in all tumors except superficial bladder cancer and particularly carcinoma in situ (CIS) of the bladder (Terry and Rosenberg, 1982). Here the use of local immunotherapy with intravesical BCG has been effective even when other intravesical chemotherapeutic agents have failed (Lamm, 1987; Soloway and Perry, 1987).

The mechanism of the antitumor action of BCG has remained unclear, largely due to the complexities of the immune response to this organism which involves stimulation of both cellular (Lefford, 1975; Youmans, 1975) and humoral (Spector et al., 1982; Winters and Lamm, 1983) systems. The answer is of vital interest, firstly to allow optimisation of treatment regimens including the question of maintenance treatment and secondly in the hope of extending effective immunotherapy to other tumor types (Hudson et al., 1987).

There are three major theories as to the broad mechanism of action of BCG (Lamm, 1987):
1. A specific immune response to BCG also stimulates non-specific immune mechanisms which then destroy tumor cells.

2. A specific immune response to BCG stimulates specific antitumor immune mechanisms, e.g. by cross reaction between BCG and tumor antigens (Minden et al., 1974).
3. The local antitumor action of BCG is simply due to the "toxic" effects of severe inflammation leading to ischaemia and sloughing of superficial tumor cells.

Much work has been done on the interactions between BCG and the immmune system. There has been a concentration on the systemic effects of therapy (Davies, 1982; Thatcher et al., 1979). However, many early rodent experiments with subcutaneous implantation of chemically induced tumors, well reviewed by Bast suggested that the antitumor action of BCG was due to a local immune response and that direct contact between vaccine and tumor cells was required for effective tumor cell killing which was not due to direct toxic action but rather required the interaction of BCG with a functioning host immune system (Bast et al., 1974). In particular the cellular immune system appeared to be most important with athymic animals failing to develop anti-tuberculous immunity or mount antitumor responses. More recently it has been shown that congenitally athymic (nude) mice fail to respond to intravesical BCG given for the treatment of the experimental MBT2 bladder tumor and that moreover the administration of syngeneic T-lymphocytes could restore antitumor activity (Ratliff et al, 1987). It has also been shown that the helper subset of T-lymphocytes appear to be critical for antitumor reponses and that anti-tumor activity can be transferred from one experimental animal to another by BCG sensitised splenocytes with this phenotype in the absence of any other immunocompetent cell or BCG organism (Davies and Sabbadini, 1982). These cells had to be injected at the same site as the tumor showing that their activity was local. However, these cells are not capable of direct tumor cell killing. There activity is mediated rather by release of various lymphokines including Interleukin-2 and Interferon-gamma (Smith, 1980; Trinchieri et al., 1977). Interleukin-2 has been found in the urine in increased amounts after intravesical BCG therapy (Haaff et al., 1987) and is responsible for activation of cytotoxic T-lymphocytes and B-lymphocytes (Bich-Thuy et al., 1985; Farrar at al., 1981). Interferon-gamma formerly also known as Macrophage Activating Factor (MAF) is responsible for macrophage activation where it has been shown to enhance macrophage induced tumor killing in vitro (Gore et al., 1986). It is also involved in the generation of natural killer cells from precursor cells (Gidlund et al., 1978). This activity is increased systemically by BCG therapy but the current evidence suggests that natural killing is not responsible for the local antitumor effects response in patients with extensive carcinoma in situ and/or super- ficial bladder tumor undergoing BCG therapy in out depart- ment (Thatcher and Crowther, 1978; Thatcher et al., 1979). Preliminary results have been reported previously (El-Demiry et al., 1987).

SUBJECTS AND METHODS

Eighteen patients were entered for treatment with BCG: 16 males and 2 females, mean age 63.3 years (range 44-80 years). This high risk group consisted of 17 patients with extensive carcinoma in situ (9 primary and 8 secondary) and 1 patient with widespread G2 pTa tumor which had been unresponsive to three other chemotherapeutic agents. the associated tumors in the cases with secondary carcinoma in situ were all high grade tumors with lamina propria invasion in 4 cases. One patient refused further treatment or follow-up after 2 instillations and is not evaluable. The mean follow-up is 24 months (range 3-32 months).

These patients were all treated in one center but they form part of a Scottish Urological Group Trial of BCG therapy. Briefly the protocol is a standardised course of investigation which includes a cystoscopy with histological and urinary cytological assessment prior to treatment, between the fourth and fifth instillation, 2 weeks after completion of therapy and then 3 monthly for 2 years.

BCG-therapy

Evans BCG (Glaxo Danish Strain) was obtained as a lyo- philised preparation , 60 mg wet weight of this preparation containing $1-5 \times 10^9$ colony forming units of BCG were suspended in 60 ml of saline and instilled into the bladder via a urethral catheter which was then removed. Patients were instructed to retain the BCG solution for 2 hours if possible. The instillation of BCG was repeated weekly for 8 weeks.

Bladder biopsies

Four quadrant "cold cup" biopsies and biopsies of any abnormality were taken at every cystoscopy for routine histopathology and a further 2 similar biopsies were snap frozed in liquid nitrogen for immunohistochemical analysis. Samples were then stored at -70°C until cryostat sections 5-10 um thick were cut, air dried and fixed in acetone. They were then either stained immediately or stored dehydrated in aluminium foil at -20°C until used.

The following controls were used:
1. Normal bladder biopsies from multiorgan transplant donors.
2. Post instillation biopsy from 2 patients who had undergone intravesical Mitomycin-C therapy 8 weeks previously.
3. Chronically inflamed bladder biopsies from bladder cancer patients which showed radiation cystitis, follicular cystitis or non-specific chronic inflammation on microscopy.

Immunohistochemical staining technique

For this study we initially used, in the first 7 patients, an indirect immunoperoxidase method (Prescott et al., in preparation) but later changed to a streptavidin-biotin immuno-alkaline phosphatase technique because of the often intense endogenous peroxidase activity of polymorphs in the biopsies (El-Demiry et al., 1986). We used commercially available well defined murine primary monoclonal antibodies raised against the cell surface markers of the Class I Major Histocompatibility (MHC) antigen also called HLA-ABC and the Class II MHC antigen also called HLA-DR, T-lymphocytes (T3) and their subsets helper (T4) and suppressor/cytotoxic (T8), macrophages, B-lymphocytes, Natural Killer Cells (HNK and Tc-receptor) and the T-lymphocyte Interleukin-2 receptor.

ASSESSMENT OF RESULTS

Biopsies were examined by light microscopy by two observers. All cell counts were made at x320 magnification and all figures quoted refer to cells/high power field (HPF) - area = 0.07 mm^2. Results are expressed both semiquantitatively and in the case of T-lymphocyte parameters also quantitatively.

RESULTS

Seven patients failed to complete the course of BCG because of side effects. Fourteen of 16 patients (94%) evaluable at 3 months after their final instillation had a complete response as defined by negative cystoscopy and negative urinary cytology. The 2 early failures and 4 initial responders developed recurrent tumors so that at one year the complete response rate was 7 of 13 or 54%. Carcinoma in situ responded in all cases except one.

Routine histology

Routine H&E staining of bladder mucosal biopsies showed that all 17 patients developed a marked round cell inflammatory response with 16 patients developing typical non-caseating epithelioid granulomas and sloughing of urothelial cells. In all except one of these 16 patients the granulomas had disappeared by 6 months after treatment together with the majority of the inflammatory infiltrate.

Immunohistochemistry

The results of immunohistochemical analysis are summarised in Tables 1 and 2. For the first 7 patients semi-quantitative analyses only were made between pre-treatment and 3 months post-treatment biopsies.

In all 17 cases, BCG treatment induced strong uniform expression of HLA-DR antigen by the urothelial cells. This was usually as intense as (or more intense than) the expression of similar epitopes by macrophages in these biopsies. In 5 of 8 biopsies examined by the alkaline phosphatase technique 3 months after completion of therapy we found that the urothelium was still uniformly strongly positive, the remaining 3 cases were patch ly positive. At 6 months after therapy this had reduced to 3 positive, 2 patchily positive and 3 negative. HLA-DR antigen was not expressed by the carcinoma in situ in a cystectomy specimen removed 6 months after treatment or by any of the recurrent tumors.

TABLE 1. Semiquantitative analysis of MHC antigen expression by urothelium and mononuclear cell infiltration in study groups.

| | Normal bladder | Bladder tumor patients | | | Chronic inflammation |
		Pre-treatment	BCG treatment	Post Mitomycin-C	
Urothelial cells					
HLA-ABC	++	+ or +/-	++	++	++
HLA-DR	-	- or +/-	++	-	- or +/-

- not expressed, +/- patchy expression, + weak expression, ++ strong expression

Infiltrate					
T-cell	+	++	++++	+	
B-cell	-	+	++	-	
Macrophage	+	++	+++	+	VARIABLE
NK-cell	-/+	+/-	+/-	+/-	
Dendritic/ID-cell	+	+	+	+	
Predominant site	Epithelium	Submucosa	Submucosa	Submucosa	Submucosa

- range + to ++++ (normal to intense infiltration)

TABLE 2. T-cells in the submucosa of normal bladder and neoplastic bladder

	Normal bladder	Pre-treatment	Post BCG treatment
Subset analysis mean T4/T8 ratio	0.68	4.96	3.13
Mean Interleukin-2 receptor expression	-	9%	28.2%
Class II MHC* (HLA-DR expression	-	+	++

* not expressed quantatively because of other cell types also expressing this antigen.

The predominant cell in the mononuclear cell infiltrate was the T-lymphocyte. As well as infiltrating the urothelium these cells formed the bulk of suburothelial cellular aggregates found in both treated and untreated bladders and were the main constituent cells of the peripheral cuffs of granulomas. The submucosal T-cell infiltration in normal bladders (mean 1.36, range 1.1-1.64 cells/HPF) was increased in the untreated neoplastic biospies (mean 38.8, range 3.2-101 cells/HPF). Measurement of the T-cell infiltrate between the aggregates and granulomas showed a further increase after BCG therapy (mean 139, range 64-272 cells/HPF) which was declining by 6 months after treatment (mean 81.3, range 2.3-259 cells/HPF). Further T-cell analysis (Table 2) showed that unlike the findings in normal bladder the vast majority of these cells were of the helper (T4) variety and that by their expression of Interleukin-2 receptors and HLA-DR many of these were in an immunologically active state. This activation was increased by BCG. The excess of helper T-cells begins to decline at 6 months after treatment when the mean T4:T8 ratio falls to 1.16 (range 0.5-1.98).

Macrophages and B-lymphocytes formed the bulk of the remainder of the cellular infiltrate. The macrophages were widespread, scattered throughout the epithelium with T-cells and throughout the lamina propria as well as

intimately involved with T-cells in suburothelial aggregates and granulomas. B-lymphocytes were almost exclusively
confined to germinal follicles in the lamina propria.

Natural killer (NK) cells were identified only in
small numbers and when found were almost always HNK+ Fc+
(high NK activity) rather than HNK+ Fc- (lower NK
activity).

DISCUSSION

We found that intravesical BCG induced a marked mononuclear cell infiltrate in the bladder wall which consisted
predominantly of T-lymphocyts in agreement with the
findings of Guinan in the rat (Guinan et al., 1986). There
were also increases in the infiltration of all other cell
types including B-lymphocytes (which are not present in the
normal bladder) (El-Demiry et al., 1986) but with the
exception of natural killer cells which remained sparse in
post-treatment biopsies. The inflammatory reaction had
largely settled by 6 months after treatment.

This inflammatory infiltrate was paralelled in time by
the novo expression of the HLA-DR antigen on tumor cells
which was apparent in the mid treatment biopsy specimens
and persisted for 3-6 months after treatment. The expression was very intense and occured in all patients examined.
This is the first study to demonstrate that BCG treatment
directly alters the phenotype of tumor cells. Such "aberrant" expression of HLA-DR antigen may have implications
for the mechanism of antitumor activity of BCG.

The initiation of both humoral and cell mediated
immune responses requires interaction between antigen
presenting cells and helper T-lymphocytes (Ratliff et al.,
1986). Antigen presenting cells always express HLA-DR antigen which is recognised by T-lymphocytes in association
with processed antigen (Unanue et al., 1984; Shimonkevitz
et al., 1983). Under normal circumstances, expression of
this antigen is confined to cells of the immune system,
vascular endothelium and a few areas of epithelium (Daar et
al., 1984). The restriction of this important immune
recognition antigen to a few cell types has been proposed
as the main defence against auto-immune reactions (Mason,
1985). Controversely "abberant" HLA-DR expression by epi-

thelia is found in conditions where auto-immune aetiology has been demonstrated as in for instance Hashimotos thyroiditis (Bottazo et al., 1983). In fact it has been shown that such HLA-DR expressing thyrocytes can present antigen to T-lymphocytes in vitro (Londei et al., 1984).

If human specific antigens exist in bladder cancer, and there is evidence to suggest that they do, then intense aberrant expression of HLA-DR antigen by tumor cells may allow direct presentation of tumor antigen to T-lymphocytes (Ben-Aissa et al., 1985; Koho et al., 1984). This would bypass the usual requirement that the cell be first recognised as "foreign" by macrophages and undergo processing before macrophage presentation of processed antigen to T-cells. There is some evidence from other tumors that HLA-DR expression may result in enhanced antitumor immune responses. Guerry found increased lymphoproliferative response in vitro to HLA-DR positive malignant melanoma cell lines taken from early disease compared with HLA-DR negative lines (Guerry et al., 1984). Moreover the use of anti HLA-DR serum blocked this response.

The next question is how does BCG therapy result in aberrant HLA-DR expression. Such aberrant expression also occurs in other conditions not usually ascribed an auto-immune aetiology such as gastritis without auto-antibodies and the dermal tuberculin reaction (Scheynius and Tjerlund, 1984; Spencer et al., 1986). These have in common a local accumulation of T-lymphocytes as is often the case with solid tumors where aberrant expression occurs to a greater or lesser degree (Durrant et al., 1987; Ferguson et al., 1985). The expression of HLA-DR by bladder urothelium has not been extensively studied. Normal urothelium is HLA-DR negative as is urothelium acutely inflammed by E. coli infection, at least in the rat experimental model (Daar et al., 1984; Hjelm, 1984). There are no published figures for expression by bladder tumors but we find that this occurs, usually weakly and heterogeneously in approximately one third (unpublished observations).

Thus aberrant HLA-DR expression may be related to T-lymphocyte infiltration. Gamma-Interferon, a lymphokine released by activated T-lymphocytes, has been shown to be a potent inducer of HLA-DR expresion by both normal and neoplastic cells (Basham and Merigan, 1983; Schwartz et al., 1985). We found large numbers of activated helper T-lymphocytes in our biopsies which would be expected to produce Interleukin-2 as found by Haaff and Interferon-gamma (Haaff et al., 1987). Interferon-gamma production by peripheral blood mononuclear cells is elevated in bladder cancer patients in general (Shapiro et al., 1984).

If the "aberrant" HLA-DR expression by bladder tumor cells is as seems likely related to exposure to Interferon-gamma released by T-lymphocytes in response to BCG therapy then another point becomes clear. Recent evidence suggests that some BCG antitumor activity may be due to release of a monocyte cytolytic factor (Nkamura et al., 1987). It has been shown that monocytes can be activated to kill tumor cells by Interferon-gamma in the presence of muramyl dipeptide (a constituent of the BCG cell wall) (Gore et al., 1986). Therefore Interferon-gamma release may also contribute to non-specific antitumor mechanisms.

ACKNOWLEDGEMENT

We are grateful to Evans Medical Ltd for supplies of the BCG used in this study.

REFERENCES

Basham TY, Merigan TC (1983). Recombinant Interferon increases HLA-DR synthesis and expression. J Immunol 130: 1492-1494.

Bast RC, Zbar B, Borsos HJ (1974). BCG and cancer (2 parts) N Engl J Med 290: 1413-1420 and 1458-1469.

Ben Aissa H, Paulie S, Koho H, Biberfeld P, Hansson Y, Lundblad ML, Gustafson H, Jonsdottir I, Perlman P (1985). Specificities and binding properties of 2 monoclonal antibodies against carcinoma cells of the human urinary bladder. Brit J Cancer 52: 65-72.

Bich-Thuy LT, Fuaci AS (1985). Direct effect of Interleukin-2 on the differentiation of human B-cells which have not been pre-activated in vitro. Eur J Immunol 15: 1075-1079.

Bottazo GF, Pujol-Borrell R, Hanagusa T (1983). Role of aberrant HLA-DR expression and antigen presentation in induction of endocrine auto-immunity. Lancet II: 1115-1118.

Daar AS, Fuggle SV, Fabre JW, Ting A, Morris PJ (1984). The

detailed distribution of MHC Class II antigens in normal human organs. Transplantation 38: 293-297.

Davies M (1982). Bacillus Calmette-Guérin as an antitumor agent. The interaction with cells of the mammalian immune system. Biochem Biophys Acta 651: 143-174.

Davies M, Sabbadini E (1982). Mechanisms of BCG action. 1 The induction of non-specific helper cells during the potentiation of auto-immune cell mediated cytotoxic responses. Cancer Immunol Immunother 14: 46-53.

Durrant LG, Ballentyne KC, Armitage NC, Robins RA, Marksman R, Hardcastle JD, Baldwin RW (1987). Quantitation of MHC antigen expression on colorectal tumors and its association with tumor progression. Brit J Cancer 56: 425-432.

El-Demiry MIM, Hargreave TB, Bussuttil A, James K, Chisholm GD (1986). Immunohistochemical identification of lympho-cyte subsets and macrophages in normal human urothelium using monoclonal antibodies. Brit J Urol 58: 436-442.

El-Demiry MIM, Smith G, Ritchie AWS, James k, Cumming JA, Hargreave TB, Chisholm GD (1987). Local immune responses after intravesical BCG treatment for carcinoma in situ. Brit J Urol 60: 543-548.

Farrar WL, Johnson HM, Farrar JJ (1981). Regulation of the production of immune Interferon and cytotoxic lymphocytes by Interleukin-2. J Immunol 126: 1120-1125.

Ferguson A, Moore M, Fox H (1985). Expression of MHC products and leukocyte differentiation antigens in gynaecological neoplasms: an immunohistochemical analysis of the tumor cells and infiltrating leucocytes. Brit J Cancer 52: 551-563.

Gidlund M, Orn A, Wigzell H, Senik A, Gresser I (1978). Enhanced NK activity in mice injected with Interferon and Interferon inducers. Nature (London) 273: 759-761.

Gore S, Lopez-Berestein G, Fidler IJ (1986). Potentiation of direct antitumor cytotoxicity and production of tumor cytolytic factors in human blood monocytes by human recombinant Interferon-gamma and muramyl dipeptide derivatives. Cancer Immunol Immunother 21: 93-99.

Guerry D, Alexander MA, Herlyn MF, Zehnegebot LM, Mitchell KF, Zmijewsky CM, Lusk EJ (1984). HLA-DR histo-compatibility leucocyte antigens permit cultured human melanoma cells from early but not advanced disease to stimulate autologous lymphocytes. J Clin Invest 3: 267-271.

Guinan P, Shaw M, Ray V (1986). Histopathology of BCG and Thiotepa treated bladders. Urol Res 14: 211-215.

Haaff EO, Catalona WJ, Ratliff TL (1987). Detection of Interleukin-2 in the urine of patients with superficial bladder tumors after treatment with intravesical BCG. J Urol 136: 970-974.

Hjelm EM (1984). Local cellular immune response in ascending urinary tract infection: occurrence of T-cells, immunoglobulin producing cells and Ia expressing cells in rat urinary tract tissue. Infect Immun 44: 627-632.

Hudson MA, Ratliff TL, Gillen DP, Haaff EO, Dresner SM, Catalona WJ (1987). Single course versus maintenance Bacillus Calmette-Guérin therapy for superficial bladder tumor: a prospective randomised trial. J Urol 138: 295-298.

Koho H, Paulie S, Ben-Aissa H, Jonsdottir I, Hansson Y, Lundblad ML, Perlman P (1984). Monoclonal antibodies to antigens associated with transitional cell carcinoma of the human urinary bladder. 1. Determination of the selectivity of six antibodies by cell-ELISA and immunofluorescence. Cancer Immunol Immunother 17: 165-172.

Lamm DL (1987). BCG immunotherapy in bladder cancer. In "Urology Annual," Norwalk Conneticut/Los Altos: Appleton and Lange, pp 67-86.

Lefford MJ (1975). Delayed hypersensitivity and immunity in tuberculosis. Am Rev Dis 111: 373-377.

Londei M, Lamb JR, Bottazo GF, Feldman M 81984). Epithelial cells expressing aberrant MHC Class II determinants can present antigen to cloned human T-cells. Nature (London) 312: 639-641.

Mason DW (1985). The possible role of Class II major histocompatibility comples antigen in self tolerance. Scand J Immunol 21: 397-400.

Minden P, McClatchy JK, Wainberg M, Weiss DW (1974). Shared antigens between Mycobacterium bovis (BCG) and neoplastic cells. J Natl Canc Inst 53: 1325-1331.

Nakamura K, Chiao JW, Nagamatsu GR, Addonizio JC (1987). Monocyte cytolytic factor in promoting monocyte mediated lysis of bladder cancer cells by Bacillus Calmette-Guérin. J Urol 138: 867-870.

Prescott S, James K, Busuttil A, Hargreave TB, Chisholm GD, Smyth JF. HLA-DR expression by high grade superficial bladder cancer treated with BCG. (In preparation).

Ratliff TL, Gillen D, Catalona WJ (1987). Requirement of a thymus dependent immune response for a BCG mediated antitumor activity. J Urol 137: 155-158.

Ratliff TL, Shapiro A, Catalona WJ (1986). Inhibition of murine bladder tumor growth by Bacillus Calmette-Guérin:

lack of a role for natural killer cells. Clin Immunol Immunopath 41: 108-115.

Scheynius A, Terlund U (1984). Human keratinocytes express HLA-DR antigens in the tuberculin reaction. Scand J Immunol 19: 141-147.

Schwartz R, Momburg F, Moldenhauer G, Dorken B, Schirrmacher V (1985). Induction of HLA class II antigen expression on human carcinoma cell lines by IFN-gamma. Int J Cancer 35: 245-250.

Shapiro A, Ratliff Tl, Kelley DR, Catalona WJ (1984). Heightened Interferon-gamma production by mononuclear cells from bladder cancer patients. Cancer Res 44: 3140-3143.

Shimonkevitz R, Kappler J, Marrack P, Grey HM (1983). Antigen recognition by H2 restricted T-cells. J Exp Med 158: 303-316.

Smith KA (1980). T-cell growth factor. Immunol Rev 51: 337.

Soloway MS, Perry A (1987). Bacillus Calmette-Guérin for the treatment of superficial transitional cell carcinoma of the bladder in patients who have failed Thiotepa and/or Mitomycin-C. J Urol 137: 871-873.

Spector WH, Marianayagam Y, Ridley MJ (1982). The role of antibody in primary and re-infection BCG granulomas of rat skin. J Path 36: 41-57.

Spencer J, Pugh S, Isaacson PG (1986). HLA-D region antigen expression on stomach epithelium in the absence of auto-antibodies. Lancet II: 983.

Terry WD, Rosenberg FA (1982). Immunotherapy of human cancer. In "Excerpta Medica New York Proufaca," New York: Elsevier North Holland.

Thatcher N, Crowther D (1978). Changes in non-specific lymphoid (NK-, K-, T-cell) cytotoxicity following BCG immunisation of healthy subjects. Cancer Immunol Immunother 5: 105-107.

Thatcher N, Swindell R, Crowther D (1979). Effects of repeated Corynebacterium parvum and BCG therapy on immune parameters: a weekly sequential study of melanoma patients. Clin Exp Immunol 36: 227-236.

Trinchieri G, Santoli D, Knowles BB (1977). Tumor cell lines induce Interferon on human lymphocytes. Nature 270: 611-613.

Unanue ER, Beller DI, Lu CY, Allen PM (1984). Antigen presentation - comments on its regulation and mechanisms. J Immunol 132: 1-5.

Winters WD, Lamm DL 81983). Antibody responses to Bacillus Calmette-Guérin during immunotherapy in bladder cancer patients. Cancer Res 41: 2672-2676.

Youmans GP (1975). Relation between delayed hypersensitivity and immunity in tuberculosis. Am Rev resp Dis 111: 109-118.

EORTC Genitourinary Group Monograph 6:
BCG in Superficial Bladder Cancer, pages 107–122
© 1989 Alan R. Liss, Inc.

MECHANISMS OF ACTION OF INTRAVESICAL BCG FOR BLADDER CANCER

Timothy L. Ratliff

Department of Surgery, Washington University School of
Medicin and The Jewish Hospital of St. Louis, St.
Louis, Missouri, USA

SUMMARY

Though superficial bladder cancer patients have been
treated with intravesical BCG since 1976 the mechanisms of
action remain unknown. Evidence points towards an immune
mechanism of BCG induced antitumor activity. Although
specific antitumor immunity may play a role in BCG immunotherapy, additional work is needed to more clearly define
this possibility. Several investigators have noted a clinical association between favorable response to BCG therapy
and a systemic response delayed type hypersensitivity (DTH)
to BCG antigen indicated by conversion to a positive
purified protein derivative (PPD) skin test. Additional
animal studies have in turn documented evidence of specific
binding between BCG and fibronectin (FN) found in the
urothelial basement membrane which appears necessary for
the development of both the DTH response and antitumor
activity. Other studies have suggested which cellular
components of the immune system and lymphokines may be
involved in the antitumor response.

Further work will be needed to better understand BCG
mechanisms as these findings may be important to other
forms of cancer therapy. Questions of immune suppression,
genetic influence on the immune response and immuno-
competence at the time of surgery may assume increasing
importance. A strong effort will therefore be needed to
better understand these mechanisms so that patients may be
selected, treated and followed in a more effective manner.

INTRODUCTION

The treatment of recurrent superficial transitional cell carcinoma (TCCA) of the bladder by the intravesical instillation of BCG appears to provide an effective means of inhibiting tumor recurrence. The mechanisms by which intravesical BCG inhibit tumor growth are not known. Intravesical BCG for superficial bladder cancer has been termed by some as a form of immunotherapy (Lamm, 1985) but others have suggested that non-immune mechanisms may be involved (Connoly, 1983).

Understanding the mechanisms by which BCG works could be far reaching. This knowledge could provide a basis for developing immunotherapy protocols for bladder cancer therapy. Furthermore, a clear understanding of these mechanisms could lead to therapy without the need for treating with viable, potential infective bacteria.

This manuscript will discuss available evidence concerning potential mechanims of action and define areas in which further investigations are needed.

FACTORS AFFECTING THE INITIATION OF ANTIBLADDER TUMOR ACTIVITY

It is clear from the studies performed to date that BCG is retained and internalized after intravesical instillation. As a result, patients express systemic immunological responses to BCG antigens and granulomatous inflammation is observed in the bladder. Thus, the events surrounding the retention and internalization of BCG are important to our understanding of the initiation of the antitumor response. Our studies on the initiation events suggest that in the mouse tumor model BCG attachment to fibronectin (FN) exposed on the bladder wall is a requisite step for the development of an immunological response and for the expression of both delayed type hypersensitivity and antitumor activity within the bladder.

Fibronectin is a dimeric glycoprotein found in blood, body fluids, and connective tissue matrices. It plays an important role in the function of cell adhesion, cell motility and the interaction between cells and connective tissues of the basement membranes. The molecule is composed of two disulfide bonded 210-250 kd subunit polypeptides and possesses several specific binding sites, including sites specific for a number of macromolecules, including collagen, fibrin, heparin sulfate, dextran sulfate, DNA and bacteria (Hynes and Yamada, 1982).

FIBRONECTIN AND ITS ROLE IN INITIATION OF BCG MEDIATED ANTITUMOR ACTIVITY

Our clinical studies involved histological analysis of BCG attachment to mouse bladders (Ratliff et al., 1987). BCG was instilled into normal bladders and bladders damaged by electrocautery. Acid Fast stains demonstrated attachment of BCG in cauterized bladders only. Quantitative experiments verified the histologic observations. Minimal BCG attachment (mean $< 10^2$ colony forming units) was noted in normal bladders in contrast with the mean of 1.42×10^4 colony forming units/bladder in bladders damaged by electrocautery.

To investigate the proteins to which BCG attached, the binding of BCG to various inflammatory and extracellular matrix proteins comprising the fibrin clot was tested. BCG was found to bind in vitro to surfaces coated in vivo with extracellular matrix proteins but not to control albumin coated coverslips. BCG also bound to coverslips coated with purified plasma FN, but not other purified extracellular matrix proteins including laminin, fibrinogen and Type IV collagen. BCG attachment to surfaces coated with either a mixture of extracellular matrix proteins or purified FN was inhibited by antibodies specific for FN. In addition BCG attachment to cauterized bladders in vivo was inhibited by anti-FN antibodies. These results demonstrated that FN mediated the attachment of BCG to coated surfaces and more importantly that it apparently acted as the primary component mediating attachment within the bladder.

Further studies confirmed the initial hypothesis. Evidence was obtained suggesting that FN mediated attachment was the necessary first step for the expression of both an immune response and antitumor activity. In a recent study delayed type hypersensitivity (DTH) to mycobacterial antigens was quantified by measuring accumulation of ^{125}I-UDR in the bladder after instillation of BCG as described by Thomas (Thomas and Schrader, 1983). Significant delayed type hypersensitivity was measured (mononuclear cell accumulation verified histologically) in BCG sensitized mice treated intravesically with BCG. Inhibition of BCG attachment to the bladder wall by blocking FN-mediated BCG attachment inhibited the expression of DTH response in sensitized mice.

The necessity of BCG binding to FN for the expression of antitumor activity also was tested. C3H/HEJ mice were anesthetized and cauterized. MBT-2 tumors were implanted in cauterized mice and BCG treatment was initiated 24 hrs later and weekly thereafter. In a second group of mice FN-mediated BCG attachment was inhibited. Inhibition of FN-mediated BCG attachment blocked BCG mediated antitumor activity.

Binding between BCG and soluble FN also has been demonstrated (J. Aslanzadeh, unpublished). This binding was found to be similar to the binding interaction described for staphylococci and streptococci and that binding was most likely receptor mediated, rapidly saturable (reaching equilibrium in 3 minutes) and essentially irreversible. Scatchard analysis of the FN/BCG interaction demonstrated approximately 8,000 to 15,000 receptors per bacterium with an association constant of $9.0 \times 10^{-9} M$. The Scatchard plot provided a straight line suggesting that one receptor class was present.

In contrast to previous observations with Staphylococcus aureus which showed enhancement of soluble FN binding in the presence of sodium chloride, soluble FN binding to BCG was inhibited by the presence of as little as 0.15 M NaCl. NaCl in concentrations up to 0.5 M did not inhibit BCG attachment to FN-coated surfaces. In addition BCG binding to soluble FN was optimal at an acidic pH, with a lower level of binding occurring at neutral or basic pH. Since we observed that binding of soluble FN to BCG prior to intravesical instillation inhibits attachment of BCG to the bladder wall, the potential of blocking BCG attachment to the bladder wall by soluble FN is present. These findings suggest that a diluent for BCG should have a neutral or basic pH and should be supplemented with at least 0.15 M NaCl. Such a diluent would decrease the potential inhibition of BCG attachment to the bladder wall by minimizing the binding of soluble FN to BCG.

The method of internalization of BCG once attached is not known. We have observed ingestion of BCG by mouse and human bladder tumor cells in vitro. The ingestion process is time dependent and inhibited by cytochalasin-B and incubation at 4°C. Internalized BCG appears to be contained within lysosomal structures. The fate of the bacteria once internalized and the physiological role of the ingestion process remain to be established.

The attachment of BCG to the bladder wall via FN may be important to the antitumor activity of BCG for several reasons. It may function in a passive manner as an attachment matrix mediating retention of BCG and allowing induction of an immune response to the organism. The expression of this anti-BCG immune response within the bladder may then eliminate the tumors. FN may also play a more active role in the induction of the immune response and expression of antitumor activity. Since FN may be opsonic, it may direct BCG to macrophages or urothelial cells for ingestion and/or antigen processing and presentation to the immune system. Furthermore, by entering the macrophage complexed to BCG, FN could become the target of the immune response as and altered self antigen.

In summary a requisite first step in the initiation of an immune response is introduction of the antigen to the immune system. Results of our recent experiments suggest that FN plays an important role in this process. FN, which is preferentially distributed throughout the basement membrane of the bladder urothelium, appears to mediate attachment of BCG to areas of disrupted mucosa. This attachment has been demonstrated in both in vivo and in vitro conditions. It appears to be receptor mediated, is relatively irreversible, and is blocked by pretreatment with anti-FN antibodies. Not only has BCG/FN binding been demonstrated to occur at sites of disrupted urothelium but this binding has also been demonstrated as necessary for the development of DHT and antitumor activity.

EFFECTOR MECHANISMS

Cancer immunotherapy may be defined as an immunological response which leads to the destruction of the tumor. The response may be directed against antigens present on a tumor (specific immunotherapy) or the response may be initiated by recognition of BCG antigens which results in a cascade of non-specific immunological events leading to tumor destruction (non-specific immunotherapy).

NON-IMMUNOLOGIC MECHANISMS

Non-immunologic mechanisms include either a direct toxic effect of BCG organisms for tumor cells or inflammation in the absence of antigenic recognition. There are no published reports that show direct toxicity of BCG to bladder tumor cells. In our own studies we have observed no toxic effects of BCG for the mouse bladder tumor, MBT-2, or the human bladder cancer cell line, T-24, during in vitro co-culture (T.L. Ratliff, unpublished). Moreover, intravesical BCG therapy for bladder tumors implanted in immunodeficient mice (athymic nude mice) did not inhibit tumor growth. These animals received the same exposure to BCG as immunologically intact mice. If direct toxicity were a primary mechanism, one would expect to observe antitumor activity in the immune deficient mice.

Acute inflammation resulting in cystitis is a second non-immunologic mechanism. Intravesical BCG therapy induces inflammation but is of a chronic nature. Inflammation also is induced by chemotherapeutic agents used in intravesical therapy such as Adriamycin which has been shown to be inferior to BCG.

To determine whether inflammation alone mediated antitumor activity Lamm and associates treated MBT-2 mouse bladder tumors intralesionally with BCG cell wall skeletons (Lamm et al., 1982a). The cell wall skeletons had no effect on MBT-2 growth suggesting that chronic inflammation alone is not sufficient for antitumor activity.

Experiments using the L-10 hepatoma tumor model provide direct evidence that acute and chronic inflammation alone do not inhibit tumor growth. Hanna showed that neither vaccinia virus, oxazolone nor turpentine inhibited L-10 growth (Hanna et al., 1972). Acute inflammation for each compound was histologically documented and characterized leaving no doubt that acute inflammation alone was not the mechanism of action of BCG in the L-10 model. Moreover, non-viable BCG were not effective in this model suggesting that chronic inflammation alone was not sufficient for mediating antitumor activity.

Other studies offer indirect evidence that non-immuno-logic inflammation is not associated with BCG induced anti-tumor activity. In the L-10 model, BCG was not effective in guinea pigs with depressed T-lymphocyte responses (Zbar et al., 1971). It is well documented that acute as well as chronic inflammation with granuloma formation occurs in the absence of immunologic recognition but such a response is not sufficient in the L-10 model for mediation of antitumor activity. We have observed similar results using the MBT-2 mouse bladder tumor in athymic nude mice. No antitumor activity was observed in the absence of a T-lymphocyte response, however, adoptive transfer of BCG sensitized spleen cells restored BCG induced antitumor activity (Ratliff et al., 1987).

In conclusion, considerable evidence exists suggesting that immunologic mechanisms are associated with the anti-tumor activity of BCG but no published data suggests non-immunological mechanisms. One may conclude based on the available evidence that immunologic mechanisms appear more likely to be associated with effective intravesical BCG therapy.

IMMUNOLOGIC MECHANISMS

The participation of immunologic mechanisms in intra-vesical BCG therapy is suggested by indirect data from several research groups, however, definitive evidence is lacking for both clinical and animal studies.

Immunological mechanisms are divided into two catego-ries, specific and non-specific responses which were defined above. The specific response is further divided into antibody (humoral) and cellular mechanisms. The rela-tive roles of these mechanisms will be examined below.

SPECIFIC IMMUNOLOGICAL MECHANISMS

Involvement of specific immunologic responses either humoral of cell-mediated in the elimination of bladder tumors dictates the presence of recognizable antigenic determinants on bladder tumor cells. Indirect but suggested evidence for the presence of tumor associated antigens on both human and mouse bladder tumors has been provided by several investigators (Bubenik et al., 1970; Grossman, 1985; Guinan et al, 1978; Hakala et al., 1974; Helstrom et al., 1982; Morales et al., 1980; Soloway et al., 1978).

HUMORAL MECHANISMS

Data examining the potential role of antibodies in intravesical BCG therapy are practically non-existent. It is well known that BCG has an adjuvant effect on antibody production to antigens of diverse origin including syngeneic tumors (Rook, 1983). Whether antibodies to bladder tumors are produced after BCG therapy remains to be established.

Winters studied patients receiving BCG for serum antibodies recognizing BCG antigens (Winters and Lamm, 1981). These antibodies were shown to increase during combined intravesical and intradermal BCG therapy. Winters and Lamm suggested that antibodies recognizing BCG antigens may cross-react with bladder TCC antigens. There are reports suggesting that some tumor cells do possess antigenic determinants cross-reactive with BCG antigens (Minden et al., 1974), however, Winters and Lamm provided no evidence that cross-reactive antibodies were present in BCG therapy patients. This is the only published data concerning humoral mechanisms which represents a hypothetical possibility with little supporting evidence. A recent report by Haspel and associates documents the production of antibodies reactive with colon carcinoma cells after administration of a BCG-tumor cell vaccine to tumor-bearing patients (Haspel et al., 1985). This report provides further evidence supporting the potential for antibody production in bladder cancer patients.

CELL MEDIATED MECHANISMS

There are no clinical data implicating the presence of a specific T-lymphocyte response to tumor associated antigens in bladder cancer patients treated with BCG. Only limited data in bladder tumor models are available.

Reichert suggested that long-term immunity was induced in mice bearing the mouse bladder tumor MBT-2, treated with intralesional BCG (Reichert and Lamm, 1984). Mice surviving the initial treatment course were rechallenged with MBT-2 tumors and only 56% developed tumors. Additional intra-lesional BCG did not enhance the antitumor effect. These experiments suggested the presence of a specific response to MBT-2 antigens, however, the experiments lack appropri-ate tumor specificity controls and do not directly demon-strate the presence of immune cells with specificity for MBT-2 cells. Since the response was not defined, these data could support the presence of either a cellular or humoral response. Additional studies must be performed to confirm this preliminary observation and identify the immunologic mechanisms.

Other tumor models for which BCG therapy has been tested have shown variability in the development of specific cellular responses to tumors (Bartlett et al., 1972). Studies on the role of specific cellular responses in the L-10 guinea pig hepatoma model show that specific cellular responses are present (Zbar et al., 1972). Guinea pigs that eliminated tumors after intralesional BCG treat-ment expressed long-term resistance to L-10 tumors. Mice receiving only L-10 tumor cells did not inhibit the growth of a second tumor challenge. Furthermore, the growth inhibitory activity of BCG-treated L-10 immune mice was specific for the L-10 tumor since the growth of anti-genically distinct tumors were not inhibited by the L-10 sensitized animals.

Studies on other tumor models show that antitumor immunity, i.e., recognition of tumor associated antigens by syngeneic hosts, is not required for effective BCG mediated antitumor activity, although, T-cell responses to BCG were required (Bartlett et al., 1972). Taken together the data show that either or both tumor antigen recognition and re-cognition of BCG antigens may be important in BCG mediated antitumor mechanisms depending on the tumor model being studied. Thus, it is a distinct possibility that specific antitumor immunity may be associated with destruction of bladder tumors. Additional work is needed to more clearly define the role of tumor specific immunity in the bladder tumor.

NON-SPECIFIC IMMUNOLOGICAL MECHANISMS

Non-specific immunological mechanisms involve the antigenic recognition of BCG antigens which result in the initiation of a cascade of events that ultimately kill bladder tumor cells. The mechanisms can include either lymphokine or non-specific cell-mediated tumor cell killing.

CLINICAL STUDIES

Clinical studies suggest a link between a patient's response to BCG antigens and response to therapy. Lamm and associates have shown that a delayed cutaneous hypersensitivity (DTH) response to purified protein derivative (PPD) correlates well with the therapeutic response to BCG (Lamm et al., 1982b). Only 1 of 17 (6%) patients who converted from PPD negative to PPD positive after BCG therapy developed recurrent tumors while 38% of those either remaining negative or who were PPD positive upon entering therapy developed tumor recurrence.

Kelley and associates also reported a correlation between PPD responsiveness and therapeutic efficacy (Kelley et al., 1986). A significant correlation ($P < .0006$) was observed between a DTH to PPD and treatment results. Among patients who were initially PPD positive (5 patients) and those who converted their skin tests to positive (25 patients), tumor persisted or recurred in only 6 of 30 patients (29%). In contrast, tumors persisted or recurred in 21 of 32 (66%) who did not convert their PPD skin test.

Kelley and associates further showed that granulomatous inflammation in bladder biopsy specimens obtained 6 weeks after completion of therapy also significantly correlated ($P < .003$) with a favorable response to therapy (Kelley et al., 1986).

Taken together these results suggest that a DTH-induced inflammatory response is closely associated with response to intravesical BCG therapy, however, the data are only suggestive and more direct evidence is needed to establish a firm link.

PRECLINICAL STUDIES

As stated above, the mechanism by which BCG treatment for bladder cancer inhibits tumor growth is not known. However, a considerable body of evidence, specifically those clinical studies showing an association between development of DTH by measuring PPD conversion and a favorable prognosis, implicates and immunological mechanism for this antitumor activity. This section will discuss some of the work which has been attempted to characterize the effector response of the BCG induced immunologic mechanism.

Pang showed that an intraperitoneal injection of 10 mg (10^8 CFU) BCG induced regression of subcutaneously implanted MBT-2 tumors in 50 to 90% of treated mice (Pang and Morales, 1982). Analysis of the peritoneal exudate cells revealed that BCG induced non-specific cytotoxic cells expressed a natural killer cell phenotype. This data led Pang and Morales to suggest that natural killer cells were associated with the antitumor activity of BCG. No attempts were made, however, to identify the lymphoid cells infiltrating the regressing tumor nor were specific studies reported to determine whether cured mice could reject subsequent MBT-2 challenge.

Shapiro and associates reported a significant correlation between augmentation of natural killer cell activity of splenocytes and effficacy of intravesical BCG therapy (Shapiro et al., 1983). In this murine model MBT-2 tumor cells were implanted intravesically. The level of both natural killer cell activity and antitumor activity were dependent upon the dose of BCG. Moreover in a second series of experiments, depressed natural killer cell activity was associated with a lack of antitumor activity. These results supported the hypothesis presented by Pang and Morales linking natural killer cell activity with BCG mediated antitumor activity, however, direct evidence linking natural killer cells to BCG mediated antitumor activity remained lacking.

Ratliff and associates performed further experiments in attempts to provide more direct evidence linking natural killer cell activity to the antitumor affects of BCG (Ratliff et al., 1986). Antiasialo GM serum, which has been demonstrated to abrogate natural killer cell activity without significantly altering T-lymphocyte, B-lymphocyte

or macrophage responses was administered to mice prior to
initiation of BCG therapy and at 5 day intervals throughout
therapy. Natural killer cell activity was demonstrated to
be depressed in the spleen and iliac lymph nodes throughout
therapy. The depression of NK-activity had no effect on BCG
mediated antitumor activity. These data provide the most
direct evidence to date that natural killer cells are not
the primary mechanism of BCG mediated antitumor activity,
however, antiasialo serum is not specific for natural
killer cells. More specific methods of abrogating natural
killer cell activity need to be developed to confirm the
observation. In addition locally infiltrating cells
conceivably could escape the effects of antiasialo GM and
would remain undetected in an analysis of splenocyte and
lymph node cell cytotoxicity. Although more definitive data
are needed, the data suggest that BCG mediated killer cell
modulation is independent of the antitumor mechanisms.

Other animal tumor models have been studied which
suggest that the non-specific immunologic mechanism are
associated with BCG mediated antitumor activity. Bartlett
showed that both immunogenic and non-immunogenic tumors
were rejected when injected together with BCG while a
contralateral injection of BCG had no effect on tumor
growth (Bartlett et al., 1972) . Bartlett demonstrated that
a DTH reponse to BCG without concomitant development of
tumor specific immunity mediated inhibition of tumor
growth. These data suggest that bystander killing, i.e.,
the non-specific killing of tumor cells by mononuclear
cells activated by a specific reponse to BCG, is important
in tumor rejection. Studies in other systems, however, have
shown that the development of DTH response alone is not
sufficient for inhibition of tumor growth. Injection of PPD
or dinitrophenyl poly-L-lysine in the tumors of immunized
animals was not sufficient to induce tumor regression even
though a DTH response to these antigens developed.
Injection of soluble factors induced a DTH inflammatory
response indistinguishable from the BCG induced response
during the first 4 days. After this time interval, the BCG
response became chronic with the development of granulomas
while the response to the other stimuli receded. These
results suggest that granuloma formation with its
accompanying chronic macrophage response is required for
effective inhibition of tumor growth.

Histological and ultrastructural studies strongly

implicated cells of the macrophage-monocyte lineage in antitumor activity of BCG. These results show that macrophages are the primary infiltrating cells and suggest that the cytopathic effect of activated macrophages is mediated both at the primary tumor site and in regional lymph nodes by non-phagocytic mechanisms involving direct cell surface contact. In this regard macrophages isolated from animals injected with BCG and tumor cells have been shown to be cytotoxic in vitro. However, direct evidence implicating macrophages as an effector cell is lacking.

Ratliff demonstrated that the antitumor activity of intravesical BCG therapy may require a thymus dependent immune response (Ratliff et al., 1987). Intravesical BCG was demonstrated to have no antitumor activity when administered to athymic nude mice bearing MBT-2 tumors. However, adoptive transfer of BCG sensitized splenocytes (1 spleen equivalent per mouse, i.v.) immediately prior to the first BCG treatment transferred delayed type hypersensitivity of intravesical BCG.

These results do not identify the specific aspect of thymus dependent response associated with antitumor activity. Several T-lymphocytes responses could mediate an antitumor response including cytolytic T-lymphocytes, production of cytotoxic lymphokines, helper T-lymphocyte activity associated with antitumor antibody production and lymphokine mediated activation of non-specific cell mediated cytolytic mechanisms. Additional studies will be required to identify these participating responses.

Little data is available concerning the role of lymphokines in the inhibition of bladder tumor growth by BCG. Haaff and asssociates found that Interleukin-2, a T-lymphocyte derived growth factor, was present in urine specimens of BCG treaeted patients only after BCG instillation (Haaff et al., 1986). Detectable Interleukin-2 levels were present for prolonged periods (at least 7 hours) showing that the potential exists for prolonged exposure of bladder tumors to cytotoxic and cytostatic lymphokines.

In vitro experiments have shown that bladder tumor cells are susceptible to the antiproliferative properties of Interferon-gamma (a T-cell derived lymphokine). Whether lymphokines such as Interferon-gamma, lymphotoxin or Tumor Necrosis Factor are actively involved in the antitumor activity of BCG remains to be established. Similar hypothetical potential mechanisms can be presented for lymphokine activated killer cells and other non-specific mechanisms.

REFERENCES

Bartlett GL, Zbar B, Rapp HJ (1972). Suppression of murine tumor growth by immune reaction to the Bacillus Calmette-Guérin strain of Mycobacterium bovis. J Natl Can Inst 48: 245-257.

Bubenik J, Perlman P, Helmstein K, Moberger G (1970). Cellular and humoral immune responses to human urinary bladder carcinomas. Int J Can 5: 310-316.

Connolly JG (1983). Letter to the Editor, RE.: Immunotherapy of superficial bladder cancer. J Urol 130: 368.

Grossman HB (1985). Tumor markers in urology. Semin Urol 3: 10-17.

Guinan P, McKiel C, Flanigan M, Bhatti R, Pessis D, Ablin RJ (1978). Cellular immunity in bladder cancer patients. J Urol 119: 747-749.

Haaff EO, Catalona WJ, Ratliff TL (1986). Detection of Interleukin-2 in the urine of patients with superficial bladder tumors after treatment with intravesical BCG. J Urol 136: 970-974.

Hakala TR, Castro A, Elliot A (1974). Humoral cytotoxicity in human transitional cell carcinoma. J Urol 111: 382-385.

Hanna MG, Zbar B, Rapp HJ (1972). Histopathology of tumor regression after intralesional injection of Mycobacterium bovis. II . Comparitive effects of vaccinia virus, oxzazolone and turpentine. J Natl Can Inst 48: 1697-1707.

Haspel MS, McGabe RP, Pomato N (1985). Generation of tumor cell-reactive human monoclonal antibodies using peripheral blood lymphocytes form activily immunized colorectal carcinoma patients. Can Res 45: 3951-3961.

Hellstrom I, Rollins N, Settle S (1982). Monoclonal antibodies to two mouse bladder cancer antigens. Int J Cancer 29: 175-180.

Hynes RO, Yamada KM (1982). Fibronectins: Multifunctional modular glycoproteins. J Cell Biol 95: 369-377.

Kelley DR, Haaff EO, Becich M, Lage J, Bauer WC, Dresner SM, Catalona WJ, Ratliff TL (1986). Prognostic value of purified PPD skin test and granuloma formation in patients treated with intravesical BCG. J Urol 135: 268-270.

Lamm DL, Reichert DF, Harris SC (1982a) Immunotherapy of murine transitional cell carcinoma. J Urol 128: 1104-1108.

Lamm DL, Thor DE, Stogdill VD, Radwin HM (1982b). Bladder cancer immunotherapy. J Urol 128: 931-935.

Lamm DL (1985). Bacillus Calmette-Guérin immunotherapy for bladder cancer. J Urol 134: 40-47.

Minden P, McClatchy JK, Wainberg M (1974). Shared antigens between Mycobacterium bovis (BCG) and neoplastic cells. J Natl Can Inst 53: 1325-1329.

Morales A, Djeu J, Herberman RB (1980). Immunization by irradiated whole cells or cell extracts against an experimental bladder tumor. Invest Urol 17: 310-313.

Pang ASD, Morales A (1982). Immunoprophylaxis of a murine bladder cancer with high dose BCG immunizations. J Urol 127: 1006-1009.

Ratliff TL, Gillen DP, Catalona WJ (1987). Requirement of a Thymus dependent immune response for BCG-mediated antitumor activity. J Urol 137: 155-157.

Ratliff TL, Palmer JO, McGarr JA, Brown EJ (1987). Intravesical Bacillus Calmette-Guérin therapy for murine bladder tumors: initiation of the response by Fibronectin-mediated attachment of Bacillus Calmette-Guérin. Can Res 47: 1762-1766.

Ratliff TL, Shapiro A, Catalona WJ (1986). Inhibition of murine bladder tumor growht by Bacillus Calmette-Guérin: lack of a role of natural killer cells. Clin Immuno Immunopath 41: 108-115.

Reichert Df, Lamm DL (1984). Long term protection in bladder cancer following intralesional immunotherapy. J Urol 132: 570-573.

Rook GAW (1983). Immunologically important constituents of mycobacteria antigens. In Ratledge C, Stanford J (eds): "The biology of the mycobacteria", New York: Academic Press, pp 85-128.

Shapiro A, Ratliff TL, Oakley DM, Catalona WJ (1983). Reduction of bladder tumor growth in mice treated with intravesical Bacillus Calmette-Guérin and its correlation with Bacillus Calmette-Guérin viability and natural killer cell activity. Can Res 43: 1611-1613.

Soloway MS, Martino C, Hyatt C (1978). Immunogenicity of N-[-4-(5-Nitro-2-Furyl)-2-Thiazolyl] Formamide-induced bladder cancer. Natl Can Inst Mongr 49: 293-300.

Thomas WR, Schrader JW (1983). Delayed hypersensitivity in mast-cell-deficient mice. J Immun 130: 2565-2570.

Winters WD, Lamm DL (1981). Antibody responses to Bacillus Calmette-Guérin during immunotherapy in bladder cancer patients. Can Res 41: 2672-2676.

Zbar B, Bernstein ID, Bartlett GL, Hanna MG, Rapp HJ (1972). Immunotherapy of cancer: regression of intradermal tumors and prevention of growth of lymph node metastases after intralesional injection of living Mycobacterium bovis. J Natl Can Inst 49: 119-130.

Zbar B, Bernstein ID, Rapp HJ (1971). Suppression of tumor growth at the site of infection with living Bacillus Calmette-Guérin. J Natl Can Inst 46: 831-839.

PART II. CLINICAL BACKGROUNDS FOR BCG-IMMUNOTHERAPY IN SUPERFICIAL BLADDER CANCER

EORTC Genitourinary Group Monograph 6:
BCG in Superficial Bladder Cancer, pages 125–145
© 1989 Alan R. Liss, Inc.

INTRACAVITARY TREATMENT OF TRANSITIONAL CELL CARCINOMA OF
THE BLADDER: QUESTIONS AND LESSONS AFTER 27 YEARS OF
EXPERIENCE

K.H. Kurth, R. Sylvester, M. de Pauw, F. ten Kate
Department of Urology, University of Amsterdam
(K.H.K.), Department of Pathology, University of
Rotterdam (F.t.K.), the Netherlands, and EORTC Data
Center, Brussels, Belgium

Twenty seven years have elapsed since the reports by
Jones and Swinney and by Veenema about topical chemotherapy
of bladder tumors with cytostatic agents (Jones and
Swinney, 1961; Veenema et al., 1962).

Today, as twenty seven years ago, intravesical treatment is given therapeutically in case of incompleted transurethral resection (Ta and T1 lesion) or as an alternative
prior to a more radical approach for the treatment of
carcinoma in situ. Whereas the latter indication became
generally accepted (Edsmyr, 1984; Glashan, 1982; Jakse,
1984) to eradicate carcinoma in situ, urologists in Europe
were more reluctant to apply or to examine the therapeutic
activity in case of papillary Ta-T1 lesions. Only more
recently the apparant need to examine the therapeutic
activity of a drug before it is given prophylactically, led
to phase II studies using a marker lesion for the
examination of the ablative efficacy of the drug.

Although progression of a superficial lesion to a
muscle-invasive bladder tumor cannot be excluded during an
8 weekly course of intracavitary treatment, the likelihood
of such a progression is very small as long as there is no
combined papillary and flat lesion (carcinoma in situ).
Therefore the fear for the development of muscle invasive
disease during intracavitary treatment should be even less
in patients with papillary lesions than in patients with
carcinoma in situ where chemo- or immunotherapy is accepted
for definitive treatment.

Intravesical chemotherapy and immunotherapy are exerted because of their potential to reduce the high percentage of recurrent tumor by destroying floating tumor cells after TUR and the cytotoxic activity of the drugs on microscopically present and macroscopically unrecognized tumorous lesions. Intracavitary treatment was started as a clinical experiment, it gained acceptance because of its superiority when compared with TUR alone in prospective randomized studies, but for many urologists it is still questionable if all patients need an inconvenient and expensive treatment.

Questions to the usefulness of chemotherapy and, if given, how it should be given were repeatedly formulated in the past by experts in this field (Bouffioux et al., 1985; Pavone-Macaluso, 1980; Schulman et al., 1984) (Table 1).

TABLE 1.

---

1. What is the most active drug?
2. What is the best time for initiation of therapy (pre- or intra-operative, immediately after TUR or after closure of the epithelial defect)?
3. What is the optimal time for the drug to be kept in the bladder?
4. What is the ideal time between each instillation?
5. What dose should be given at each instillation?
6. How long should the drug be administered?
7. In what liquid and what volume should if be dissolved?
8. May all the tumors benefit from the treatment?
9. What is the influence of diureses and urinary pH?
10. What is the possible role of adjuvants favoring the superficial penetration of the drug into the epithelium?

(C. Bouffioux, 1985)

IS THERE THE BEST CHEMOTHERAPEUTIC AGENT?

There is no evidence from the EORTC protocols 30782 and 30790 that any of the drugs used (Adriamycin, Cisplatinum, Thiotepa, Epodyl) is superior in preventing recurrent tumors. Mitomycin-C was not examined by the EORTC in a comparative protocol examining different drugs. However, prophylactically applied in a randomized trial Engelmann found no significant differences between Mitomycin-C, Adriamycin and VM-26 (Engelmann et al., 1982).

Thus, from drugs widely used, as Adriamycin, Thiotepa, Epodyl and Mitomycin-C, none came out as a superior drug. This does not mean that a patient who showed no response to one drug may not react to another drug (Prout et al., 1982). 5/14 Patients who failed after treatment with Thiotepa showed complete response using Mitomycin-C.

Other drugs like 5-FU and Bleomycin were never examined in a large randomized study and it is therefore unproved whether or not these drugs are possibly similar active as the agents mentioned above.

Intracavitary treatment has much similarity with an in vitro assay with the disadvantage of no ideal circumstances for the production of cytotoxicity. Switching from chemotherapy to immunotherapy may be meanful, however, this has been examined prospectively only by few authors. Soloway treated patients who had failed Thiotepa and/or Mitomycin-C with BCG and observed complete remission of the marker lesion or conversion of urine cytology to normal in 50% of the patients (Soloway and Perry, 1987). For the evaluation of an alternative approach we need more of those phase II studies.

SHOULD THE FIRST INSTILLATION BE GIVEN EARLY AFTER ENDOSCOPIC RESECTION OR DELAYED?

This question had been examined in two parallel EORTC protocols (30831, 30832). Mitomycin-C and Adriamycin were used, patients were randomized for immediate instillation after TUR or instillation 1 to 2 weeks after surgery.

Analyzing the recurrence rate (number of positive cystoscopy during study devided by the total months of follow-up multiplied with 12 to express recurrence rate per year), no significant differences were found in favor of one of the treatment arm. There is, however, a slight tendency for better results in patients treated by early instillation (Table 2).

TABLE 2. Comparison early versus delayed instillation (p = not significant) (Kurth et al., 1988b)

| | Adriamycin | |
	Early	Delayed
Patients with follow-up	188	178
Mean follow-up (months)	12	12.3
Percent with recurrence	17	26
Recurrence rate per year	0.25	0.35
Tumor rate per year	0.68	0.67

EORTC 30832, 03-87

Analysis of subgroups has not yet been performed and a significant difference in favor of early instillation cannot be excluded (Kurth et al., 1988a). Pre-operative instillation was applied by Mishina and the results were compared with post-operative instillation (Mishina et al., 1982). Different dosages were used and patients were not randomly allocated to one or the other treatment arm. In this study pre-operative instillation did not show a prophylactic effect on recurrences.

WHAT IS THE OPTIMAL TIME FOR THE DRUG TO BE KEPT IN THE BLADDER?

In most studies an instillation time of one or two hours is recommended. To our knowledge there is only one study referring to differences in instillation time. Therefore, the instillation time recommended in different treatment schedules reflects what is desirable from the standpoint of an author, but has not taken enough in account what is achievable in elderly patients. Eksborg decided for a practical approach (Eksborg et al., 1980). The chemotherapeutic agent to be instilled was first dissolved in a container (plastic bag) fixed several centimeters above the level of the patient in supine position. During the intracavitary treatment the bag remained connected with the catheter. Whenever the patient had detrusor activity the instillation fluid ran back into the plastic bag and was re-instilled if the time schedule for contact was not yet achieved.

WHAT IS THE IDEAL TIME BETWEEN EACH INSTILLATION?

For most therapeutic studies weekly instillations were applied and this was adopted also for prophylactic purposes. Generally, four consecutive weekly instillations are followed by montly instillations. Burk randomized patients into three treatment groups (Burk et al., 1983) of which the first group received instillations with Adriamycin 50 mg once a week for three months, the second group received instillations by 2-weeks intervals for six months, and the third group received one instillation every month for one year.

The frequency of drug induced cystitis was 19.8% in patients treated with an instillation once a week for three months and 11% in the group receiving the 2-weekly instillations for six months. Although the initial percentage of recurrent tumor was at the lowest level after completion of the instillation therapy in group one, the percentage of recurrence was similar after one year in all three treatment arms with 38.1%, 31.3%, and 32.4% respectively.

Schulman instilled Adriamycin 50 mg twice during the first week, then weekly during the first month and thereafter monthly for one year (Schulman et al., 1983). Of the patients 26.3% presented with chemical cystitis, being severe enough to go off-study in 20.8%. This frequency of chemical cystitis after intracavitary treatment is much higher than reported by others (Kurth et al., 1984).

The recurrence rate seemed more favorable than the recurrence rate observed in other studies, but as this was not a randomized study no conclusions can be drawn regarding the possible enhanced prophylactic effect. The same can be stated for the studies reported by several others (England et al., 1981; Flüchter et al, 1982; Gavrell et al., 1978).

WHAT DOSE SHOULD BE GIVEN AT EACH INSTILLATION?

We recently performed a study to examine absorption of drugs after intravesical administration (Mross et al., 1987). Prior to instillation an aliquot of the solution was kept for drug analysis. To our surprise the mean dose of the drug instilled in patients who should have received

30 mg was 26.7 mg (range 21.4 - 31.2 mg)), and for patients who should have received 50 mg the mean dose was 45.8 mg (range 37-56.6 mg) (Table 3).

TABLE 3. Epi-Dox concentration (mean ± S.D. and range) in samples following 30 and 50 mg dosages

| | Dose of Epi-Dox | |
	30 mg (N=17)	50 mg (N=15)
Instillation fluid U1 (mg)	26.7 ± 2.3 21.4 - 31.2	45.6 ± 5.8 37.0 - 56.6
Recovered instillation fluid U2 (mg)	20.8 ± 4.9 8.5 - 31.0	36.6 ± 5.8 22.8 - 45.4
Irrigation fluid U3 (mg)	1.4 ± 0.2 0.1 - 6.75	1.4 ± 0.8 0.31 - 3.54
Initial urine voided U4 (mg)	0.03 ± 0.04 0.002 ± 0.14	0.29 ± 0.37 0.004 ± 1.97

It would not be feasible to perform this kind of investigations in a large randomized study, however, one may express some doubts on the significance of findings in a study where the dose differed minimally. Only few phase I-II dose response studies for topical treatment of superficial bladder tumors were executed (De Furia et al., 1980; Kurth et al., 1988b). At least three drugs, Mitomycin-C, Adriamycin, and Epirubicin, seem to have a dose response curve and are apparently more active at higher dose (Kurth et al., 1988b; Melloni and Pavone Macaluso, 1980).

HOW LONG SHOULD THE DRUG BE ADMINISTERED?

In the aforementioned EORTC protocols 30831 and 30832 patients were randomized after six months of treatment for another six monthly instillations or for no further instillations. A preliminary analysis examining the recurrence rate as endpoint did not yield any significant differences between the treatment arms (Kurth et al., 1988c) (Table 4).

TABLE 4. Comparison instillation for 6 months (nm) versus instillation for 12 months (m), p = not significant (Kurth et al., 1988b)

	Adriamycin	
	No Maintenance	Maintenance
Patients with follow-up	147	146
Mean follow-up (months)	14.5	14.5
Percent with recurrence	24	19
Recurrence rate per year	0.28	0.22
Tumor rate per year	0.59	0.41

EORTC 30832, 03-87

These observations are in agreement with the results reported by Huland (Huland et al. 1988). The authors examined the effect of prolonged instillation treatment with Mitomycin-C 20 mg (group 1, 2, and 3) and of Adriamycin 50 mg (group 4). Group one was treated every two weeks during the first year, every four weeks in the second year, and every three months in the third year. Group two was treated every week for eight weeks, and then every four weeks in the first, the second and the third year. Group three was treated every week for twenty weeks. Group four was treated with Adriamycin 50 mg according to the schedule of group one (every two weeks in the first year, four-weekly in the second year and three-monthly in the third year.

After a mean follow-up of twenty months no significant differences between the four treatment arms were observed. Thus, in this preliminary report weekly instillation for twenty weeks was as good as instillation for three years.

IN WHAT LIQUID AND IN WHAT VOLUME SHOULD THE DRUG BE DISSOLVED? WHAT IS THE INFLUENCE OF URINARY pH?

The effects of pH on the antitumor activity of six cytostatic agents - Cisplatin, Doxorubicin, Ethoglucid, Mitomycin-C, Thiotepa, and VM-26 - were tested in vitro

(Jauhiainen et al., 1985). The activity of these drugs was determined on the Walker 256 carcinosarcoma cell line, by using the ATP-bioluminescence method. Cytostatics were incubated at different pH (5.0-7.4) for two and four hours. The activity of the cytostatics was not effected by pH, although Mitomycin-C had somewhat lower activity at pH 5 at four hours. The authors concluded since the pH of normal urine is within the range used in this test, the use of buffer solutions (phosphate buffered physiological saline solution pH 7.4) during the intravesical instillation therapy is not necessary. However, buffering may help to avoid chemical cystitis. Groos and Masters examined the relationship between osmolality and cytotoxicity (Groos and Masters, 1986). Their study indicates that the in vitro cell kill is enhanced when antitumor agents are instilled in a solution that lowers the osmolality of the resultant drug solvent mixture. The drug should be dissolved in distilled water rather than in saline and the commercial preparation of some drugs should be modified to reduce the influence of additives on the osmotic value of the instilled fluid. The drugs with an enhanced cytotoxicity in hypo-osmolar media were Thiotepa, Mitomycin-C, Cisplatinum, Doxorubicin and Epirubicin. The cytotoxicity effect was measured in media of six different osmolalities using a human bladder cancer cell line measuring inhibition of colony forming cells. Reducing osmotic value from 590 to 125 mOsm/kg the in vitro cytotoxicities of the drugs increased significantly. These results are in agreement with data reported by Levin (Levin and Moskovitz, 1986). These authors compared the effect of distilled water on ex-foliated tumor cells from transitional bladder carcinoma with the effect of chemotherapeutic agents dissolved in saline or in distilled water.

Regarding the volume for dissolving the drug it seems useful to use as little as needed. Finally one should make sure that the total amount of the drug is instilled into the bladder and nothing is left in the catheter, the syringe or the bag.

It is not without importance what kind of container is used for dissolving the drug. From drugs like Doxirubicin, Mitomycin-C and Fluoruracil it is known that they are more stable in plastic containers than in glass containers. The T-90 value for Doxorubicin in glass is 40 hours whereas in plastic containers there is no apparent decrease even after

48 hours (Benvenuto et al., 1981). Epodyl mixed with water in aluminumfoil cups lost nearly 50% of its concentration in five minutes time, whereas it is stable in glass cups (Larsen, 1980).

MAY ALL THE TUMORS BENEFIT FROM THE TREATMENT?

There is no doubt, that primary tumors behave better than recurrent tumors (Table 5) and solitary tumors do much better than multiple tumors (Table 6). Surprisingly, the size of the tumor had no significant impact on the recurrence rate (Table 7).

TABLE 5. Prognostic factor: primary versus recurrent (mean follow-up 20 months)

	Overall	Primary	Recurrent
Number of patients	371	253	118
Pts. with recurrence	162	93	69
Percent recurrence	44	37	58
Recurrence rate/year	0.44	0.32	0.69
Tumor rate/year	1.17	0.75	2.06

primary versus recurent $p < 0.000$ EORTC 30790, 05-85

TABLE 6. Prognostic factor: number of tumors at entry (mean follow-up 20 months)

	1 tumor	> 1 tumor
Number of patients	155	216
Pts. with recurrence	52	110
Percent recurrence	34	51
Recurrence rate/year	0.26	0.58
Tumor rate/year	0.58	1.65

1 tumor versus > 1 tumor $p < 0.000$ EORTC 30790, 05-85

TABLE 7. Prognostic factor: tumor size (mean follow-up 20 months)

	Overall	< 1 cm	< 3 cm	> 3 cm
Number of patients	370	128	148	94
Pts. with recurrence	162	61	59	42
Percent recurrence	44	48	40	45
Recurrence rate/year	0.44	0.45	0.44	0.43
Tumor rate/year	1.17	1.35	1.03	1.14

<1 cm versus > 3 cm p = not significant

EORTC 30790, 05-85

Looking at a prognostically favorable group with a single tumor and comparing results achieved with cytostatic agents or TUR alone, adjuvantly treated patients do significantly better (Table 8).

TABLE 8. Prognostic factor: 1 tumor at entry treatment (mean follow-up 20 months)

	Overall	ADM	Epodyl	Control
Number of patients	155	67	59	29
Pts. with recurrence	52	22	13	17
Percent recurrence	34	33	22	59
Recurrence rate/year	0.26	0.26	0.13	0.55
Tumor rate/year	0.58	0.56	0.26	1.29

ADM versus Epodyl p = not significant   EORTC 30790, 05-85
ADM versus Control p = 0.02
Epodyl versus Control p < 0.000

The same is true for patients with multiple tumors. The recurrence rate per year is significantly higher is patients not treated adjuvantly (Table 9). Adjuvant treatment also significantly lowered the recurrence rate in patients with a primary or recurrent tumor (Table 10).

TABLE 9. Prognostic factor: 4 tumors at entry treatment
(mean follow-up 20 months)

	Overall	ADM	Epodyl	Control
Number of patients	85	38	34	13
Pts. with recurrence	51	23	17	11
Percent recurrence	60	61	50	85
Recurrence rate/year	0.73	0.65	0.56	1.50
Tumor rate/year	2.55	2.60	1.20	6.20

ADM versus Epodyl p = not significant   EORTC 30790, 05-85
ADM versus Control p = 0.02
Epodyl versus Control p = 0.03

TABLE 10. Prognostic factor: treatment recurrent patients
(mean follow-up 20 months)

	Overall	ADM	Epodyl	Control
Number of patients	118	48	45	25
Pts. with recurrence	69	27	20	20
Percent recurrence	58	56	49	80
Recurrence rate/year	0.69	0.59	0.52	1.25
Tumor rate/year	2.06	2.04	1.14	4.01

ADM versus Epodyl p = not significant   EORTC 30790, 05-85
ADM versus Control p = 0.02
Epodyl versus Control p = 0.012

However, if one calculates the mean interval between
recurrent tumors and analyses prognostic factors in the
EORTC protocol 30790 the likelihood to develop a recurrent
tumor (irrespective of the treatment applied) in one year
time is very high for the recurrent tumors, T1 lesions,
multiple tumors or tumors with a high grade (G2-G3).
However, the likelihood to develop a recurrent lesion over
the next three years is very low in a unifocal, primary low
stage - low grade lesion (Table 11).

TABLE 11.

Tumor characteristics	Recurrence rate	Interval between recurrences
Ta	2.6	39 (months)
Ta G1 (primary)	1.9	54 (months)
Tx solitary and primary	1.6	64 (months)
Tx G3 recurrent and multiple	17.7	6 (months)

EORTC 30790, 05-85

Thus, in conclusion, even patients with a good prognosis have some benefit from adjuvant chemotherapy. The likelihood of developing a recurrent lesion is very low for those patients. Adjuvant chemotherapy or immunotherapy therefore may be reserved for patients with less favorable prognostic factors.

DOES INTRAVESICAL CHEMOTHERAPY PREVENT INVASIVE BLADDER CANCER?

To answer this question long-term follow-up studies are needed. Looking to the final analysis from EORTC protocol 30790 (unpublished observations) the uncorrected survival curve shows no difference in survival for patients adjuvantly treated or not treated (Figure 1).

Out of 421 patients analyzed, 75 patients have died. More patients (9%) died of cardiovascular disease rather than of a malignant disease (Table 12). Out of 391 patients, 46 developed a muscle invasive bladder tumor. Interestingly, most of the patients developed progression during the treatment (32/46, Table 13). The lack of significant difference in survival between adjuvantly and not-adjuvantly treated patients is in contrast to what has been reported by others.

In the study of Huland all patients were adjuvantly treated and the frequency of progression was compared with a historical control (Huland et al., 1988). It can therefore not be stated undoubtly, that adjuvant chemotherapy lowers the frequency of invasive bladder cancer. This seems to be the case for patients treated with BCG as reported recently (Herr, 1988).

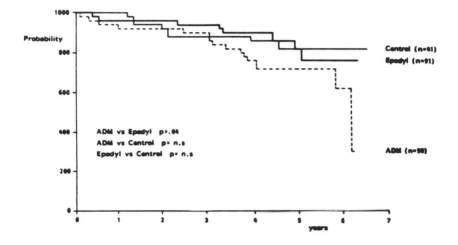

Figure 1. Uncorrected survival: Ta category EORTC 30790, 1988 .

TABLE 12. Cause of death

	Mal. Dis.		Cardiovasc.		Other		Total	
	No.	%	No.	%	No.	%	No.	%
ADM	10	6	16	9	4	2	30/180	17
Epodyl	13	8	15	9	4	2	32/169	19
Control	2	3	8	11	3	4	13/ 72	18
Total	25	6	39	9	11	3	75/421	(18)

EORTC 30790, 1988

TABLE 13. Increase in T category > T1

	No		During Treatment		At Any Time		Total
	No.	%	No.	%	No.	%	
ADM	145	88	12	7	20	12	165
Epodyl	137	88	12	10	19	12	156
Control	63	90	5	7	7	10	70
Total	345	88	32	8	46	12	391

EORTC 30790, 1988

However, most of the patients (73%) who were random-ized for TUR alone in EORTC 30790 were adjuvantly treated after they went off-study. Therefore, in this study patients with immediate adjuvant treatment are compared with patients primary allocated to TUR alone, but in the majority treated later on with some form of chemotherapy. Furthermore, the survival curves are uncorrected and one cannot totally exclude small differences if they are corrected for death by other cause (Figure 1).

IS THERE A RELATION BETWEEN THE TENDENCY TO PRESENT FRE-QUENT RECURRENCES AND THE POTENTIAL TO DEVELOP INVASIVE DISEASE? WHAT IS THE IMPACT OF REVIEW PATHOLOGY?

An answer is given in Table 14.

TABLE 14. Prognostic factors at entry on study

	P-value	
	First Recurrence	Survival
T-category (L) (Ta vs T1)	.05	.04
T-category (R) (Ta vs T1)	.003	.006
Size (1 cm vs > 1 cm)	not signif.	not signif.
Number of tumors (1 vs > 1)	.0000	.28
Grade (L) (G1 vs G2-3)	.001	.03
Grade (R) (G1 vs G2-3)	.001	.004

(L = local pathology)   EORTC 30790, 1988
(R = review pathology)

The number of tumors, a most important prognostic factor for the development of new recurrences is not important for the survival, whereas the T-category and G-category have a strong impact on both new recurrences and survival. This is especially true if the tumors are classified and graded by a review pathologist. Agreement for the T-category between local and review pathologist was achieved in T1 lesions in only 44.2% and for the Ta lesions in 84.5%. Agreement for G-category was found in 59.1% (Tables 15 and 16).

TABLE 15. Over- and underclassification of tumor stage by the local institution based on review pathology

	T1 (%) (N=131)	T1 (%) (N=175)
Overclassified	68 (51.9)	1 (0.6)
Underclassified	4* (3.0)	21 (12.0)
CIS	1 (0.7)	4 (2.3)
Tx		1 (0.6)
Agreement local vs review	58 (44.2)	148 (84.5)

* In all 4 patients tumor extended into the bladder muscle.

TABLE 16. Over- and underclassification of tumor grade by the local institution based on review pathology*

Overclassified	: G1	3/135	(2.3%)
	G2	12/113	(10.6%)
	G3	6/26	(23.0%)
	Total	21/274	(7.6%)
Underclassified	: G0	32/ 32	(100.0%)
	G1	64/135	(47.7%)
	G2	26/113	(23.0%)
	Total	122/280	(43.5%)
Agreement local vs review:	G1	67/135	(50.0%)
	G2	75/113	(66.3%)
	G3	20/ 26	(76.9%)
	Total	162/274	(59.1%)

* two classified as Gx by local institution
  one classified as Gx by review pathologist

Because we expect a better survival for low-grade and low-stage tumors (and a highly significant difference when survival for Ta and T1 tumors is compared) the findings of the review pathologist in Table 14 fit better in what we expect from the natural course of disease.

The question "How should intravesical chemotherapy be given?" cannot be answered based on clinical reports. Therefore a wide open field for further studies still exists.

WHAT HAPPENS TO THE DRUG?

Doxorubicin, Epirubicin, 5-FU and Mitomycin-C showed only minor absorption after intravesical instillation (Eksborg et al., 1979; Engelmann and Jacobi, 1985; Jacobi and Kurth, 1980; Kurth et al., 1985; Leissner et al., 1978; Mross et al., 1987; Wajsmann et al., 1984). The amount of Thiotepa absorbed from the bladder and the plasma levels of the drug showed wide variation among patients with normal bladders and those with abnormal bladder mucosa. At a concentration of 60 mg/60 ml of Thiotepa normal bladder mucosa permitted an average passage of 90% of the instilled Thiotepa. Disseminated papillary tumors of the bladder or necrosis of the bladder mucosa after fulguration or transurethral resection of a very large papillary tumor led to increase of the absorption to nearly 100%. Serum levels of Thiotepa showed an increase corresponding with the absorbed amount of the drug from the bladder (Lunglmayer, 1971). It is well known that drugs with a lower molecular weigth like Thiotepa are more absorbed than drugs with a molecular weight above 300. Attempts to enhance the oncolytic activity of a cytostatic agent by combining it with various adjuvant may increase systemic absorption and toxicity. It cannot be excluded that once absorbed into the circulation an anticancer drug may exert a carcinogenic effect. The resorbed drug may have a direct carcinogenic genetic effect at a different site or it may cause sufficient immunosuppression to allow the development of a second tumor (Newling, 1985). Therefore the use of potentiators of chemotherapeutic agents intravesically applied may not be harmless.

IN CONCLUSION

The superior chemotherapeutic agent for intravesical chemotherapy is not yet identified.

Early instillations do not yet deliver better results than delayed instillation.

The optimal time for the drug to be kept in the bladder is not yet defined.

Intensive and frequent chemotherapy increases the local toxicity, but it has not yet been shown to be superior.

The highest concentration of the drug that the bladder will tolerate should be administered as long as there is no important absorption of the drug into the circulation.

Drugs used for prophylactic intracavitary treatment should have proven therapeutic activity (phase II studies).

There are risks in the administration of intravesical drugs.

Drugs are absorbed in low amount through the intact urothelium.

Anticancer drugs are carcinogenic and may have distant and/or late effects.

Short- or long-term intracavitary treatment should be based on individual parameters such as known prognostic factors.

Prevention of tumor progression is an important aim of intravesical chemo- and immunotherapy. It can, however, only be studied in patients with long-term follow-up. There are up to now no convincing data in large randomized studies showing a lower risk of tumor progression in patients adjuvantly treated with cytostatic agents.

In future studies the value of sequential and combined treatment may be examined. One may use potentiators which do not increase systemic toxicity, one may look for immunotherapeutic agents with less local toxicity than exerted by BCG and finally one should look for cellular immunity in

those patients receiving long-term intravesical chemotherapy.

REFERENCES

Benvenuto JA, Anderson Rw, Kerkhof K, Smith RG, Loo TL
(1981). Stability and compatibility of antitumor agents
in glass and plastic containers. Am J Hops pharm 38:
1914-1918.
Bouffioux Ch (1985). Intravesical chemoprophylaxis of
superficial transitional cell carcinoma of the bladder.
When should the drug be given? In Schröder FH, Richards B
(eds): "Superficial Bladder Cancer," Part B, EORTC
Monograph 2, New York: Alan R. Liss, pp 47-55.
Burk K, Troller RM, Pittner P (1983). Rezidivprophylaxe bei
oberflächlichen Harnblasenkarzinomen. Urologe 22:
332-336.
Edsmyr F, Andersson L, Esposti P (1984). Intravesical
chemotherapy of carcinoma is situ in bladder cancer.
Urology (suppl.) 23: 37-39.
Eksborg S, Ehrsson H, Andersson I (1979). Reversed-phase
liquid chromatographic determination of plasma leverls of
Adriamycin and Adramycinol. J Chromatography 164:
479-486.
Eksborg S, Nilson SO, Edsmyr F (1980). Intravesical instillation of Adriamycin. A model for standardization of the
chemotherapy. Eur Urol 6: 218-220.
Engelmann UH, Frohneberg D, Jakse G, Bauer HW, Jacobi GH
(1982). Die intravesikale Rezidiv Chemoprophylaxe des
oberflächlichen Harnblasentumors. Fortschritte Urologie
und Nephrologie 19: 32-35.
Engelmann UH, Jacobi GH (1985). Intravesical Adriamycin
instillations - what happens to the drug? In Schröder FH,
Richards B (eds): "Superficial Bladder Tumors, Part B,"
EORTC GU-Group Monograph 2, New York: Alan R. Liss.
England HR, Flynn JT, Paris AMI, Blandy JP (1981). Early
multiple-dose adjuvant Thiotepa in the control of
multiple and rapid T1 tumor neogenesis. Br J Urol 53:
588-592.
Flüchter Sh, Harzmann R, Hlobil H, Bichler KH (1982). Lokale Chemotherapie des Harnblasenkarzinoms mit Mitomycin.
Urologe (A) 21: 24-28.
De Furia MD, Bracken RB, Johnson DE (1980). Phase I-II
study of Mitomycin-C topical therapy for low-grade,
low-stage transitional cell carcinoma of the bladder: an

interim report. Cancer Treatment Reports 64: 225-229.

Gavrell GJ, Lewis RW, Meehan WL, LeBlanc GA (1978). Intra-vesical Thiotepa in the immediate post-operative period in patients with recurrent transitional cell carcinoma of the bladder. J Urol 120: 410-411.

Glashan RW, Riley A (1982). Intravesical therapy with Adriamycin in urothelial dysplasia and early carcinoma in situ. Can J Surg 25: 30-32.

Groos E, Masters JRW (1986). Intravesical chemotherapy: studies on the relationship between osmolality and cyto-toxicity. J Urol 136: 399-402.

Herr H (1988). Treatment of superficial bladder cancer: an overview. In Frohmüller (ed): "Uro-Oncology," New York: Alan R. Liss, in press.

Huland H, Klöppel G, Otto U, Feddersen I, Brachmann W, Hubmann H, Kaufmann J, Knipper W, lantzius-Beninga F (1988). Cytostatic intravescial instillation in patients with superficial bladder carcinoma for prevention of recurrent tumors. Acta Medica: 147-158.

Jacobi Gh, Kurth KH (1980). Studies on the intravesical action of topicaly administered g^{3}H-Doxorubicin hydro-chloride in men: plasma uptake and tumor penetration. J Urol 124: 34-37.

Jakse G, Hofstädter F, Marberger H (1984). Topical Doxoru-bicin hydrochloride therapy for carcinoma in situ: a follow-up. J Urol 131: 41-42.

Jauhiainen K, Kangas L, Käpyla H, Alfthan O (1985). Intra-vesical cytostatics: pH-dependence of antitumor activity. Urol Res 13: 19-21.

Jones HC, Swinney J (1961). Thiotepa in the treatment of tumors of the bladder. Lancet 2: 615-618.

Kurth KH, Schröder FH, Tunn U, Ay R, Pavone Macaluso M, Dalesio O, Ten Kate FJW, and members of the EORTC GU-Group (1984). Adjuvant chemotherapy of superficial transitional cell bladder carcinoma: preliminary results of an EORTC randomized trial comparing Doxorubicin Hydro-chloride, Ethoglucid and transurethral resection alone. J Urol 132: 258-262.

Kurth KH, De Wall JG, Van oosterom AT, De Jong EAJM, Tjaden UR (1985). Plasma levels during intravesical instillation of Mitomycin-C. In Schröder FH, Richards B (eds): "Super-ficial Bladder Tumors, Part B," EORTC GU-Group Monograph 2, New York: Alan R. Liss.

Kurth KH, Bouffioux C, Sylvester R, De Pauw M, and members of the EORTC GU-Group (1988a). Early and delayed instil-lation with and without maintenance of either Adriamycin or Mitomycin-C in patients with superficial transitional carcinoma of the bladder. Acta Medica. 159–164.

Kurth KH, Mross K, Ten Kate F, Weissglas G, Carpentier PJ, Boeken Kruger CGD, Blom J, Groen JM, Van Caubergh RD, Van Aubel O (1988b). Phase I-II study of intravesical Epirubicin in patients with carcinoma in situ of the bladder. In Fromüller H (ed): "Uro-Oncology," New York: Alan R. Liss, in press.

Kurth KH, Bouffioux C, Sylvester R, De Pauw M, and members of the EORTC GU-Group (1988c). Is there an optimal treatment scheme for adjuvant intravesical therapy? Preliminary analysis of an EORTC protocol comparing early and delayed instillation with and without maintenance of either Adriamycin or Mitomycin-C in patients with superficial transitional carcinoma of the bladder. In "Progress and Controversies in Oncological Urology II," EORTC GU-Group Monograph 5, New York: Alan R. Liss, pp 525–532.

Larsen J (1980). Inactivation of Epodyl in aluminium foil cups as a cause of ineffective treatment of non-invasive bladder tumors. Scand J Urol Nephrol. 14: 239–242.

Leissner KH, Gustavsson, Nilsson S, Almersjö O (1978). General resorption of intravesically instilled 5-Fluorouracil. J Urol 120: 407–409.

Levin DR, Moskovic B (1986). Distilled water versus chemotherapeutic agents for transitional bladder carcinoma. Eur Urol 12: 418–421.

Lunglmayer G, Czech K (1971). Absorption studies on intraluminal Thiotepa for topical cytostatic treatment of low-stage bladder tumors. J Urol 106: 72–74.

Melloni D, Pavone Macaluso M (1980). Intravesical treatment of superficial urinary bladder tumors with Adriamycin. In Pavone Macaluso M, Smith PH, Edsmyr F (eds): "Bladder tumors and other topics in urological oncology," New York: Plenum, pp 317–320.

Mishina T, Oda K, Murata S, Ooe H, Mori Y, Takahashi T (1982). Mitomycin-C bladder instillation therapy for bladder tumors. J Urol 114: 217–219.

Mross K, Maessen P, Van der Vijgh WFJ, Bogdanowicz JF, Kurth KH, Pinedo HM (1987). Absorption of 4-Epi-Doxorubicin after intravesical administration in patients with transitional cell carcinoma in situ of the bladder. Eur J Clin Oncol 23: 505–508.

Newling DWW (1985). Superficial bladder cancer - the need for long-term follow-up of clinical trials. In Schröder FH, Richards B (eds): "Superficial Bladder Tumors, Part

B," EORTC GU-Group Monograph 2, New York: Alan R. Liss.

Pavone Macaluso M, Ingargiola GB (1980). Local chemotherapy in bladder cancer treatment. Oncology (suppl.) 37: 71-76.

Prout Jr GR, Griffen PP, Nocks BN, De Furia MD, Daly JJ (1982). Intravesical therapy of low-stage bladder carcinoma with Mitomycin-C: comparison of results in untreated and previously treated patients. J Urol 127: 1096-1098.

Schulman CC, Denis L, Oosterlinck W, De Sy C, Hantrie M, Bouffioux C, Van Cangh PJ, Van Erps P (1983). Early adjuvant Adriamycin in superficial bladder carcinoma. World J Urol 1: 83-88.

Schulman CC (1984). Intravesical chemotherapy in the management of superficial bladder tumors. In Kurth, Debruyne, Schröder, Splinter, Wagener (eds): "Progress and Controversies in Oncological Urology," EORTC GU-Group Monograph 1, New York: Alan R. Liss, pp 275-285.

Soloway MS, Perry A (1987). BCG for treatment of superficial TCC of the bladder in patients who have failed Thiotepa and/or Mitomycin-C. J Urol 137: 871-873.

Veenema RJ, Dean AL, Roberts M, Fingerhut B, Chowhury RK, Tarassoly H (1962). Bladder carcinoma treated by direct instillations of Thiotepa. J Urol 88: 60-63.

Wajsman Z, Dhafir RA, Pfeffer M, McDonald S, Block A, Dragone N, Pontes E (1984). Studies of Mitomycin-C absorption after intravesical treatment of superficial bladder tumors. J Urol 132: 30-33.

EORTC Genitourinary Group Monograph 6:
BCG in Superficial Bladder Cancer, pages 147–152
© 1989 Alan R. Liss, Inc.

THE EXPERIENCE WITH INTRAVESICAL BCG-IMMUNOTHERAPY IN THE MANAGEMENT OF SUPERFICIAL BLADDER CANCER IN THE UNITED KINGDOM

Mell R.G. Robinson

Department of Urology, Pontefract General Infirmary, Frairwood, Pontefract, England

The first paper suggesting that the Bacillus Calmette-Guérin (BCG) was of value in the treatment of superficial bladder cancer was reported by Morales (Morales et al., 1976). Following this, several studies in North America have demonstrated the efficacy of BCG intravesical therapy in the prophylactic and therapeutic control of carcinoma in situ (TIS), and Ta and T1 (UICC TNM classification, 1978) bladder neoplasms (Brosman, 1982; Herr et al., 1985; Lamm et al., 1980).

Shortly after Morales original report, Douville reported 6 patients with recurrent papillary bladder tumors who were treated therapeutically (i.e. without prior resection of the tumor) with BCG abdominal scarification and intravesical instillation (Douville et al., 1978). Four patients were completely cleared of tumor but all 4 responders had severe systemic toxic reactions. Two of these were so severe that they required hospitalisation and anti-tuberculous drugs. The toxicity of BCG cancer immunotherapy can be severe and life-threatening. Rosenberg reported persistent fever and severe liver function abnormalities after a single injection of living BCG into malignant melanomas and we observed widespread interstitial granulomas found at post-mortem in patients who received intratumoral freeze-dried Glaxo BCG immunotherapy for carcinoma of the prostate (Rosenberg et al., 1978). These lesions were found in the lungs, liver, bone marrow, spleen and heart and although they were usually asymptomatic they were observed to persist for months after immunotherapy (Robinson and Rigby, 1981).

Because of the observed toxicity, and because of the level of knowledge at that time concerning the mode of action of BCG in the destruction of superficial bladder tumors the Yorkshire Urological Cancer Research Group and the Institute of Urology, London began in 1978 a study of intravesical BCG in the treatment of non-invasive bladder cancer (Robinson et al., 1980; Robinson and Rigby, 1981). Our objectives were to document the histological changes produced in the tumor and normal bladder epithelium and the treatment toxicity.

Following a report by Martinez-Pineiro that intravesical BCG alone was as effective as combined intradermal and intravesical therapy we decided to use intravesical Glaxo BCG only. We gave 1 ampule of Glaxo freeze-dried vaccine diluted in 50 ml normal saline weekly for 4 weeks and then monthly for 11 months. Twenty-seven patients with T1 NX MX recurrent bladder tumors were studied. Twenty-one patients had only a cysto-urethroscopy and biopsy before the first 4 instillations of BCG and 6 patients had all their tumors resected before treatment. Cysto-urethroscopies were repeated at 1 month and 3 months thereafter. At each follow-up cystoscopy biopsies were taken of the tumor surface, tumor base, normal epithelium and of any epithelium which appeared abnormal.

Granulomatous lesions with multinucleated giant cells, lymphocytes and plasma cells were observed in biopsies from 10 of the 27 patients. They were found in the subepithelium, not usually near malignant epithelial cells. Tumor necrosis in association with granulomas was not observed. Of the 21 patients whose tumors were not originally resected tumor regression was observed in 4, no change in 10 and progression in seven. Severe symptomatic toxicity was observed in 2 of the 27 patients. Both had persistent pyrexia and abnormal liver function tests. One, who had a good tumor response did not respond to anti-tuberculous therapy with Isoniazid but did respond to Ethambutol and Rifampicin. The other patient did not receive anti-tuberculous drugs and his tumor rapidly progressed to T4 category raising the question of tumor enhancement by BCG therapy.

We concluded from these results that BCG-Glaxo was not effective in the control of non-invasive bladder tumors and that toxicity could be severe. Unfortunately our observations, together with the non-availability of strains of BCG other than Glaxo (Evans) strain seems to have discouraged other investigators in the United Kingdom from studying BCG in the management of bladder cancer. Recently, however, El-Demiry using 60 mg wet weight of Evans BCG (Glaxo Danish strain) containing $1\text{-}5\times10^9$ colony forming units in the treatment of carcinoma in situ has demonstrated, using a panel of monoclonal antibody probes in an indirect immunoperoxidase technique, a predominance of T-cells of helper/inducer phenotype ($T4^+$), beta-lymphocyte ($B1^+$) and macrophages (Leu $M3^+$, 3.9^+) in bladder biopsies after BCG therapy. Their results suggest that the components of an active immune response are present in carcinoma in situ and are enhanced by BCG therapy (El-Demiry et al., 1987). In addition Kaisary has compared intravesical Glaxo and Pasteur strains of BCG in the management of multiple superficial bladder carcinomas (Kaisary, 1987). He reports a resolution of 63.6% of tumors in 11 patients treated with the Glaxo strain and a 90% resolution of 10 patients treated with the Pasteur strain at 12 and 24 months respectively. His patients were initially given 6 weekly instillations of BCG and complete responders then continued BCG therapy at monthly intervals. Partial responders received a further 6 weekly instillations followed by montly instillations and non-responders were withdrawn from the study.

The encouraging results for both strains of BCG from Kaisary's study have stimulated the superficial bladder cancer working party of the Medical Research Council (MRC) to initiate a phase II comparative study of BCG-Pasteur versus BCG-Glaxo in multiple recurrent bladder cancer. The objectives of this study are to compare the response of residual superficial bladder tumors to Evans BCG or to Pasteur BCG, to observe the recurrence rate after subsequent 24 months of prophylactic instillations and to compare incidents of adverse reactions between the 2 BCG strains. The patients will be allocated at random to either BCG-Pasteur strain or Evans BCG (Glaxo strain). As in Kaisary's study at each instillation 60 mg wet weight Evans BCG (Glaxo strain) will be given in 100 ml of normal saline (1×10^9 - 5×10^9 colony forming units) or 120 mg wet weight BCG-Pasteur strain in 100 ml of normal saline (4.8×10^8 - 9.6×10^8 colony forming units) will be administered at each instillation.

It may be concluded that because of our disappointing initial results with Glaxo-BCG, study of the management of

superficial bladder cancer by intravesical BCG immunotherapy in clinical trials has not been so readily under-
taken by clinicians in the United Kingdom as by those in
North America. Stimulated, however, by the scientific
studies of El-Demiry and associates and the clinical
experience of Kaisary the Medical Research Council is now
promoting a renewed interest in this important treatment
for superficial bladder cancer.

REFERENCES

Brossman SA (1982). Experience with BCG in patients with
  superficial bladder carcinoma. J Urol 128: 27-30.
Douville Y, Pelouze G, Roy R, Charrois R, Kibrite A, Martin
  M, Dionne L, Coulonval L, Robinson J (1978). Recurrent
  bladder papillomata treated with Bacillus Calmette-
  Guérin: a preliminary report (phase I trial). Cancer
  Treat Rep 62: 511-522.
El-Demiry MIM, Smith G, Ritchie AWS, James k, Cumming JA,
  Hargreave TB, Chisholm GD (1987). Local immune responses
  after intravesical BCG treatment for carcinoma in situ.
  Brit J Urol 60: 543-548.
Herr HW, Pinsky CM, Whitmore Jr WF, Sogani PC, Oettgen HF,
  Melamed MR (1985). Experience with intravesical Bacillus
  Calmette-Guérin therapy of superficial bladder tumors.
  Urology 25: 119-123.
Kaisary AV (1987). Intravesical BCG therapy in the
  management of multiple superficial bladder carcinomas.
  Comparison between Glaxo and Pasteur strains. Br J Urol
  59: 554-558.
Lamm DL, Thor DE, Harris SC, Reyna JA, Stogdill VD, Radwin
  HM (1980). Bacillus Calmette-Guérin immunotherapy of
  superficial bladder cancer. J Urol 124: 38-43.
Martinez-Pineiro JA (1978). Introduction of immunology and
  immunotherapy of bladder tumors. In Pavone-Macaluso M,
  Smith PH (eds.): "Bladder tumors and other topics in urological oncology," New York: Plenum Publishing Co. Ltd.
Morales A (1976). Adjuvant immunotherapy in superficial
  bladder cancer. In Bailor JC, Weisberg EH (eds.): "Workshop on genito-urinary cancer immunology. NCI Monograph
  49," Washington DC: US Department of Health, Education
  and Welfare, pp 315-319.
Robinson MRG, Richards B, Adib R, Akdas A, Rigby CC, Pugh
  RCB (1980). Intravesical BCG in the management of cell
  tumors of the bladder: A toxicity study. In Pavone-

Macaluso M, Smith PH, Edsmyr F (eds.): " Bladder tumors and other topics in urological oncology," New York: Plenum Press, pp 171.

Robinson MRG, Rigby CC (1981). Intravesical BCG therapy for Ta and T1 bladder tumors: Histopathological and toxicity in bladder cancer. In Oliver RTD, Hendry WF, Bloom HJG (eds.): "Principles of combination therapy," London: Butterworths, pp 287-295.

Rosenberg SA, Seipp C, Sears HF (1978). Clinical and immunologic studies of disseminated BCG infection. Cancer 41: 1771-1780.

UICC (1978). TNM classification of malignant tumors. Third ed., Geneva: IUCC.

EORTC Genitourinary Group Monograph 6:
BCG in Superficial Bladder Cancer, pages 153–160

INTRAVESCIAL BCG THERAPY IN PATIENTS WITH SUPERFICIAL BLADDER TUMORS

Adolphe Steg, Michael Belas, Christian Leleu, Laurent Boccon-Gibod
Dept. of Urology (A.S., M.B, C.L.), Hôpital Cochin,
Dept. of Urology (L.B.G.), Hôpital Bichat, Paris, France

We report here our experience with superficial bladder tumors treated with intravesical instillations of Bacilllus Calmette-Guérin (BCG). Since 1983, we have treated 200 patients (165 males and 35 females). Their mean age has been 66.3 year (range, 32–87); 68 (34%) have been over 70, and 11 (5.5%) over 80.

Follow-up has been longer than 1 year in 158 patients (79%) and longer than 2 years in 50 patients (25%).

Treatment began 3 weeks after transurethral resection (TUR). We instilled 150 mg of BCG-Pasteur (Institute Pasteur, Paris) once a week for 6 weeks and once every 2 weeks for the next 3 months. In 61 patients, therapy was maintained thereafter by monthly instillations for the next 18 months.

Our analysis of results will concern mainly the 158 patients who were monitored for more than a year.

CATEGORIZATION OF PATIENTS

Patients were divided according to pathologic findings into four 4 groups: stage Ta, stage T1, primary carcinoma in situ (CIS), and stage Ta or T1 associated with CIS (Table 1).

TABLE 1. Patients categorization by tumor and follow-up

	No. of patients	No. followed for over 1 year
Stage Ta	82	61
Stage T1	52	43
Primary CIS	34	30
Stage O or A associated with CIS	32	24
Total	200	158

Stage Ta tumors

Among 82 patients with stage Ta tumors (papillary tumor strictly confined to the epithelium), 61 had a follow-up of over a year (74.4%) and 22 a follow-up of over two years (26.8%); mean follow-up was 22.2 months. All but two patients had at least one recurrence before BCG therapy began.

TABLE 2. Tumor response, recurrence and progression in 61 patients with stage Ta tumors who have been followed for over a year

Result	No.	%
Complete response	45	73.8
Recurrence	11	18.0
Progression	5	8.2

There was no recurrence in 45 patients, and the recurrence rate (number of recurrences per 100 patient months) dramatically decreased after BCG therapy (Table 3). However, these figures have to be interpreted cautiously, because the mean follow-up is much longer before than after BCG therapy and recurrences will probably increase with time. Nevertheless.

TABLE 3. Tumor recurrence in patients with stage Ta tumors before and after BCG therapy

Treatment status	Tumor recurrence rate	Mean follow-up, months
Before BCG	9.54	53.3
After BCG	1.04	22.2

The 11 patients who had recurrences after BCG therapy were free of tumor longer after BCG than before BCG (increase of the tumor-free interval).

In five patients, tumor progressed to muscle invasive disease.

In 1986, we analyzed the results of our first 39 patients, and we concluded that BCG probably seems to prevent muscle invasion, because none of the patients developed muscle invasive disease. That impression was not confirmed when more patients had been treated (Table 4).

In seven patients with diffuse bladder papillary tumors, TUR was incomplete and BCG was used for treatment of residual tumors. Results are presented in Table 5. If a first course of BCG has failed, a second course of BCG might be useful.

Stage T1 tumors

In the 53 patients whose papillary tumors had invaded the lamina propria, 43 were followed for more than a year (82.7%) and 10 had a follow-up for more than 2 years (19.2%). The mean follow-up has been 17.6 months. The results in the 43 patients are summarized in Table 6.

TABLE 4. Stage Ta: Comparison of results in 1986 and 1988

Result	1986: 39 patients No.	(%)	1988: 61 patients No.	(%)
Complete Response	32	82	45	73.8
Recurrence	7	18	11	18
Progression	0	0	5	8.2

TABLE 5. Results of further BCG treatment in residual stage 0 with residual tumors (N=7)

Result	After 6 instillations	After 12 instillations
No tumor	4 (57.1%)	6 (85.7%)
Decrease of tumor	3	0
Recurrence	0	1

TABLE 6. Tumor recurrence and progression in 43 patients with stage T1 tumors who have been followed for over a year (N=43)

Result	No.	%
Complete response	27	62.8
Recurrence	8	18.6
Progression	8	18.6

The percentage of complete response in stage T1 tumors was lower than in patients with stage Ta tumors (62.8% versus 73.8%) and the rate of progression considerable higher (18.6% versus 8.2%).

However, one must consider that the group with stage T1 tumors is not homogeneous. Of the 43 patients, there were 37 in whom muscle was seen in the specimen and was free of invasion (stage T1 tumors), and six in whom the lamina propria was invaded, but the muscle was not seen in TUR material. In these patients muscle might well have been invaded, in other words, these could be T2 tumors. When one considers those two groups, separately, the unfavorable results have occurred at a higher rate in the patients who possible had a T2 tumor (Table 7). For that reason, we consider that, when the lamina propria is invaded, BCG therapy is indicated only if muscle is seen in the specimen which is not invaded.

TABLE 7. Recurrence and progression of T1 tumors with or without complete staging requirements.

Result	Stage T1 with muscle in specimen (N=37)		Stage T1 without muscle in specimen (N=6)	
	No.	%	No.	%
Complete response	25	67.6	2	33.3
Recurrence	8	21.6	0	0
Progression	4	10.8	4	66.7

Primary carcinoma in situ (CIS)

We have treated 34 patients with primary CIS, i.e., intra-epithelial, flat, high-grade carcinoma in patients with no concomitant tumor or history of any other type of bladder tumor. Follow-up has been over a year in 30 patients (88.2%) and over 2 years in 14 (41.2%). The mean follow-up has been 15.4 months. The results are presented in Table 8.

TABLE 8. Tumor recurrence and progression in 30 patients with primary carcinoma in situ who have been followed for over a year.

Result	No.	%
Complete response	23	76.7
Recurrence	2	6.7
Progression	5	16.7

Tumors did not recur in 23 patients; 19 were controlled with cystoscopy and TUR, and four with no complaints and regular negative cytologic findings did not accept endoscopic control. Two patients had a recurrence -- one in the bladder and one in the urethra. In five patients, tumors progressed to muscle invasion, in all but one in the urethra.

Superfical tumors associated with CIS

Among our 200 patients, we have isolated the cases in which superficial bladder tumors (15 stage Ta and 17 stage T1) were associated with concomitant carcinoma in situ. Such an association has been demonstrated to have an unfavorable prognosis.

Ten of the 15 patients with stage Ta tumors and 14 of the 17 with stage T1 tumors have been followed for over a year. The results are shown in Table 9. When treated with BCG, superficial tumors associated with CIS do not behave differently from isolated tumors: BCG seems to suppress the unfavorable outcome.

TABLE 9. Tumor recurrence and progression in 24 patients with superficial tumors associated with CIS who have been followed for over a year

| | Stage Ta + CIS (N=10 mean follow-up 16.4 months | | Stage T1 + CIS (N=14) mean follow-up 16.7 months | |
	No.	%	No.	%
Complete response	8	80	12	85.7
Recurrence	1	10	1	7.1
Progression	1	10	1	7.1

SIDE EFFECTS

The analysis of side effects is based on 2,420 instillations in 158 patients. The most common side effect has been cystitis. Only 10% of the patients did not experience any local reaction. All others had symptoms of bladder irritation (dysuria, frequency, or hematuria) after BCG instillations. Symptoms lasted more than 6 hours in 38% of the patients. In less than 10%, symptoms lasted 2-3 days. Generally, the patients found relief with symptomatic medication. However, in seven patients (4%), bladder irritation was such that BCG treatment had to be discontinued.

A febrile reaction has also been very common and has resolved with anti-pyretics and fluids. In 4% of the patients, temperature rose to over 38°C and subsided with Isoniazid (150 mg/day) given for 3 days.

COMPLICATIONS

One patient had cervical lymph node enlargement, which disappeared with anti-tuberculous drugs.

Profuse hematuria was observed in two patients. In one, it was treated with total cystectomy after failure of all other treatments. This patient had been treated earlier with radiation therapy.

Three patients had epididymitis, of whom two patients had 2 typical granulomatous lesions and three patients had arthritis, which was successfully treated with Isoniazid.

Four patients had a retracted bladder. In three the bladder recovered normal capacity after treatment; in one, total cystectomy was performed.

We observed BCG-itis in five patients. This means severe disseminated BCG infection characterized by high fever, broncho-pulmonary lesions, granulomatous hepatitis, and in one patient intramedullary granulomatosis. In three patients a traumatic urethral catheterization with bleeding might have favored BCG dissemination. All five patients reacted favorably to specific treatment with Isoniazid, Rifampicin and Prednisone during 3 months. The severe systemic side effects, due to intravesical BCG administration are subject of a separate paper reported elsewhere in this volume.

EORTC Genitourinary Group Monograph 6:
BCG in Superficial Bladder Cancer, pages 161–169
© 1989 Alan R. Liss, Inc.

BLADDER TUMORS INVADING THE LAMINA PROPRIA (STAGE T1):
INFLUENCE OF ENDOVESICAL BCG THERAPY ON RECURRENCE AND
PROGRESSION

Laurent Boccon-Gibod, Christian Leleu, J.M. Herve,
Michael Belas, Adolphe Steg
Dept. of Urology (L.B.G.), Hôpital Bichat, Dept. of
Urology (C.L., J.M.H., M.B, A.S.), Hôpital Cochin,
Paris, France

SUMMARY

We treated 47 patients with transitional cell bladder
carcinoma invading the lamina propria (stage T1) from 1984
to 1986 with complete transurethral resection followed by
one to three courses of endovesical BCG instillation and
followed them for 14-64 months with cystoscopic and endoscopic tests and bladder biopsy. Complete response was
achieved in 64%, and 36% had recurrences (recurrence rate
per 100 month/patient, 2.2); 21% progressed to muscle
invasion. Duration of treatment, tumor size or type (solid
versus papillary), and presence of carcinoma in situ bore
no relation to the final result. A history of previous T1
bladder tumor appeared associated with a higher risk of
progression, although not statistically significantly. The
results were compared with those obtained by transurethral
resection alone in a similar group of 50 patients treated
from 1982 to 1984 and followed for 12 to 100 months. Of
these 90%, had recurrence, and 34% progressed to muscle
invasion, with a recurrence rate per 100 month/patient of,
9.2. In light of the limits of a non-randomized historical
comparison, it appears that endovesical BCG therapy favorably alters the recurrence pattern of T1 bladder cancer.

INTRODUCTION

Transitional cell carcinoma (TCC) of the bladder
invading the lamina propria (stage T1), although incorpo-
rated in superficial bladder tumors, has more unfavorable

prognosis than more superficial lesions: after transurethral resection (TUR), 40-70% of T1 tumors recur, and
30-40% progress to muscle invasion, with its life-threatening implications (Dalesio et al., 1983; England et al.,
1981; Green et al 1984; Heney et al., 1982; Jakse et al.,
1987; Kurth et al., 1984; Lutzeyer et al., 1982; Steg et
al., 1979). Endovesical Bacillus Calmette-Guérin (BCG)
therapy has been shown to reduce markedly the recurrence
and progression rates of superficial TCC (Brosman, 1985;
Badalament et al., 1987; Haaff et al., 1985; Haaff et al.,
1986; Herr et al., 1986; deKernion et al., 1985; Lamm,
1985; Reynolds et al., 1985; Schellhammer et al., 1986;
Steg et al., 1986). However, its impact on stage T1 TCC of
the bladder has seldom been specifically addressed. We
report here our experience with prophylactic endovesical
BCG after complete TUR of stage T1 TCC in 47 patients
followed for 14-60 months, and we compare their outcome
with that of 50 similar patients treated with TUR alone in
the 2 years preceding BCG therapy.

PATIENS AND METHODS

Our study compared two groups of patients with T1
bladder TCC treated during the years 1982-1986 (see Tables
1 and 2).

Group A consisted of 50 patients (45 men and 5 women),
42-84 years old (mean, 67), who were treated with TUR alone
in 1982-1984. Of the 50, 25 had primary T1 bladder TCC (23
grade 3, 2 grade 2), and 25 had recurrent tumor (16 T1, 9
Ta, all grade 3) after initial T1 bladder TCC. The patients
were treated with complete TUR and followed for 12-100
months (mean, 34) with cytologic and endoscopic tests,
biopsy, or TUR at regular intervals.

Group B consisted of 47 patients (39 men and 8 women),
32-86 years old (mean, 65), who were treated in 1984-1986
with TUR followed by endovesical BCG (Institute Pasteur,
Paris France). Of the 47, 15 had primary T1 bladder TCC (14
grade 3, 1 grade 2), and 32 had recurrent tumor (18 T1, 12
Ta; all grade 3) after initial T1 bladder TCC treated with
TUR only (26) or TUR followed by topical chemotherapy,
using Epodyl (6). Endovesical BCG therapy was given as
follows: 150 mg of fresh BCG-Pasteur, two ampules, each
containing 75 mg of BCG containing 10^6 colony-forming

units, were instilled via an urethal catheter in the
bladder diluted with 50 mg of saline and kept in the
bladder for 90 minutes.

Treatment was given in three phases: induction, one
instillation per week for 6 weeks (8 patients); re-induction, one instillation bi-weekly for 12 weeks (39
patients). After induction or re-induction a number of
patients received maintenance therapy , one instillation
per month for 1 year (22 patients). No particular reason,
other than the personal choice of the attending urologist,
dictated these variations.

Patients were followed for 14-64 months (mean, 27) and
4 weeks after each treatment period they underwent cysto-
endoscopy under anesthesia, with collection of bladder
washings for urinary cytology, random mucosal biopsies and
resection of any visible tumor or suspicious area. Complete
response was assumed if endoscopic and cytologic tests and
random biopsies, all yielded negative findings; recurrence,
if a new tumor appeared; and progression if muscular
invasion or metastatic disease was evident.

TABLE 1. Characteristics of patient groups

Characteristics	Group A (TUR alone)	Group B (TUR + BCG)
Number of patients	50	47
Age, years	42-84 (mean, 67)	32-86 (mean, 65)
Sex ratio, male/female	45/5	39/8
Period	1982-1984	1984-1986
Follow-up, months	12-100 (mean, 35)	14-64 (mean, 27)

TABLE 2. Tumor characteristics of patient groups

	Group A TUR	Group B TUR + BCG	CHI^2*
Tumor size:			
> 3 cm	30	28	0.01
< 3 cm	20	19	
Number of tumors:			
< 2	27	20	1.49
> 2	23	27	
Type of tumors:			
Papillary	42	39	0.01
Solid	8	8	
History:			
Primary	25	15	2.73
Recurrence	25	32	

* all non-significantly differences

Statistical analysis generated actuarial recurrence-free and progression-free survival curves. Qualitative variables were compared with the CHI-squared test, and survival rates were compared with the log-rank method and the Mantel test.

RESULTS

Group A

Of the 50 patients, five (10%) remained tumor-free during follow-up, and 45 (90%) had recurrence, the recurrence rate per 100 month/patient was 9.22. Five patients had recurrence at a lower stage (Ta), and 17 (34%) at the same stage (Ta); 23 (51%) progressed either locally to muscle invasion (17) with (4) or without (13) distant metastases or distant metastases only (6).

Group B

Most of the patients complained of minor side effects
lasting 2 days after each instillation (pain and urgency in
76%; fever in 38%; and haematuria in 21% of the patients
respectively) Usually these side effects responded to
symptomatic treatment.

Of the 47 patients, 30 (64%) achieved complete
response, and remained tumor-free during follow-up. The
recurrence rate per 100 month/patient was 2.2. Seventeen
patients (36%) had recurrences. Progression to muscle invasive disease was encoutered in 10 (21%) of the patients.

Statistical analysis showed that tumor characteristics
(size, number, type, and solid versus papillary), presence
or absence of CIS elsewhere in the bladder, and duration of
therapy were unrelated to clinical outcome (data not
shown).

DISCUSSION

Until recently, TCC invading the lamina propria of the
bladder has been included in the group of superficial tumors. It has a more unfavorable prognosis than TCC limited
to the mucosa: recurrence rates after TUR range from 40 to
70%, and progression to life-threatening muscle invasion
occurs in 30-40% of cases. The frequency of carcinoma in
situ associated with normal looking bladder mucosa partially explains these prognostic features (Heney et al., 1982).

Endovesical prophylaxis with BCG has shown a remarkable efficacy in the treatment of superficial bladder
carcinoma with or without carcinoma in situ, as well as in
pure CIS (Haaff et al., 1985; Kavoussi et al., 1988).
However, most published reports have pooled data on T1 and
Ta tumors and CIS, and the real impact of BCG on T1 lesions
has seldom been specifically addressed. Lamm (1985) and
Reynolds (1985) reported 44 patients with T1 tumors randomized to TUR alone versus TUR plus BCG; the recurrence and
progression rates decreased from 65 and 8% to 16 and 3%
respectively.

Our data were not generated by a randomized controlled
study, but they do confirm two salient points:

- TUR alone is unable to keep TCC from invading the lamina propria: 90% of the patients have recurrences, and half of them will progress to muscle invasive disease potentially associated with metastatic disease (Fig. 1).
- Adjuvant treatment with endovesical BCG reduces the recurrence rate after TUR from 9.2 to 2.2 per 100 month/patients. Of the patients 64% remain tumor-free with a mean follow-up of 34 months, and 20% progress to muscle invasion with or without metastatic disease (Fig. 1).

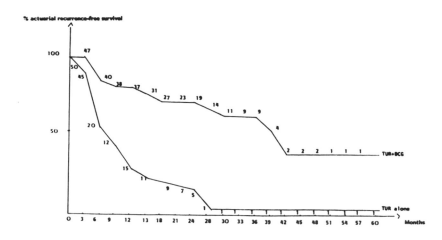

Figure 1. T1 bladder cancer TUR versus TUR + BCG. Percentage of actuarial recurrence-free survival versus follow-up in months.

Alltogether, 70% of the patients will have their T1 TCC controlled with a "bladder-saving" procedure, and the disease will remain unaffected by BCG in 30%. It should be noted that the proportion of Ta, T1, and T2-T3 recurrences was the same in both groups. Thus, although BCG reduced the recurrence potential of T1 tumors, it probably did not affect the biologic characteristics of the recurrent tumor itself. Size, number, type, and presence or absence of CIS were not determinants of recurrence and progression. BCG is known for its remarkable efficacy in the treatment of CIS (Brosman, 1985; Catalona et al., 1987; Herr et al., 1986; deKernion et al., 1985), and none of our patients had recurrence of pure CIS. Although it did not reach statistical significance the risk of progression seems to be higher in recurring than in primary cases. In contrast to observations by others (Haaff et al., 1986; Kavoussi et al., 1988), we found no relationship between results and duration of therapy. Also Badalament could not demonstrate a difference in results in patients treated with or without maintenance therapy (Badalament et al., 1987). However, if a tumor recurs at the same stage after a 6 week induction course of BCG, a reinduction treatment of six instillations over a period of 12 weeks is advisable. As half the recurrences are associated with progression, the presence of a T1 recurrence after two courses of BCG should lead to a re-evaluation of therapy.

Although it was not a prospective randomized study, we felt that our historical comparison offered a valuable, if preliminary, insight into the potential benefit of BCG therapy after TUR of T1 bladder TCC. The two groups of patients were treated at the same institution over a specific period (1982-1984 and 1984-1986), during which neither the senior urologists in charge, the pathologist, the referral patterns, nor the TUR technique changed markedly. Statistical analysis showed the two groups to be equivalent with respect to age, sex ratio, and tumor characteristics (Tables 1 and 2).

In conclusion, BCG therapy after complete TUR of T1 bladder TCC dramatically affects recurrence and progression rates and allows bladder preservation in 70% of the cases. It is hoped that further progress in immunochemistry and cytogenetics will help to make it possible to select the non-responders early, so that they can be offered other adequate forms of therapy.

REFERENCES

Badalament RA, Herr HW, Wong GY, Gnecco C, Pinsky CM, Withmore Jr WF, Fair WR, Oettgen JF (1987). A prospective randomized trial of maintenance versus nonmaintenance intravesical Bacillus Calmette-Guérin therapy of superficial bladder cancer. J Clin Oncol 5: 441.

Brosman SA (1982). Experience with BCG in patients with superficial bladder carcinoma. J Urol 128: 27-30.

Brosman SA (1985). The use of BCG in the therapy of bladder carcinoma in situ. J Urol 134: 36-39.

Catalona WJ, Hudson MA, Gillen DP, Andriole GL, Ratliff T (1987). Risks and benefits of repeated courses of intravesical Bacillus Calmette-Guérin therapy for superficial bladder cancer. J Urol 137: 220.

Dalesio O, Schulman CC, Sylvester R, de Pauw M, Robinson M, Denis L, Smith P, Viggiano G (1983). Prognostic factors in superficial bladder tumors. A study of the European Organization for Research on treatment of cancer: Genito-Urinary Tract Cancer Co-operative Group. J Urol 129: 730-733.

England HR, Paris AMI, Blandy JP (1981) The correlation of T1 bladder tumor history with prognosis and follow-up requirements. Brit J Urol 53: 593-597.

Green DF, Robinson MRG, Glashan R, Newling D, Dalesio O, Smith PH (1984) Does intravesical chemotherapy prevent invasive bladder cancer? J Urol 131:133.

Haaff EO, Dresner SM, Kelley DR, Ratliff TL, Shapiro A, Catalona WJ (1985). The role of immunotherapy in the prevention of recurrence and invasion of urothelial bladder tumors: A review. World J Urol 3: 76.

Haaff EO, Dresner SM, Ratliff TL, Catalona WJ (1986). Two courses of intravesical Bacillus Calmette-Guérin for transitional cel carcinoma of the bladder. J Urol 136: 820.

Heney NM, Nocks BN, Daly JJ, Prout GR, Newall JB, Griffin PP, Perrone TL, Szyfelbein WA (1982). Ta and T1 bladder cancer: location, recurrence and progression. Brit J Urol 54: 152.

Herr WH, Pinsky CM, Whitmore Jr WF, Pranod JR, Sogani C, Oettgen HF, Melamed MF (1986). Long-term effect of intravesical Bacillus Calmette-Guérin on flat carcinoma in situ of the bladder. J Urol 135: 265-267.

Jakse G, Loidi W, Seeber G, Hofstadter F (1987). Stage T1, grade 3 transitional cell carcinoma of the bladder: An unfavorable tumor? J Urol 137: 39.

Kavoussi LR, Torrence RJ, Gillen DP, Hudson MA, Haaff EO, Dresner SM, Ratliff TL, Catalona WJ (1988). Results of 6 weekly intravesical Bacillus Calmette-Guérin instillations on the treatment of superficial bladder tumors. J Urol 139: 935.

deKernion JB, Huang MY, Limand R (1985). The management of superficial bladder tumor and carcinoma in situ with intravesical. J Urol 133: 598.

Kurth KH, Schröder FH, Tunn U, Ay R, Pavone Macaluso M, Debruyne F, de Pauw M, Dalesio O (1984). Adjuvant chemotherapy of superficial transitional cell bladder carcinoma: preliminary results of a European Organization for Research on Treatment of Cancer randomized trial comparing doxorubicin hydrochloride, ethoglucid and transurethral resection alone. J Urol 132: 258.

Lamm DL (1985). Bacillus Calmette-Guérin immunotherapy for bladder cancer. J Urol 134: 40.

Lutzeyer W, Rubben H, Dahm H (1982). Prognostic parameters in superficial bladder cancer: An analysis of 315 cases. J Urol 127: 250-252.

Reynolds H, Stogdill VD, Lamm DL (1985). Disease progression in BCG treated patients with transitonal cell carcinoma of the bladder. J Urol 133: 392A.

Schellhammer PF, Ladaga LE, Fillion MB (1986). Bacillus Calmette-Guérin for superficial transitional cell carcinoma of the bladder. J Urol 135: 261.

Steg A, Allouch G, Desligneres S (1979). Les facteurs de risques des Tumeurs de Vessie au stade A: Description d'un nouveau paramètre. Ann Urol 13: 221.

Steg A, Leleu C, Boccon-Gibod L, Debre B (1986). Traitement des tumeurs superficielles et des carcinomes in situ de vessie par la BCG thérapie intra-vésicale. Ann Urol 20: 26.

EORTC Genitourinary Group Monograph 6:
BCG in Superficial Bladder Cancer, pages 171–185
© 1989 Alan R. Liss, Inc.

LONG-TERM EFFECT OF INTRAVESICAL BACILLUS CALMETTE-GUÉRIN (BCG) TICE STRAIN ON FLAT CARCINOMA IN SITU OF THE BLADDER

D.J. Reitsma, P. Guinan, D.L. Lamm, O.P. Khanna, S.A. Brosma, J.B. DeKernion, R.D. Williams, G. Sipmson, M.G. Hanna Jr.
Organon Teknika, Bionetics Research Institute (D.J.R., G.S., M.G.H.), Rockville; University of Illinois (P.G.), Chicago; WV University School of Medicine (D.L.L.), Morgantown; Div. of Urology Hahnemann University (O.P.K.), Philadelphia; Kaiser Permanente (S.A.B.), Los Angeles; Div. of Urology, UCLA Medical Center (J.B.D.), Los Angeles; Dept. of Urology, University of Iowa Hospital and Clinics (R.D.W.), Iowa City, USA

INTRODUCTION

There were 40,500 new cases of bladder cancer in the United States in 1986. In the same year, 10,600 people died from this disease, making it the eighth ranking cause of cancer death among males and the fourteenth among women (Lewis, 1987).

Carcinoma in situ (CIS) is defined as a diffuse presence of highly anaplastic malignant cells within the confines of the urothelial lining. The lamina propria reveals no specific abnormalities. At cystoscopy, the lesion may look like normal bladder mucosa or it may present as a red velvet-like area. If CIS is associated with overt bladder tumors, it signifies a field change and the need for more aggressive therapy. Although CIS has the histological characteristics of a high-grade malignancy, the time at which it will transform from a non-invasive superficial cancer to an invasive one is unpredictable. A period of non-progressive behaviour (Utz et al., 1980) may precede subsequent invasion (Utz et al., 1970). As with other types of bladder cancer, invasion of the muscular wall of the bladder signifies the potential for metastasis and the need for cystectomy (Marshall et al., 1956; Masina, 1965).

Although CIS is generally diffuse, if the lesion is small and located away from the bladder orifices, resection and/or fulguration of the involved areas may be considered adequate therapy. Between 48% and 70% of the patients thus treated develop tumor recurrences (Johnson and Boileau, 1982), so that additional treatment is neccesary to prevent new tumors or new recurrences following surgery (Richie et al., 1985).

Intravesical chemotherapy appears to be able to limit recurrence by destroying wandering tumor cells which might remain in contact with damaged epithelium after TUR. It can also exert cytotoxic effects on areas of CIS or unstable urothelium (Schulman et al., 1980). The efficacy of three chemotherapeutic agents has been defined in many clinical trials: Thiotepa has an overall complete response rate of 29%; Doxorubicin generates an overall complete response rate of 38%; Mitomycin-C averages complete response rates of 48%.

BCG has long been known to be a potent stimulator of the immune system (Biozzi et al., 1954). Although BCG immunotherapy proved highly effective in animal tumor models, its effect has not been substantiated in the treatment of most human cancers despite initial successes (Bast et al., 1974). The exception is in the treatment of bladder cancer.

Recent studies using intravesical BCG for the treatment of bladder cancer report complete response rates of 20% to 100%, the overall rate being 61%. For the treatment of CIS, the complete response rate being 69% (Tables 1 and 2). These rates compare favorably to those obtained with chemotherapy and have surprised many oncologists because of widespread skepticism accorded the notion of BCG immunotherapy.

The most common adverse effects of BCG are irritative bladder symptoms in nearly all patients, hematuria in about half the patients, and a flu-like syndrome in just over a quarter. A serious but uncommon (less than 1%) side effect has been systemic BCG infection (Lamm et al., 1986).

A major misconception is that BCG used in immunotherapy is generic and that substrains will perform similarly. There are several differences in the properties of BCG vaccines. These properties are biological as well as physical,

TABLE 1. All stages of bladder malignancy-response rate as percentage of complete remissions induced by BCG: Recent major clinical investigations

Reference (first author)	Total # Patients	Complete Remission	% Compl. Rem.
DeKernion, (1985)	63	39	62
Brosman, (1985 1984)	113	85	75
Schellhammer, (1986)	28	20	71
Morales, (1979)	20	12	60
Staino-Coico, (1985)	22	12	54
Douville, (1978)	6	4	67
Haaff, (1986) Kelley, (1986)	61	48	79
Soloway, (1987)	30	15	50
Merguerian, (1987)	13	11	85
Catalona, (1987)	100	65	65
Herr, (1985)	1	1	100
Martinez-Pineiro, (1984)	12	5	42
Robinson, (1980)	10	2	20
Huffman, (1985)	15	4	27
Brosman, (1982)	39	20	51
Herr, (1986)	71	49	69
Lamm, (1985)	30	14	47
Katsushi, (1985)	43	35	81
Hudson, (1987)	41	29	71
Badalament, (1987)	93	38	41
Mydlo, (1986)	29	11	38
Total	922	563	61%

TABLE 2. BCG therapy for carcinoma in situ

Reference (first author)	Number	Complete Response	Complete Response Percentage
Kelly, (1985)	12	8	66
Schellhammer, (1986)	28	20	71
Staiano-Coico, (1985)	22	12	55
Haaff, (1986)	19	13	68
Morales, (1984)	17	10	59
Herr, (1986)	71	49	69
Katsushi, (1986),			
Lamm, (1985)	43	35	81
Hudson, (1987)	1	5	45
Mydlo, (1986)	25	10	40
DeKernion, (1985)	19	15	79
Brosman, (1985)	33	31	94
Total	300	208	69

and may result in differences in levels of efficacy. The number of colony forming units (CFU) per intravesical treatment is a salient feature of any BCG vaccine, best seen by comparing BCG-Glaxo with BCG-Tice or BCG-Connaught. As described by Robinson, BCG-GLaxo (which has approximately 15×10^6 CFU per ampule) has a 20% complete response rate in bladder cancer (Robinson et al., 1980) while BCG-Tice or BCG-Connaught, with published complete response rates greater than 70% in bladder cancer, have approximately 6×10^8 CFU per ampule. When one compares weight per ampule to colony forming units per ampule for various sources of BCG, other differences become obvious. These correlate to specific activity based on content of subcellular particles and process ingredients. Table 3 defines these variables. In comparing Glaxo and Armand Frappier sources with Tice, Pasteur, or Connaught sources, there is a discordance between the ratio of number of CFU to weight per ampule. Originally, all BCG sources were prepared for immunization against tuberculosis. Viable as well as subcellular material would contribute effectively towards immunization. On the other hand, in intravesical therapy, it appears that intact organisms may be the key essential component for the antitumor effect. It is not clear whether subcellular components contribute to adverse reactions during intra-vesical therapy. The only recommendation at this time can be to use preparations which have a high number of CFU for moderate-to-low weight per ampule. In this respect, Tice or Connaught sources as presently manufactured would be most suitable.

TABLE 3. BCG, strain, weight, and strength

	Strain	Weight/Ampule	Colony Forming Units (CFU)
1.	Tice	50 mg	$2-8 \times 10^8$ CFU
2.	Pasteur	75 mg	6×10^8 CFU
3.	Connaught	40 mg	$8-32 \times 10^8$ CFU
4.	Armand Frappier	120 mg	10^7 CFU
5.	Glaxo	75 mg	$8-26 \times 10^6$ CFU
6.	Moreau	100 mg	2×10^9 CFU

Although a prospective randomized study of BCG in the treatment of CIS is desirable, it is infeasible because BCG is now considered by most urologists to be the treatment of choice for CIS of the bladder (DATTA, 1988). We, therefore, undertook a retropective study of the use of BCG-Tice in the treatment of bladder cancer.

MATERIALS AND METHODS

Patients had been treated under six INDs which are summarized in Table 4. These INDs had many features in common. The most important shared aspect was the use of an induction plus maintenance treatment schedule. One ampule of BCG-Tice was used per intravesical instillation; the dose was sometimes reduced due to side effects. Investiga-tors who had used BCG-Tice were identified from IND files at the FDA, from files at the National Cancer Institute, and from published literature. Only the CIS patients were evaluated for efficacy. Patient data had generally not been recorded on case report forms and were sometimes incomplete. At our request, investigators copied the relevant parts of their patient's medical files and sent them to us for data abstraction. Data retrieval was continued until mid-1987.

TABLE 4. BCG-Tice series: summary of study features

No.	Investigator (Study #)	Indications	TREATMENT SCHEDULE FOR CARCINOMA IN SITU			
			Induction	Maintenance	Dose (mg)	Route
1)	Guinan (1883)	• CIS • Prophylaxis	qwk X 6	qmo X 12	50	Intravesical
2)	Lamm (1414)	• CIS • Prophylaxis • Invasive Dx	qwk X 6	at 8,10,12 wk 6 mo; q6mo X 4yr	.5 and 50 mg	Percutaneous Intravesical
3)	Khanna (2951)	• Low risk • High risk/CIS	qwk X 6	qmo X 12, q3mo X 8, q6mo X 4	50	Intravesical
4)	Brosman (1111	• CIS Existing tumor • Prophylaxis	qwk to CR	q2wk X 3mo, qmo X 2yr	50	Intravesical
5)	Dekernion (1571)	• CIS Existing tumor • Prophylaxis	qwk X 8	qmo X 12	50	Intravesical
6)	Williams (2427)	• CIS • Prophylaxis	qwk X 6	qmo X 12	50	Intravesical

Since patients were treated from 1979 through 1987 by more than 100 urologists, it was virtually impossible to obtain original pathology slides for review. Therefore, the diagnosis of CIS was based on original pathology reports. Cytology date were not obtained on some patients, making it impossible to document an otherwise complete remission (CR: no recurrence of tumor and a negative cytology) using standard response criteria. If such patients would otherwise have been classifiable as CR by cystoscopy or biopsy, they were distinguished in the retrospective analysis by the term CRNC (complete remission no cytology) and analyzed separately.

In the course of analysis, we encountered a group of patients considered by their urologists to have recurrent

CIS but for whom baseline biopsy was not positive for CIS. These patients had a history of CIS documented by previous biopsies. The results of this group (designated presumed CIS) are described separately.

Information regarding adverse reactions was gathered by the abstractors reviewing the medical records. In some instances, adverse reactions and side effects had been recorded on IND-specific patient record forms.

RESULTS

Patient data

Records were obtained on 153 CIS patients. Demographic data across the various INDs are uniform and are consistent with the known age distribution in cases of bladder cancer (Table 5).

Pathology records

Eighty percent of patient records were found to have copies of pathology department biopsy reports documenting baseline diagnosis. Another 9% of patients had baseline diagnosis described in other documents such as in hospital and physician notes and in letters to referring physicians. In some cases, signed IND case report forms or signed query forms were used as evidence. Nine percent of patients were considered CIS positive by cystoscopic examination only as described in similar documents. Prebaseline diagnosis was similarly documented for the presumed CIS group.

Response rates

The response rates for CIS patients are shown in Table 6. Table 7 documents the response rates for the presumed CIS patients. The response rates for both groups are similar: 73.9% of the CIS patients attained an initial CR or CRNC while 65.5% of the presumed CIS attained CR or CRNC. At a mean follow-up time of 17.9 ± 13.3 months, the number of CIS patients still in remission had dropped to 65.5% while the total remission rate for the presumed CIS patients had declined to 62.1%.

TABLE 5. Demografic data

Variable	Guinan (#1883) n = 71	DeKernion (#1571) n = 30	Lamm (#1414) n = 23	Khanna (#2951) n = 15	Williams (#2427) n = 9	Brossman (#1111) n = 5	All Centers n = 153
Center							
Sex:							
Male	63	25	18	14	8	4	132
Female	8	5	3	1	1	1	19
Not Stated	–	–	2	–	–	–	2
Total	71	30	23	15	9	5	153
Age (Mean ± SD) (yrs):							
CIS Patients	67.3 + 10.6	68.7 + 9.4	69.3 + 8.3	72.9 + 9.2	70.0 + 7.3	73.0 + 5.5	68.8 + 9.7
(Range)	(38–97)	(46–81)	(54–85)	(54–86)	(55–79)	(69–81)	(38–97)
Presumed CIS Patients	68.7 + 11.1	65.9 + 7.9	56.3 + 13.5	62.5 + 2.1	68.7 + 13.1	64	64.1 + 10.8
(Range)	(50–83)	(53–80)	(39–75)	(61–64)	(48–84)	–	(39–83)

Response rate in primary chemotherapy failure

CIS patients. A total of 36 patients had previously failed intravesical chemotherapy with one or more agents, primarily Thiothepa and/or Mitomycin-C. Subsequent patient BCG response data were adequate for evaluation in 35 patients. Initially, 21 of the 32 (65.6%) achieved CR or CRNC status. The current response categorization was available for 35 patients with 22 (62.9%) still in remission (CR or CRNC) at their last evaluation. Mean follow-up period for these 22 patients was 17.1 ± 10.2 months at study termination.

Presumed CIS patients. A total of six presumed CIS patients had previously failed intravesical chemotherapy. Of these, three achieved an initial remission (CR or CRNC) on BCG and four of the six were categorized as CR or CRNC status at their last evaluation. Mean follow-up period for these four individuals was 33.2 ± 24.4 months at study termination.

EXTENDED FOLLOW-UP OF CR/CRNC CATEGORY

In view of the good response rate in both the CIS and presumed CIS groups at close of study, we felt it was important to try to extend the follow-up period for those patients in the CR/CRNC category until mid-1988. Information on these patients was obtained from their physicians by mail or by telephone and confirmed on signed query forms.

CIS group

Of the 78 CR/CRNC patients (Table 6), seven were lost to follow-up by mid-1988 and eigth had died of causes unrelated to BCG or CIS. Of the remaining 63 patients, two patients had failed during the past year, and 61 (56.3%) were still in CR/CRNC. Mean follow-up for the CIS group in CR/CRNC was extended from 17.9 ± 13.3 months to 27.3 ± 13.6 months.

Presumed CIS group

Of the 18 patients in CR/CRNC in mid-1987, one was subsequently lost to follow-up and there were four deaths unrelated to BCG or CIS. Fifty percent were still in CR/CRNC due to four treatment failures during the past year. For the presumed CIS group, follow-up increased from a mean of 19.8 ± 15.5 months to 30.9 ± 14.0 months.

TABLE 6. Response rates CIS patients

	Initial Response	Response at Close of Study Mid-1987
CR documented cytologically	47 (39.5%)	43 (36.1%)
CR without confirmatory cytology	41 (34.4%)	35 (29.4%)
Total CR/CRNC remissions	88 (73.9%)	78 (65.5%)

Total CIS population: 123

Response not classifiable due to inadequate data: 4

TABLE 7. Response rates presumed CIS patients

	Initial Response	Response at Close of Study Mid-1987
CR documented cytologically	14 (48.3%)	15 (51.7%)
CR without confirmatory cytology	5 (17.2%)	3 (10.3%)
Total CR/CRNC remission	19 (65.5%)	18 (62.1%)

Total population presumed CIS: 30

Response not classifiable due to inadequate data: 1

DURATION OF BCG-TICE TREATMENT

Mean duration of treatment for the CIS group was 11.1 months ranging from a mean of 6.1 to 20.8 months across all IND centers. Mean duration of induction treatment required to produce an initial remission was 5.6 (3.8 to 10.4) months. For the presumed CIS group, the mean duration of BCG treatment was 12.0 months ranging from a mean of 10.3 to 12.9 months. Mean duration of induction treament required to produce an initial remission was 6.8 months (4.0 to 8.3 months).

The adverse reactions found were tabulated on Table 8 and the results of a large survey (Lamm et al., 1986) are listed for comparison.

TABLE 8. Adverse reactions to BCG

	All Substrains (Lamm, 1981) Percentages	Tice BCG (this survey) Percentages
Irritated bladder dysuria/cystitis	91	65
Frequency	90	48
Hematuria	43	27
Fever/flu/malaise ($< 102^O$F)	28	13
Fever ($> 103^O$F)	3.9	8
Nausea/vomiting	8	3
Systemic BCG infection	0.9	<1
Major hematuria	0.5	2

DISCUSSION

Always an issue when interpreting a retrospective study is whether the treatment group represents the disease population as a whole. Site audits revealed no missing date, and the demographic figures on the six INDs showed uniformity and are consistent with the known age distribution in cases of bladder cancer. Furthermore, the results reported here for BCG-Tice in CIS lie within the literature for BCG in the treatment of CIS. Therefore, we feel confident that these results are valid and can be used to assess various aspects of the use of BCG-Tice to treat bladder cancer.

The response rates for the most frequently used chemotherapeutics in local bladder cancer therapy (Thiotepa, Doxorubicin, and Mitomycin-C) vary from 29% to 48%. The initial CR/CRNC response rate for intravesical treatment with BCG-Tice was 74.9% with 56.3% of patients in the CIS group still in CR/CRNC at a mean follow-up of 27.3 months. The initial response rate in the presumed CIS may have decreased slightly over time. The presumed CIS may have included more advanced or more aggressive cases of CIS as suggested by the fact that the treating urologists did not deem it necessary to document recurrence histologically.

It is significant that a new treatment in oncology has achieved a therapeutic impact comparable and even superior to standard therapy in a major cancer. It is remarkable that its magnitude of effect is only slightly diminished as second line therapy. The response rate for primary treatment of CIS in this survey was 74.9% whereas the response rate in the group of 32 patients evaluable for BCG treatment after failing prior chemotherapy was 65.6%. The mechanism of action of BCG in human bladder cancer is still somewhat speculative, but it is probably immune mediated. This mechanism is clearly different enough from that of chemotherapy to allow for the achievement of efficacy approaching that of previously untreated patients.

As would be expected, the incidence of adverse effects varies considerably from study to study. The survey performed by Lamm indicates the high frequency of side effects, most are related to inflammation of the bladder and presumably also to the development of an immune response in the bladder wall. The percentage of side effects found in our study is much lower than that reported by the Lamm survey. One explanation is that side effects were underreported in patient medical records in our study. However, this is only plausible for the mildest side effects. Physicians were aware that they were using an experimental treatment protocol and were therefore more likely to note any side effects and adverse reaction. Furthermore, if significant irritative or other bladder symptoms occurred, symptomatic drug therapy was usually prescribed and duly recorded. It is probable that BCG-Tice actually causes fewer side effects and adverse reactions than most other BCG substrains.

Mild-to-moderate side effects are common and are usually treated by symptomatic medication. Side effects seem less common when using BCG-Tice for intravesical treatment of bladder cancer than for the overall incidence from other substrains of BCG. When using BCG, the potentially most serious side effect seen during intravesical therapy is systemic BCG infection. This has been reported in less than 1% of cases and is usually associated with catheter traumatization. However, it is amenable to standard antituberculous regimens if infection is recognized early and treatment is initiated in a timely fashion.

The treatment schedule used was generally that of an induction period of 6 weekly intravesical instillations of BCG-Tice followed by a maintenance period of 12 monthly instillations. If a remission was not induced initially, a second induction period generally followed. The BCG treatment durations found in this survey for both study populations, CIS and presumed CIS, vary from the prescribed regimens. This difference is more apparant than real as some INDs did not call for an exact 6-week/12-month schedule, but instead prescribed a more gradual transition from the induction to the maintenance period. The overall numbers are also compromised somewhat by those patients requiring a re-induction period and by the fact that a number of patients were still completing the protocols at the close of study. Based on our results, however, we can state that a highly acceptable remission rate and duration is obtained if the 6-week induction and 12-month maintenance schedule is used.

CONCLUSION

This is the first time since the introduction of Cisplatin that a new anti-cancer treatment has achieved a success rate that surpasses that of accepted standard therapy in one of the common cancers. BCG-Tice is a biological response modifier (BRM) and has a totaly different mechanism of action. Its use (intravesical instillations) is similar to that of standard intravesical chemotherapy. Side effects are mainly due to inflammation of the bladder. The only potentially serious side effect (BCG infection) is uncommon and treatable. BCG-Tice should be considered for first line local therapy in CIS of the bladder.

ACKNOWLEDGEMENT

Data abstraction and analysis for this survey were performed by the Oxford Research International Corp., Clifton, MJ. C. Richardson (Bionetics Research Institute) supervised the logistics of this project and co-operated in the statistical analysis.

REFERENCES

Bast RC, Zbar B, Borsos T, Rapp HJ (1974). BCG and cancer (2 parts) N Engl J Med 290: 1413-1420 and 1458-1469.
Biozzi G, Benacerraf B, Grumback F (1954). Etude de activite: granulopexique du systeme reticulo-endothelial au cours de l'infection tuberculeuse expermentale de la souris. Ann Instit Pasteur 87: 291.
Diagnostic and Therapeutic Technology Assessment (DATTA) (1988). J Am Medical Assoc. 259: 14, 2153-2155.
Johnson De, Boilieau MA (1982). Bladder cancer: overview. In Johnson De, Boileau MA (eds): "Genito-urinary tumors fundamental principles and surgical techniques," New York: Grune and Stratton, pp 399-447.
Lamm DL, Stogdill VD, Stogdill BJ, Crispen RG (1986). Complications of Bacillus Calmette-Guérin immunotherapy in 1278 patients with bladder cancer. J Urol 135: 272.
Lewis A (1987). Unpublished communication. Research report: bladder cancer. National Cancer Isntitute, Washington, DC, pp 1-29.
Marshall VF, Holden J, Ma KT (1956). Survival of patients with bladder carcinoma treated by simple segmental resection. Cancer 9: 568.

Masina F (1965). Segmental resection for tumors of the urinary bladder: ten-year follow-up. Br J Surg 52: 279.

Richie JP, Shipley WU, Yagoda A (1985). Cancer of the bladder. In DeVita JR VT, Hellman S, Rosenberg SA (eds): "Cancer principles and practice of oncology," Philadelphia: JB Lippincott Co, pp 915–928.

Robinson MRG, Richards B, Adib R, Akdas A, Rigby CC, Pugh RCB (1980). Intravesical BCG in the management of cell tumors of the bladder: A toxicity study. In Pavone-Macaluso M, Smith PH, Edsmyr F (eds): " Bladder tumors and other topics in urological oncology," New York: Plenum Press, pp 171.

Schulman CC, Denis LJ, Wauters E (1980). Intravesical Cis-platinum in bladder tumors: toxicity study. In Pavone-Macaluso M, Smith PH, Edsmyr F (eds): " Bladder tumors and other topics in urological oncology," New York: Plenum Press, pp 355.

Utz DC, Hanash KA, Farrow G (1970). The plight of the patient with carcinoma in situ of the urinary bladder. J Urol 101: 160–169.

Utz DC, Farrow GM, Rife CC, Segura JW, Zincke H (1980). Carcinoma in situ of the bladder. Cancer 45: 1842.

EORTC Genitourinary Group Monograph 6:
BCG in Superficial Bladder Cancer, pages 187–192
© 1989 Alan R. Liss, Inc.

INTRAVESICAL INSTILLATION OF BCG IN CARCINOMA IN SITU OF THE URINARY BLADDER. EORTC PROTOCOL 30861

Gerhard Jakse and Members of the EORTC-GU Group.

Urologische Klinik und Poliklinik, Klinikum rechts der Isar, Technische Universität München, München, FRG

INTRODUCTION

Carcinoma in situ (CIS) of the urinary bladder can be considered as a precursor lesion of invasive cancer. This lesion will be detected most often by the clinician simultaneously with a papillary or solid tumor elsewhere in the bladder. The time taken for progression from CIS to invasive cancer varies from several months to 77 months (Jakse, 1980). Patients with symptomatic CIS who are treated inadequately by fulguration and transurethral resection of the visible lesion and radiotherapy will die within 2 years in a significant number of cases due to progressive disease (Utz, 1970).

Morales et al. reported in 1976 a decrease in the recurrence rate of 9 patients with Ta, T1 TCC treated with intravesical and percutaneous Bacillus Calmette-Guérin (BCG). Since then several studies have clearly demonstrated the efficacy of BCG in preventing tumor recurrences as well as in the treatment of CIS (Brosman, 1985; Herr, 1983; Kelley et al., 1985; deKernion et al., 1985, Lamm, 1985; Schellhamer et al., 1984). In these studies the usual dosage was 120 mg or 50 mg of BCG diluted in 50 ml of saline. Four different strains are supposed to be effective and were used: BCG-Connaught, BCG-Frappier, BCG-Pasteur and BCG-Tice. The most often used regimen is one instillation per week for six weeks. Intradermal BCG scarification does not seem to be necessary since similar results are obtained by intravesical BCG alone (Herr, 1983).

OBJECTIVES OF THE PROTOCOL

Although there is an increasing amount of studies showing the efficacy of BCG in CIS there are still several questions which are not answered at the present time. The EORTC protocol 30861 addresses the following questions: what is the number of instillations needed to achieve complete remission (CR), what percentage of CR can be obtained by the proposed treatment, how is the rate of recurrence and progression after CR, how serious are the side effects and is it possible to determine prognostic factors.

SELECTION OF PATIENS

The patients should have a good performance status (WHO: 0-2) and CIS has to be proven by biopsy. All visible tumor has to be resected. No abnormal urothelium should be present in the prostatic urethra. Bladder capacity below 150 ml, chronic urinary tract infection, previous tuberculosis, previous irradation of pelvic organs, concurrent TCC T2 or more, and other cancer except of the skin are exclusion criteria.

DESIGN OF THE PROTOCOL

The treatment will start 7-14 days after biopsy and histological confirmation of CIS. Instillations will be given once a week for six consecutive weeks. The control cystoscopy is performed two weeks after the last instillation. At the same time selected biopsies are taken.
Urine cytology will be investigated throughout the treatment. In case of complete remission (negative biopsy and cytology) treatment is stopped. In case of persistence a second or third cycle of 6 instillations will be administered. Patients do not receive maintenance therapy in order to be able to estimate the recurrence rate.

BCG-STRAIN

BCG-Connaught is used in this protocol. It is a lyophilized vaccine which is harvested from a surface culture. One lot will be used for the whole study. The BCG will be provided by Medac, Hamburg, FRG. The vaccine is stable at 4°C for 3 years. The viability is more than 8×10^7 culturable particles per ampule.

PRELIMINARY EVALUATION

Since November 1986 66 patients are enrolled in this protocol. 25 Patients are evaluable at August 1988. Data on toxicity can be given. No responses will be reported, since it is the policy of the group to give no response rates of an ongoing study.

The Table 1 gives the occurence of bacterial cystitis, drug cystitis and fever, malaise, flu-like symptoms per instillation. Table 2 demonstrates the side effects in regard to the individual patient.

TABLE 1. Side effects given as number of occurrences per total number of instillations performed and correlated to the frequency of the side effects per patient

Side Effects	Instillations		Number of Patients					
	No	Yes (%)	1	2	3	4	5	6*
Bact. cystitis	112	4 (3)	4	–	–	–	–	–
Drug cystitis	83	33 (27)	2	5	–	–	3	1
Fever	108	8 (7)	1	2	–	–	1	–

* frequency of side effects

TABLE 2. Side effects in 25 patients with CIS treated with 6 weekly BCG-Connaught instillations

			INSTILLATION		
	NO	YES	DELAY	STOP	TOTAL
Bact. cystitis	21	4	–	–	16%
Drug cystitis	10	11	1	3	60%
Fever	20	3	1	2	20%

The percentage of side effects increases significantly with the number of instillation. Whereas patients receiving 4 instillations will have only drug cystitis in about 20%, this will increase to about 60% in case they finish their 6 weekly instillations.

PROGNOSTIC FACTORS

In a concomitant study done in collaboration with Dr. J. Feichtinger, Institute of Pathology, University of Innsbruck, Innsbruck, Austria we evaluated the local immune response in patients with CIS. The study was performed on frozen sections with various monoclonal antibodies against surface markers of lymphoid cells, such as T-helper, T-suppressor, macrophages, B-cells, NK-cells and IL-2-receptor positive cells. Results of significance are given in Table 3 comparing patients who developed a recurrent tumor after CR versus those patients who did not develop a recurrence within 12 months.

TABLE 3.

	RECURRENCE	
	Yes	No
T-helper/T-suppressor	1.8:1	3.5:1
IL-2 R positive cells	12±20	35±44
NK-cells	8±12	39±25

The respective cells were determined by means of immunohistology and counted under the microscope. The number is given by mm of urothelium investigated. Only cells in the urothelium were evaluated. The stromal reaction was not considered. However, the presence of granulomas was recorded but appeared of no significance.

SUMMARY

This is a report of an ongoing phase II study which should elucidate some of the open questions which still remain in the most effective treatment of CIS by BCG. As indicated by the preliminary results on side effects the the number of instillations or reducing the dosage (as toxic reaction to BCG could be possibly reduced by changing already shown by Dr. Pagano in this meeting), as far as there is equal efficacy.

Prognostic factors in patients with intravesical BCG have yet to be defined. A recent publication by Torrence demonstrated that granulomatous cystitis or PPD skin test are of no or borderline significance (Torrence et al., 1988). They are not considered as a prognostic indicator for the individual patient. Although the number of patients (14) evaluated by immunohistological techniques is small, we do hope that the information about the local immune response will give more insight in the mode of action of BCG as well as indicate possibly a good prognostic factor.

REFERENCES

Brosman SA (1985). The use of Bacillus Calmette-Guérin in the therapy of bladder carcinoma in situ. J Urol 134: 36-40.

Herr HW (1983). Carcinoma in situ of the bladder. Seminars in Urology 1: 15-22.

Jakse G, Hofstädter F, Leitner G, Marberger H (1980). Karzinoma in situ der Harnblase: Eine diagnostische und therapeutische Herausforderung. Urologe A 19: 93-99.

Kelley DR, Ratliff TL, Catalona WJ, Shapiro A, Lage JM, Bauer WC, Haaff EO, Dresner SM (1985). Intravesical Bacillus Calmette-Guérin therapy for superficial bladder cancer: effects of Bacillus Calmette-Guérin viability on treatment results. J Urol 134: 48-53.

de Kernion JB, Huang M, Lindner A, Smith RB, Kaufman JJ (1985). The management of superficial bladder tumors and carcinoma in situ with intravesical Bacillus Calmette-Guérin. J Urol 133: 598-603.

Lamm DL (1985). Bacillus Calmette-Guérin immunotherapy for bladder cancer. J Urol 134: 40-46.

Morales A, Eidinger D, Bruce AW (1976). Intracavitary Bacillus Calmette-Guérin in the treatment of superficial bladder cancer. J Urol 116: 180-183.

Schellhamer PF, Warden SS, Ladage LE (1984). Bacillus Calmette-Guérin in the treatment of transitional cell carcinoma of the bladder. J Urol 131: 139-143.

Torrence RJ, Kavoussi LR, Catalona WJ, Ratliff TL (1988). Prognostic factors in patients treated with intravesical Bacillus Calmette-Guérin for superficial bladder cancer. J Urol 139: 941-944.
Utz DC, Hanash KA, Farrow G (1970). The plight of the patient with carcinoma in situ of the urinary bladder. J Urol 101: 160-169.

EORTC Genitourinary Group Monograph 6:
BCG in Superficial Bladder Cancer, pages 193–205
© 1989 Alan R. Liss, Inc.

THE INFLUENCE OF TICE STRAIN BCG TREATMENT IN PATIENTS WITH TRANSITIONAL CELL CARCINOMA IN SITU

Stanley Brosman

Kaiser   Permanente   Medical   Center,   Los   Angeles,
California, USA

The potential benefits to be derived from the intra-vesical instillation of Bacillus Calmette-Guérin in the management of carcinoma in situ have been described by many investigators (Brosman, 1985; Herr et al., 1983; Morales, 1980). However, many issues remain unresolved. Some of these include the long-term results, the significance of a negative biopsy in predicting prognosis and the fate of patients who do not respond to BCG. Other problems include the optimum frequency and duration of therapy and the mechanism of action.

In order to gain more insight into the course of carcinoma in situ (CIS) in patients treated with BCG, a group of 48 patients were studied to determine their survival, disease progression and benefits from BCG therapy. There was no randomization scheme in this study.

DESIGN OF STUDY

Eligibility

A group of 48 patients, 33 men and 15 women were considered to be eligible for this study (Table 1). Their mean age was 63 years. All of the patients had a histo-logically confirmed diagnosis of carcinoma in situ made within 30 days of beginning therapy. Patients with a questionable diagnosis were excluded unless there was concurrence that the patients had carcinoma in situ by a second pathologist. Patients with a diagnosis of dysplasia or severe dysplasia were not included although there were patients who had this diagnosis on several biopsies before the pathologist made the diagnosis of carcinoma in situ. There were 29 patients who had a history of papillary or sessile transitional cell carcinoma (TCC) either separately or concurrently with CIS. The TCC was treated by TUR in all of these patients. Only seven patients had been treated with previously intravesical chemotherapy. DNA histograms (flow cytometry) were not performed because of the unavailability of this technique. The patients were not required to have a positive cytology as long as the histologic diagnosis was unequivocal. Patients were not eligible if they had received prior chemotherapy within the previous 30 days. Patients who had previously received BCG were excluded. The patients were required to have an endoscopic examination within 30 days of beginning therapy to confirm the absence of any co-existing papillary or sessile transitional cell carcinoma. The presence of these tumors excluded patients from beginning the study until the tumors were removed.

TABLE 1.

Number of patients:	:	48
Follow-up	:	35 months (range 24-66)
CIS + TCC	:	29
Duration of therapy	:	12 weeks induction
		1 year maintenance
Prior chemotherapy	:	7
Completed induction phase:		40 (83%)
Cystoscopy ± biospy	:	every 6 weeks
		every 3-6 months

Patients with other malignancies, with the exception of skin cancer, were excluded unless the cancer had been in remission for 5 years. Performance status had to be 0 or 1 and there could be no obvious disease which would limit life expectancy to less than 3 years. All of the patients were informed prior to the initiation of their BCG therapy, that the only treatment which could come closest to curing their cancer was cystectomy. They were informed that BCG therapy was not tolerated by everyone and certainly did not cure the cancer in everyone. After receiving 12 instillations a decision would be made as to the success or failure of the therapy. Patients who were judged to have failed BCG therapy were given an option of cystectomy or additional intravesical chemotherapy with another agent. They were encouraged to have cystectomy if their health permitted so. There were patients who were not eligible for cystectomy either for medical reasons or personal choice but the possible failure of intravesical BCG to eradicate or stop the progression of their disease was emphasized.

Protocol

Patients were scheduled to receive one ampule of Tice strain BCG, weekly for 12 weeks and thereafter monthly for 12 months. They were allowed to miss two consecutive weekly instillation and one monthly instillation. Although the patients needed 12 instillations of BCG before completion of the induction phase, the interval for completion of this phase varied widely. Some patients who developed very strong reactions were treated with instillations every 2-3 weeks. Most patients did not have 12 consecutive weekly instillations.

The BCG was reconstituted with 50 cc of saline and allowed to stand for 30 minutes before it was instilled. Gloves and masks were worn during the preparation of the mixture and the ampules, syringes, containers and catheter were disposed in specially marked bags.

Patients were instructed to urinate after two hours but did not have to assume any special positions while the BCG was in place. They did not remain in the clinic or office while the BCG was in the bladder. They were instructed to restrict fluids for 6-8 hours prior to the instillation. No skin testing with PPD was performed.

Patients were told about potential side effects and were asked to notify us if they developed a febrile reaction, gross hematuria or severe bladder irritative symptoms. Urine cultures were obtained prior to instillation of BCG and patients with urinary tract infection were treated with antibiotics. When the culture was negative patients were allowed to begin therapy. Urine cultures were obtained periodically depending upon the patients symptomatology. If bacteria were present, BCG was withheld until the infection was eradicated.

The development of a systemic reaction as characterized by fever more than 38°C, flu-like illness or severe bladder irritability was considered to be serious enough to begin therapy with Isoniazide hydrazide, 300 mg daily, on the day of the instillation and on the two following days. Some patients were also given non-steroidal anti-inflammatory agents, antihistamines and bladder sedatives. Patients who continued to have increasingly severe symptoms which were not controlled with these medications or who developed serious side effects were not given any additional BCG.

Cystoscopy and cytology were done 1-2 weeks after the first six instillations. Cystoscopy, cytology and bladder biopsies were performed 1-2 weeks following the 12th instillation. Cup biopsies, using local or no anesthesia, were made from sites known to be positive on previous biopsies or from suspicious areas. A biopsy from the prostatic urethra was included.

Patients with negative biopsies were put on monthly maintenance therapy. Cystoscopy and cytology was done every 3 months and biopsies were obtained every six months for two years. Patients who were thought to have an improvement in their disease received six additonal weeks of therapy and a biopsy was performed 1-2 weeks thereafter.

There were 9 patients who developed minimal or no bladder irritative symptoms and whose biopsies demonstrated persistent CIS but no inflammatory changes attributable to BCG. They were given two ampules of BCG mixed in 50 cc saline weekly until they developed symptoms of bladder irritability confirmed by the appearance of inflammatory changes in their bladder. When this occured they were treated thereafter with the standard 1 ampule dose.

Patients were considered to have a complete remission (CR) if two consecutive biopsies showed no malignancy and there was no recurrence of a papillary or sessile tumor and the urine cytology was normal. Those patients with negative biopsies but positive cytology following 12 instillations were considered to be non-responders or to have progression of CIS elsewhere in their urinary tract. Although there was a group of 5 patients who improved after the initial 12 instillations and received an additional 6 treatments, they were classified into the complete response or no response group based upon biopsies and cytology following the total of 18 instillations.

Follow-up

The patients in this study have been followed for a minimum of 24 months with a range of 24 to 66 months. The mean follow-up is 35 months. The follow-up period began after completion of 12 or 18 instillations. Although all of the BCG instillations, decisions regarding patient entry, medications, continuance on therapy, and interpretations of clincial data were made by one individual (SAB), the cysto-scopies and biopsies were performed by a large number of urologists. The clinical and laboratory data were analyzed periodically during the follow-up period.

RESULTS

Forty (83%) of the patients completed the induction phase consisting of 12 instillations of BCG (Table 2). Biopsies and cytology were negative in 28 (70%) of these patients and they were considered to have a complete response. There were seven patients in this group who received a double dose of BCG because they were thought to have no response to therapy when they were examined with cystoscopy and biopsy following six instillations. They were given 1-3 double doses before they developed an inflammatory reaction to the BCG.

There were 5 patients who were judged to have had a 50% or greater improvement and who recieved an additional six weeks of therapy. Three of these patients developed a CR and two of them were treated with a double dose of BCG.

The overall CR combining those from the 12 and 18 week instillation period was 77.5% (31 patients). There were 9 (22.5%) patients who showed no response or progression of their disease. Seven of these were failures after the 12 instillation induction phase and the other two patients were failures after receiving 18 instillations.

TABLE 2. Response to therapy in 40 CIS patients who completed 12 weekly instillations of BCG

Biopsy negative (CR)	: 28* (70%)
Improved [> 50% reduction in tumor area (PR)]:	5
Six additional weeks of therapy (CR)	: 3+
Overall CR (28+3)	: 31 (77.5%)
No response or progression (2+7)	: 9 (22.5%)

* 7 patients received double dose of BCG
+ 2 patients received double dose of BCG

There were eight patients who did not complete the induction phase, of whom five had between six to ten treatments. Three of them had complete responses.

In examining the entire group of 48 patients, there was a total of 34 (70.8%) who had a CR. Twenty of these thirty-four (59%) had no recurrence of their disease during the maintenance or follow-up period and continue to be free of tumor.

Fourteen (41%) patients in the CR group developed a recurrence of tumor (Table 3). All of the recurrences were identified within the fist 24 months of follow-up and in some patients consisted only of a positive cytology. Nine patients (64.3%) had a recurrence diagnosed within the first 12 months of the follow-up period. The recurrences were identified in the urethra and prostate in 7 patients, the upper urinary tract in 6 patients and the bladder in one patient (Table 4).

The management of the fourteen patients who developed recurrences after initially being complete responders included cystectomy (8 patients), nephro-ureterocystectomy (4 patients), TUR (1 patient), BCG infusion into the upper urinary tract in 3 patients two of whom were eventually included in the group who had nephro-ureterocystectomy (Table 5).

Five patients were treated successfully thus far but nine others have developed metastases.

TABLE 3. Duration (months) of complete response in 34 patients who had initially negative biopsies

Months	Number with Recurrences	Number without Recurrences
6	3 (8.8%)	31 (91%)
12	6 (17.6%)	25 (74%)
18	4 (12.0%)	21 (62%)
24	1 (3.0%)	20 (59%)
24	0	20 (59%)
	14 (41.0%)	20 (59%)

TABLE 4. Site of recurrence in 14 patients

Bladder	:	1
Pyelum and ureter	:	6
Urethra – prostate	:	7
		14

TABLE 5. Management of 14 patients with recurrence after initial complete response

Cystectomy	:	8
Nephro-ureterocystectomy:		4*
TUR–BCG	:	1
BCG infusion	:	3
Died with cancer	:	9/48 (18.7%)

* Includes 2 patients who failed BCG infusion

The group of 14 patients who did not respond to BCG or who failed to complete the induction phase and had persistence of their disease underwent additional therapy (Table 6). Radical cystectomy was performed in 9 patients and 5 patients were treated with chemotherapy and external beam radiation therapy. Tumor recurrence or progression developed in nine patients (64%) all of whom have either died or have distant metastases. Five patients in this group have no evidence of disease.

TABLE 6. Adjuvant therapy of 14 patients who did not complete the protocol or responded incomplete to to BCG

Cystectomy   : 9
Chemotherapy ± radiation: 5
Died of cancer   : 9/14 (64%)

Examining the entire group of 48 patients, 20 (41.7%) had a CR as a result of BCG therapy and have had no recurrence (Table 7). Ten patients who either had no response did not complete the induction phase and continued to have tumor, or were complete responders after finishing the induction phase, were eventually rendered free of tumor with a variety of treatments. Thus with or without the benefit of BCG, 30 (62.5%) patients have managed to overcome their carcinoma in situ. The other 18 (37.5%) have either died or will expire shortly as a results of their malignancy.

TABLE 7. Response in 48 CIS patients treated with BCG

No response, recurrence or progression
                          within 2 years: 28 (58.0%)
Tumor free beyond 2 years (BCG alone) : 20 (42.0%)
Died with bladder cancer   : 18 (37.5%)
BCG + adjuvant therapy   : 10 (21.0%)
Total alive without bladder cancer   : 30 (62.5%)

DISCUSSION

Although there is general agreement that CIS presents a serious form of transitional cell carcinoma, effective alternatives to cystectomy are limited to instillations of BCG, Mitomycin and Interferon-alpha (Brosman, 1985;

DeKernion et al., 1985; Herr et al., 1986; Soloway, 1985; Shortliffe et al., 1984; Torti and Lum, 1984; Lum and Torti, 1985). The most propitious manner for administering these agents has not been clearly established and the development of newer agents is awaited.

In general the success rate, as determined by the ability to render a patient biopsy and cytology negative, hovers around 70%. The results of this study support these data in that 28/40 patients who received twelve instillations were free of tumor. Whether or not these patients required as many as twelve instillations to achieve this result is not answered. Of the eight patients who did not complete this phase of the protocol, a complete remission was found in three patients receiving 6-8 instillations. This observation lends support to the opinion of Herr and associates that many patients will have a good response after six instillations. On the other side of this situation are a group of five patients who needed additional treatment beyond the twelve instillations and three of these patients achieved complete response.

It seems that we are dealing with such a complex host response/reaction to BCG that no one can predict the optimum number of instillations that would benefit each patient. A broad guideline for therapy can be established but the therapy for each patient may need to be individualized. The extent to which the patients in this study were individualized became apparent when the results were being analyzed.

The frequency of the instillations was based upon the patients tolerance to therapy. Although it was the original intent to have twelve instillations performed one week apart, there was a substantial variation from this schedule. Patients were allowed to miss no more than two consecutive weeks of therapy but many patients were receiving treatment every other week in order to minimize their adverse reactions and to allow them to receive all twelve instillations. These adverse reactions tended to occur after the first six instillations were completed.

The other major variation in the treatment schedule related to the dose of BCG. Most of the patients had an endoscopic examination after the first six instillations. If there appeared to be a minimal or no change in the bladder surface and the patients had not developed symptoms of bladder irritability, cup biopsies were made from various areas of the normal bladder and tumor. If tumor was present and the amount of inflammatory response was small, a double dose of BCG was administered weekly until clinical and/or endoscopic examination demonstrated a change in the bladder surface. Two ampules of BCG were diluted with 50 cc of saline and patients were instructed to hold this solution for $1\frac{1}{2}$ to 2 hours. There were nine patients in this study who received a double dose and none required more than three such instillations before developing an inflammatory reaction. All of these patients became biopsy and cytology negative, and they all were started on INH before beginning the double dose schedule.

The variations in dose and dosage schedule indicate that some patients may require six or fewer instillations to have an effective result while others will require more therapy. It seems unlikely that there will be a uniform schedule which will be optimum for each patient.

Another issue relates to the role of BCG in changing the natural history of this cancer. There was a 70% CR in 28 patients who completed the 12 instillation and an additional 3 patients developed a CR after having six more instillations. When these are combined the CR was 77.5%. However, if we look at the entire group of 48 patients and include the three patients with a CR who received fewer than 12 instillations, the CR rate is 70.8% (34/48) (Fig. 1). These results seem to be favorable until we begin to follow the patients for a longer period of time.

Recurrent tumor developed in fourteen of the thirty-four complete responders (41%) (Fig. 2). These recurrences were detected within the two years of follow-up and represented disease in the prostate and the upper urinary tracts in most of these individuals. In one patient with a bladder recurrence, the epithelial surface appeared normal while a tumor mass was growing in the bladder wall. This experience added to that seen in other patients receiving BCG indicates that the surface layer may be cleared of apparent disease but if tumor has already penetrated into deeper layers the therapy is likely to fail.

The outlook for patients who developed a recurrence of disease or who showed no response to BCG was poor. There were 10 patients in this group of 28 who had radical

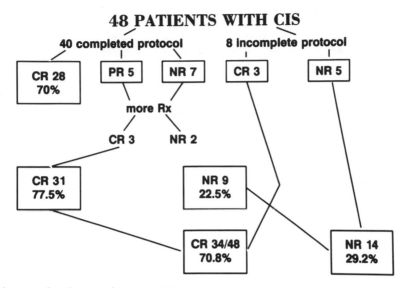

Figure 1. The role of BCG in changing the natural course of CIS.

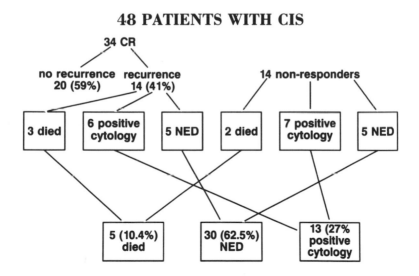

Figure 2. Fate of patients with CIS treated with BCG after initial complete response or non-response.

surgery and are still free of metastases. Eighteen other patients in this group who were treated aggressively, but too late, have died of cancer. Patients who had an initial response and recurred lived only a few months longer than those who showed no response to therapy.

Therefore only 20/48 (41.7%) of patients have remained free of cancer. There have been eighteen deaths (37.5%) and 10 patients (20.8%) have been successfully treated, thus far, with surgical therapy.

48 PATIENTS WITH CIS

no recurrence	no response or recurrence		
20	28		
(41.7%)	died	NED	positive cytology
	5	10	13
	(10.4%)	(20.8%)	(27%)

Figure 3. Long-term follow-up results in patients treated with BCG for CIS.

BCG therapy is beneficial for some patients with carcinoma in situ but the overall prognosis for patients with this disease is not good unless failures are recognized promptly, and other measures are instituted (Droller and Walsh, 1985; Stanisic et al., 1987). If we assume that 25% of our patients have invasive disease when they are initially evaluated, even though the biopsy may not disclose this information, we might predict that BCG therapy can do no better than eliminate the disease in 75% of the patients. The data in this study indicates that the means employed to reach that goal, via the number of instillations and the doses utilized, were effective for only 41.7% of the patients. Additional improvements may increase the response rate but how successful we can be is open to question.

Certainly we are delaying the time and need for surgery in many patients. Those who develop cancer in their renal pelvis or ureters would have had a recurrence even if an early cystectomy would have been performed.

Although most of the patients develop some side effects from the therapy, notably bladder irritability, there were no instances of BCG-itis or abnormal changes to the surface epithelium and localized to the bladder, BCG instillations represent a safe and effective form of therapy which is worth attempting prior to radical surgery.

REFERENCES

Brosman SA (1985). The use of Bacillus Calmette-Guérin in the therapy of bladder carcinoma in situ. J Urol 134: 36-39.

Droller MJ, Walsh PC (1985). Intensive intravesical chemotherapy in the treatment of flat carcinoma in situ: is it safe? J Urol 134: 1115.

Herr HW, Pinsky CM, Whitmore Jr WF, Oettgen HF, Melamed MR (1983). Effect of intravesical Bacillus Calmette-Guérin (BCG) on carcinoma in situ of the bladder. Cancer 51: 1323-1326.

Herr HW, Pinsky CM, Whitmore JR WF, Sogain PC, Oettgen HF, Melamed MR (1986). Long term effect of intravesical Bacillus Calmette-Guérin on flat carcinoma in situ of the bladder. J Urol 135: 265.

deKernion JB, Huang MY, Linduer A, Smith RB, Kaufman JJ: The management of superficial bladder tumors and carcinoma in situ with intravesical Bacillus Calmette-Guérin. J Urol 133: 598-601.

Lum BL, Torti FM (1985). Therapeutic approaches including Interferon to carcinoma in situ of the bladder. Cancer Treat Rev (suppl. B) 12: 45-59.

Morales A (1980). Treatment of carcinoma in situ of the bladder with BCG: a phase II trial. Cancer Immunol Immunother 9: 69.

Shortliffe LD, Freiha FJ, Hannigan JF (1984). Intravesical Interferon therapy for carcinoma in situ and transitional cell carcinoma of the bladder. J Urol. 131: 171A.

Soloway MS (1985). Follow-up data on 70 bladder cancer patients treated with intravesical Mitomycin-C. Proc Am Soc Clin Oncol 4: 96.

Stanisic TH, Donovan JM, Lebouton, Graham AR (1987). 5-year experience with intravesical therapy of carcinoma in situ: an inquiry into the risks of "conservative management". J Urol 138: 1158-1161.

Torti FM, Lum BL (1984). The biology and treatment of superficial bladder cancer. J Clin Oncol 2: 505.

EORTC Genitourinary Group Monograph 6:
BCG in Superficial Bladder Cancer, pages 207–212
© 1989 Alan R. Liss, Inc.

PERCUTANEOUS BCG PERFUSION OF THE UPPER URINARY TRACT FOR
CARCINOMA IN SITU

U.E. Studer, G. Casanova, R. Kraft, E.J. Zingg

Department of Urology, University of Bern, Inselspital, 3010 Bern, Switzerland

INTRODUCTION

Intravesical administration of Bacillus Calmette-
Guérin (BCG) is an effective therapy for flat carcinoma in
situ (Tis) of the bladder (Ackermann et al., 1986; Brosman,
1982; Catalona et al., 1987; Herr et al., 1983; deKernion
et al., 1985; Lamm, 1985). While the importance of a
systemic host reaction to intravesical instillation is
unknown and might either be a concomitant effect or a
necessity for the therapeutic efficacy of BCG (Droller,
1986; Ratliff and Gillen, 1986), the direct contact of BCG
with the diseased urothelium seems to be important:
persistence of urethral or prostatic carcinoma in situ
after successful intravesical BCG therapy has been observed
(Herr and Whitmore, 1987; Herr et al., 1986; Studer, 1987).
This prompted us to use BCG in the upper urinary tract for
carcinoma in situ.

PATIENTS AND METHODS

Between January 1986 and May 1987, 10 reno-ureteral
units of 8 patients were perfused with BCG. Their mean age
was 74 (66-86) years. All had a long history of urothelial
cancer, treated previously by repeated transurethral
resections and intravesical instillation (n=7), and/or by
radical cystectomy (n=3); one patient also underwent a
nephro-ureterectomy at the contralateral side for invasive
urothelial cancer of the renal pelvis, and two patients had
earlier an organ-preserving open resection of renal pelvis
cancer in solitary kidneys.

All patients showed positive urine cytology during follow-up examinations. In the 5 non-cystectomized patients, the multiple random biopsies of the bladder mucosa and of the prostatic urethra were negative for urothelial tumor. In all patients the ureters were intubated with 7 Fr catheters and cytology of collected urine and/or washouts was positive. In 7 of 8 patients, the ureteropyelogrammes showed no tumors.

By ultrasound control, a percutaneous nephrostomy tube was placed under local anesthesia. An unobstructed flow from the renal pelvis to the ileal conduit or the bladder was checked under fluoroscopy. 360 mg of immune BCG-Pasteur-F were dissolved in 150 ml of 0.9% saline. The flask was placed 20 cm above the kidney of the resting patient (Figure 1). After filling the pyelo-urethral system with 10-15 ml of the BCG solution, a continuous flow of approx. 1 ml per minute (= 15 to 20 drops per minute) was maintained. The perfusion was stopped after 2 hours. The patients received Ampicilline prophylactically and were kept at the hospital for one night. The perfusion was repeated at weekly intervals for a total of 6 perfusions (= 1 treatment course). If 6 weeks later cytology remained positive, a further treatment course was started.

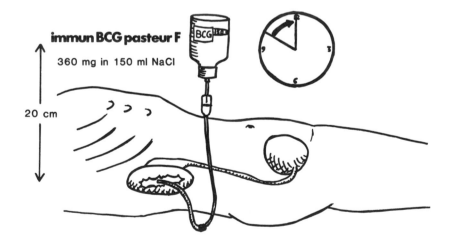

Figure 1. Percutaneous BCG perfusion.

RESULTS

Five patients had a single course of 6 BCG perfusions after which carcinoma in situ could no longer be found by cytology during an observation period of 12 to 24 months. In one of these patients, persisting papillary tumors were resected in the ureters (Table 1). Two patients had bilateral perfusions and required several courses until cytology became negative and remained so for 12 and 15 months respectively. One of these showed a recurrent bladder cancer (T1 G3) one year later. In one patient the treatment was stopped after the first perfusion because of severe septicemia.

TABLE 1.

4 patients	1 BCG course	cytology negative for 12-24 months
1 patient	1 BCG course	disappearance of CIS persistence of papillary tumor
1 patient	2 BCG courses, left 2 BCG courses, right	cytology negative for 15 months, recurrence in bladder
1 patient	3 BCG courses, left 1 BCG course, right	cytology negative for 12 months
1 patient	premature stop after 1 BCG perfusion	severe septicemia

The side effects were comparable to those seen after BCG instillation into the bladder: fever up to 38.6°C, fatigue and dysuria, pollakisuria for 1 to 3 days. No significant change in serum creatinine, no systemic spread of BCG, no major granulomatous renal masses and no urothelial cancer along the nephrostomy track have been observed so far.

DISCUSSION

A durable response of carcinoma in situ of the renal pelvis after topical BCG administration was probably first reported in 1985 by Herr (Herr, 1985). He performed renal autotransplantation with direct pyelovesical anastomosis followed by intravesical BCG.

BCG perfusion of the upper urinary tract must be considered as an experimental treatment. All the patients reported in this series had undergone previous surgery for urothelial cancer and were unwilling, unfit or unable to undergo further surgery. This is also reflected by this patient group's mean age of 74 years, and in half of the patients, a nephro-ureterectomy would have resulted in uremia, necessitating chronic hemodialysis. Despite the poor patient selection, the percutaneous BCG perfusion did not result in major complications, except for one patient who developed septicemia. Repeated fluoroscopic monitoring of proper drainage of the pyelo-ureteral system towards the bladder or ileal conduit seems to be important, as well as a low perfusion pressure produced by only slightly elevating the flask containing the BCG solution (20 cm). Fever and chills during the first night are common, and the additional risk of septicemia may require hospitalization for the first night. It is unknown if a lower dosage of BCG would show less side effects. The dosage chosen by us (360 mg in 150 ml NaCl perfused during 2 hours) is arbi-trary. It corresponds to the concentration of BCG usually used for treatment of carcinoma in situ in the bladder (120 mg BCG of the Pasteur strain dissolved in 50 ml saline).

Although never observed in our small series of patients, it is unknown if large granulomatous renal masses, which have occasionally been observed after intra-vesical BCG application, might occur more frequently when BCG is perfused through the renal pelvis (Schellhammer, 1987; Stanisic et al., 1986). The additional potential risk, that this form of treatment might spread urothelial cancer cells along the nephrostomy tube, has also never been reported.

Since multifocal carcinoma in situ is treated less frequently by radical cystectomy combined with resection of the distal ureters because of the successful use of intravesical BCG applications, it might be that carcinoma in situ of the upper urinary tract, mainly the distal ureters, may become an increasing problem in the future. According to Herr, ureteral carcinoma in situ after successful intravesical BCG therapy may occur in up to 29% of the cases (Herr and Whitmore, 1987). This high incidence stresses the need to find new organ-preserving treatment possibilities. One of these could become the BCG perfusion of the upper urinary tract, provided that our encouraging, preliminary results can be confirmed by others.

References

Ackermann D, Schnyder M, Bandelier D, Studer U (1986). Traitement des tumeurs superficielles de la vessie par le Bacillus Calmette-Guérin (BCG). J Urol (Paris) 92: 33-38.

Brosman SA (1982). Experience with Bacillus Calmette-Guérin in patients with superficial bladder carcinoma. J Urol 128: 27-30.

Catalona WJ, Hudson MA, Gillen DP, Andriole GL, Ratliff TL (1987). Risks and benefits of repeated courses of intravesical Bacillus Calmette-Guérin therapy for superficial bladder cancer. J Urol 137: 220-223.

Droller MJ (1986). Bacillus Calmette-Guérin in the management of bladder cancer (Editorial). J Urol 135: 331-333.

Herr HW, Pinsky CM, Whitmore Jr WF, Oettgen HF, Melamed MR (1983). Effect of intravesical Bacillus Calmette-Guérin (BCG) on carcinoma in situ of the bladder. Cancer 51: 1323-1326.

Herr HW (1985). Durable response of a carcinoma in situ of the renal pelvis to topical Bacillus Calmette-Guérin. J Urol 134: 531-532.

Herr HW, Pinsky CM, Whitmore Jr WF, Sogani PC, Oettgen HF, Melamed MR (1986). Long-term effect of intravesical Bacillus Calmette-Guérin on flat carcinoma in situ of the bladder. J Urol 135: 265-267.

Herr HW, Whitemore Jr WF (1987). Ureteral carcinoma in situ after successful intravesical therapy for superficial bladder tumors: incidence, possible pathogenesis and management. J Urol 138: 292-294.

deKernion JB, Huang M-Y, Lindner A, Smith RB, Kaufman JJ (1985). The management of superficial bladder tumors and carcinoma in situ with intravesical Bacillus Calmette-Guérin. J Urol 133: 598-601.

Lamm DL (1985). Bacillus Calmette-Guérin immunotherapy for

bladder cancer. J Urol 134: 40-47.

Ratliff TL, Gillen GD (1986). Requirement for thymus-dependent immune response for the inhibition of intra-vesical mouse bladder tumor growth. J Urol 135: 122A.

Schellhammer PF (1987). Letter to the Editor. Re: Intra-vesical Bacillus Calmette-Guérin therapy and associated granulomatous renal masses. Stanisic et al. J Urol 137: 315.

Stanisic TH, Brewer ML, Graham AR (1987). Intravesical Bacillus Calmette-Guérin therapy and associated granulomatous renal masses. Stanisic et al. J Urol 135: 356-358.

Studer UE, Ackermann D, Schnyder v Wartensee M (1987). Immunotherapie bei oberflächigen Harnblasentumoren. In Sommerkamp H, Altwein JE, Klippel KF (eds): "Urologische Onkologie I," München-Bern-Wien-San Francisco: W. Zuck-schwerdt Verlag, pp 129-135.

PART III. RANDOMIZED CLINICAL TRIALS WITH BCG IN SUPERFICIAL BLADDER CANCER

EORTC Genitourinary Group Monograph 6:
BCG in Superficial Bladder Cancer, pages 215–236
© 1989 Alan R. Liss, Inc.

RATIONALE FOR INTRAVESICAL CHEMOTHERAPY IN THE TREATMENT AND PROPHYLAXIS OF SUPERFICIAL TRANSITIONAL CELL CARCINOMA

Mark S. Soloway, Anne M. Jordan and William M. Murphy

Department of Urology, University of Tennessee, (M.S.S.) and department of Pathology, Baptist Memorial Hospital (A.M.J., W.M.M.), Memphis, Tennessee

Prior to embarking upon a discussion concerning the rationale for the use of intravescial chemotherapy, either in the treatment or prophylaxis for patients with superficial bladder cancer, it is important to stress the critical nature of the initial diagnostic evaluation since the information gained from this procedure will be the determining factor in regard to treatment. Adequate cytologic and histologic material must be obtained and then reviewed by the urologist and pathologist together so that an appropriate treatment plan can be determined.

The first step in the endoscopic evaluation of a patient suspected or previously determined to have a bladder tumor is to examine the excretory urogram (IVP) to outline the transitional cell epithelium of the upper urinary tract. Adequate anesthesia is critical for the diagnostic procedure. A bimanual examination is the initial step and this should include careful palpation of the prostate in the male. Any abnormality requires a biopsy to determine whether there is adenocarcinoma or transitional cell carcinoma involving the prostate.

The endoscope should be introduced under direct vision, noting any abnormality of the urethra and, more specifically, the prostatic urethra. I have helped devise an optical dilator which dilates the urethra during urethroscopy (Soloway, 1988). Following introduction of this instrument, a 24-28 Fr resectoscope sheath can be placed, thus allowing for the use of various lenses as well as transurethral resection without further changing the sheath.

Urine is collected following introduction of the sheath and this may be combined with a saline bladder washing. This specimen is promptly transferred to the cytology laboratory. The cytology is particularly helpful if high grade cells are observed in patient with only a low grade papillary tumor. This may indicate bladder, prostate, or upper tract carcinoma in situ or extension of transitional cell carcinoma into the prostatic ducts.

I use a 70 degree lens to examine the entire bladder surface, and a 12 or 30 degree lens to view the trigone and prostatic urethra. The location, appearance (papillary or sessile), and size of all tumors should be documented on an appropriate diagram which becomes a part of the patient's record. Increasingly, I have used endoscopic photography for documentation of urothelial abnormalities.

I prefer a continuous flow resectoscope for both endoscopic resection of all the obvious tumor and mucosal biopsies. Although the cold cup biopsy forceps is an excellent device for obtaining mucosal biopsies without cautery artifact; if the coagulating current is turned down, the resectoscope can obtain mucosal biopsies with little loss of cellular architecture. This is particularly useful in patients who have had prior intravesical chemotherapy with resultant fibrosis of the bladder which makes cold cup biopsies difficult.

All tumor should be resected unless the tumor extends deep into the muscle. Most superficial tumors can be entirely resected. Muscle should be included in the specimen if the appearance of the tumor suggest lamina propria or muscle invasion. Following tumor resection, I use a roller electrode for hemostasis and to cauterize the urothelium which surrounds each of the resected tumors.

Following tumor resection, the urologist should once again visualize the entire bladder with a 70 degree lens. Often tumors are missed when using the 12 degree lens with the resectoscope. A follow-up cytology is an excellent means of documenting whether all tumor has been removed. This is particularly important when there is carcinoma in situ. A post resection cytology is only helpful if the tumor is grade II or III since more than half of grade I tumors will not be detected by cytologic examination of the urine or bladder washing.

If the tumor is confined to the urothelium (Ta) or has only extended into the lamina propria (T1), I do not think CT-scans are necessary for staging. The likelihood that such tumors will have metastasized and be identified with a CT-scan is low. I do not think the cost is warranted.

The prostatic urethra should be biopsied in patients with CIS, tumor at the bladder neck, and when there is a positive cytology without obvious tumor. I prefer the resectoscope to obtain a prostatic urethral biopsy, making sure to incorporate not only the urothelium but also the prostatic ducts. It is important to know whether the tumor has extended into the duct or the prostatic stroma.

PROGNOSTIC FACTORS

After review of the cytologic and histologic material from the endoscopic tumor resection, the clinician can formulate a therapeutic plan. Tumor stage, grade, size, and multicentricity are important factors as is the patient's prior tumor history, medical status, and response to therapy. If the tumor has invaded the lamina propria, the risk of progression in stage is higher than if the tumor is confined to the urothelium. Anderstrom underscored this point with the survival analysis of patients with Ta or T1 bladder tumors (Anderstrom et al., 1980). Only 3 of 78 patients whose tumor did not invade the basement membrane died of bladder cancer in contrast to 24 of 99 with lamina propria invasion. A National Bladder Cancer Group study found that only 4% of those with Ta tumors progressed to muscle invasive tumors compared to 30% when the initial lesion was T1 (Heney et al., 1983). This National Bladder Cancer Group review contained only a few patients with carcinoma in situ.

Treatment decisions are most difficult when dealing with patients with high grade tumor. Some suggest that a G III, T1 transitional cell carcinoma is an indication for cystectomy. The advent of the continent urinary diversion has improved patient acceptance and this approach may be more attractive. Of utmost importance is to gain an under-standing of the likelihood that such a patients will die of bladder cancer if they receive intensive intravesical therapy with careful monitoring.

CARCINOMA IN SITU

The prognosis for patients with carcinoma in situ of the urinary bladder is quite variable. This represents a heterogeneous group. Carcinoma in situ is a high grade (grade III) flat transitional cell carcinoma which is confined to the urothelium (Friedell et al., 1986). If lesser degrees of cytologic abnormality are interpreted as CIS, the results of a given therapy may be artifically enhanced; thus it is important to adhere to a uniform classification system.

Patients with carcinoma in situ can be devided into several groups. Some patients are diagnosed quite early by a screening cytology. This is an uncommon presentation. More frequently, CIS is found on mucosal biopsies, either adjacent to or distant from obvious papillary tumors. Patients with diffuse, erythematous, endoscopically visible carcinoma is situ probably represent a more "advanced" stage. These patients may or may not have symptoms associated with carcinoma is situ such as dysuria, frequency, and pain.

A patient with a new diagnosis of CIS is an appropriate candidate for intravesical therapy. The indication to abandon intravesical therapy in conjunction with endoscopic resection/fulguration and proceed with cystectomy depends on the presence of associated neoplasms and response to initial intravesical treatment. The clinician does not want to delay cystectomy and risk understaging. It is critical to monitor the prostatic urethra in this group of patients. The tumor(s) in the bladder may be controlled by effective intravesical agents, however, transitional cell carcinoma may develop in the prostatic urothelium, ducts, or stroma. The incidence of transitional cell carcinoma in the prostatic urethra of patients with multifocal bladder cancer ranges from 10 to 40%, depending on whether one examines patients with superficial bladder cancer or performs step sections of bladder removed for all stages (Mahadevia et al., 1986; Montie et al., 1986).

RECURRENCE AND NEW OCCURENCES

Following initial management of a superficial tumor, the likelihood of a subsequent urothelial neoplasm ranges from 30 to over 80% and this is consistent among several series (Herr et al., 1987; Soloway, 1980). There are a number of prognostic factors which influence the likelihood of a subsequent tumor: tumor grade, stage, multiplicity, positive cytology, prior tumor history, and presence of carcinoma in situ.

There are three principal reasons for the high incidence of subsequent tumors: new occurences, true recurrences, and tumor implantation.

There is extensive evidence that bladder cancer is a field change neoplastic diathesis which can involve the entire urothelium. Bladder mapping studies have been performed by step sectioning cystectomy specimens as well as by obtaining mucosal biopsies from normal-appearing urothelium in patients being treated for superficial TCC. They indicate that preneoplastic changes are responsible for most of the "recurrences" (Farrow et al., 1976; Soto et al., 1977). In one of the first analyses of mucosal biopsies, Schade and Swinney reported a 40% incidence of carcinoma in situ (Schade and Swinney, 1973). I suspect that many of these biopsies were actually degrees of dysplasia but nonetheless, they did show that there were urothelial abnormalities distant from the obvious neoplasm. Eisenberg detected a 26% incidence of proliferative lesions adjacent to papillary tumors (Eisenberg et al., 1960). In a study from the University of Tennessee (Soloway et al., 1978), cold cup biopsies were performed every three months regardless of the presence of an evident tumor and over a one-year period, 46% of the patients had atypia, 14% carcinoma in situ, and 16% carcinoma from cystoscopically normal-appearing mucosa. The high incidence of carcinoma undoubtedly was related to biopsies taken adjacent to the tumor. There was a 38% incidence of bladder cancer in patients who had hyperplasia, atypia, or CIS in at least one of these areas distant from the initial lesion, compared to a 16% incidence in those who had normal biopsies, $p < 0.095$. Thus, some of these proliferative areas progress to neoplasia. The best term for tumors which arise from progressive growth of preneoplastic abnormalities is new occurrences rather than recurrences.

It is reasonable to conclude that new occurrences represent the primary reason for subsequent urothelial tumors following endoscopic resection of superficial bladder cancer. The role of carcinogens as an etiologic factor in bladder cancer is well documented and the entire urothelium is exposed to them. Chronic urinary tract infection, calculi, and a high residual urine have also been implicated as etiologic factors.

TRUE RECURRENCES

Following endoscopic tumor resection, there may be regrowth due to incomplete resection. These would be termed true recurrences. The likelihood of incomplete resection varies with the skill of the resectionist and the depth and grade of the tumor. It is difficult to know how frequently this occurs. A urine cytology following resection may contain tumor cells if tumor remains following endoscopic resection. I am not aware of an analysis of how often this occurs.

Another way of determining whether there has been an incomplete resection is to perform a repeat resection/ biopsy. This may be helpful for tumors which have invaded the lamina propria and the endoscopist is unsure whether all tumor has been resected or whether tumor has invaded muscle.

TUMOR IMPLANTATION

Another possible contributing factor to the high incidence of subsequent tumor following endoscopic tumor resection is implantation of tumor cells on the urothelial surface traumatized during local resection or fulguration. Although one cannot prove the existence of this phenomenon in man, laboratory studies in animals and circumstantial evidence in man suggest that this accounts for some recurrences. I have performed a series of studies using a carcinogen-induced transplantable transitional cell carcinoma (MBT-2) to study this (Soloway and Masters, 1980; Weldon and Soloway, 1975). Upon intravesical instillation, N-methyl-N-nitrosurea (NMU) produces a diffuse urothelial reaction resulting in a loss of much of the epithelium. Intravesical instillation of poorly differential transitional cell carcinoma cells following NMU results in tumor in 60% of the bladder. If the bladder is not altered by NMU prior to placement of tumor cells, only 13% of the bladder will have tumor. These tumors can only have occurred by implantation of the instilled tumor cells. In a subsequent series of studies designed to more closely approximate the clinical situation, the posterior bladder wall was cauterized prior to transurethral placement of MBT-2 cells. 54% of previously cauterized bladders contained tumor in contrast to only 12% of bladder if the same number of cells were instilled into normal bladders. In man, tumor cells exfoliate from a transitional cell carcinoma as evidenced by a positive cytology and it seems reasonable that the urothelial surface, traumatized by instrumentation and/or resection, would provide a fertile surface for implantation.

The concept of implantation or seeding of urothelial tumors in man dates back to observations by Albarran and Imbert (Albarran and Imbert, 1903). They noted the frequency of ureteral and bladder tumors coincident with tumors in the ipsilateral renal pelvis. The fact that transitional cell tumors implant in a wound after transvesical fulguration is further evidence that these cells are capable of implanting. Hinman and Kiefer emphasized iatrogenic urothelial trauma as an important factor in the high "recurrence" rate, attributing it to tumor implantation (Hinman, 1956; Kiefer, 1953).

Green and Yalowitz reviewed their experience with 100 patients undergoing concomitant transurethral resection of a bladder tumor and prostate and compared it to an equal number of patients undergoing only removal of bladder neoplasms. The recurrence rate was the same and they concluded that this was evidence against tumor implantation. The overall "recurrence" rate and the percentage of tumors located in the prostatic urethra and/or vesical neck were identical in both groups: 54 and 16%, respectively. I suggest that the incidence of subsequent tumors in their series was not insignificant and one might conclude that the trauma to the urothelium from a transurethral resection of the prostate does not alter the propensity for implantation after resection of fulguration of a bladder tumor. However, there is significant urothelial trauma associated with both procedures. Thus, their comparison does not allow for a definitive statement regarding the capability of transitional tumor cells to implant or its contribution to the high recurrence rate.

The site of recurrences in comparison to the site of initial bladder tumors may also be cited as evidence favoring the concept of implantation. Boyd and Burnand mapped the site of bladder tumors and indicated the high incidence of subsequent tumors located only in the vault of the bladder, 18% (Boyd and Burnand, 1974). In 91% of patients, the vault was at some time the site of recurrence. This was in contrast to the infrequent finding of the vault as the site of an initial tumor, 3%. They suggested that tumor cells rise toward the bladder dome and implant. These authors then proceeded with instilling a high dose of Thiotepa immediately after transurethral bladder resections and observed a dramatic decrease in the incidence of subsequent tumors (Burnand et al., 1976).

Page also contrasted the site of initial bladder tumors to the location of subsequent lesions (Page et al., 1978). Initial tumors were located within 5 cm of ureteral orifices in 77% of 56 patients, in contrast to only 20% of 25 patients with subsequent tumors at this site. No patients had the air bubble as the location of initial tumor, however, this was the site of 45% of recurrences. Trauma to the posterior wall as the result of instrumentation was thought to be a factor in inducing implantation.

THE CONCEPT OF INTRAVESICAL THERAPY

Intravesical therapy is the term used to describe the instillation of antitumor drugs directly into the bladder. It provides a relatively large amount of drug in contact with the abnormal urothelium while minimizing systemic toxicity. Unfortunately, there is a paucity of well designed studies which address the appropriate dose, concentration, and frequency of administration for each agent.

Intravesical therapy may be used for prophylaxis or treatment. When intravesical therapy is used as prophylaxis, the clinician feels that all visible tumor has been removed and a subsequent negative cytology will help confirm that high grade tumor is no longer present. Candidates for prophylaxis are patients likely to recur or progress, i.e., multifocal tumor particularly if grade II-III, invasion of the basement membrane (T1), carcinoma in situ, history of recurrences. If tumor is obviously remaining following endoscopic resection, if a follow-up cytology is positive, or if mucosal biopsies contain carcinoma, subsequent intravesical therapy would be used as treatment and a marker is present to determine its effectiveness.

An important rationale for the use of intravesical therapy is not only to prevent subsequent tumor which requires endoscopic resection, fulguration or laser treatment, but possibly more importantly, to prevent tumor progression, cystectomy, and death from bladder cancer. The effectiveness of intravesical therapy should be judged not only by the ability to obtain an initial complete response but to avoid subsequent tumors, particularly with tumor progression. Unfortunately, many studies do not have sufficient follow-up to adequately provide all of this information.

THIOTEPA

Thiotepa is an antitumor alkylating agent which has been used for intravesical therapy for over 25 years. The usual dose is 30 to 60 mg delivered in a concentration of 1 mg per ml. Thiotepa is usually instilled weekly for 6 to 8 weeks when used for treatment and weekly for 4 weeks followed by monthly instillations when used for prophylaxis. The only large dose response study compared 30 to 60 mg (1 mg/1 ml) given weekly and found no difference in efficacy or toxicity (Koontz et al., 1981).

The molecular weight of Thiotepa is 189; the lowest for the three commonly used intravesical chemotherapeutic agents. Absorbtion varies considerably and patients must have a normal leukocyte and platelet count documented prior to each instillation. Nonetheless, myelosuppression is uncommon. We have reviewed our figures and found that only 4% of 670 consecutive Thiotepa instillations were associated with myelosuppression (Soloway and Ford, 1983). When it did occur, it was never severe. On the other hand, there have been reported cases of leukemia and aplastic anemia following Thiotepa ((Silverberg and Zarrabi, 1987).

Thiotepa has been used as treatment for residual bladder cancer with a reported complete response rate of 35 to 45% (Soloway, 1980). Most trials have used Thiotepa as prophylaxis. Many of these studies used a control group and compared their recurrence rate to those receiving Thiotepa.

In virtually all of these studies, those receiving Thiotepa had a lower incidence of tumor in a given interval of time. Unfortunately, in most of these studies the dose, administration schedule, and timing of the first dose from the time of transurethral resection varied considerably.

The National Bladder Cancer Collaborative Group performed a prospective randomized study to compare Thiotepa to no intravesical therapy following endoscopic bladder tumor resection (Prout et al., 1983). The time to first recurrence was significantly longer for those patients receiving Thiotepa when compared to the non-treated control group. Interestingly, the benefit was only for those with a grade I lesion; 51% of the treated group was tumor free at two years compared to 14% of those who did not recieve Thiotepa. There was no significant benefit for patients with grade II or III tumors.

Thiotepa is relatively inexpensive. Chemical cystitis is infrequent and rarely severe. Myelosuppression can occur and blood counts must be monitored prior to each instillation.

ADRIAMYCIN

I have not had any personal experience with the use of Adriamycin for intravesical chemotherapy, and thus my remarks will be limited. Adriamycin's molecular weight is 580 and absorption with resultant myelosuppression is rare. Most of the side effects with intravesical Adriamycin are due to chemical cystitis.

A recent Southwest Oncology Group study compared intravesical Adriamycin to BCG. BCG was significantly more effective for both treatment and prophylaxis of superficial bladder cancer (Crawford et al., 1985).

Ausfeld reviewed his experience with both intravesical Adriamycin and Mitomycin-C when used as prophylaxis (Ausfeld et al., 1987). Mitomycin-C 40 mg/40 ml was instilled every other week for two months and then montly for the remainder of the year. Thus, patients who recieved Mitomycin had many more instillations than those who received Adriamycin.

This was not a randomized trial, but assuming the populations were relatively similar; the authors felt it reasonable to compare the recurrence rate. The recurrence rate was calculated as the total recurrences x100 divided by the total patient months of follow-up. It was 1.6 for Adriamycin and 0.35 for Mitomycin-C. A high percentage of patients had low grade, low stage tumors. 75% of the patients who recieved Adriamycin had a Ta tumor and 55% had grade I tumors. 75% had a solitary tumor prior to resection. In the Mitomycin-C group, 58% had a Ta lesion, 50% had a grade I tumor, and 64% had solitary tumors. Despite the low grade and low stage of most of these lesions, 52% of those with an initial Ta lesion and 67% with T1 had a recurrence in the Adriamycin group.

MITOMYCIN-C

Mitomycin-C is another commonly used systemic chemotherapeutic agent that has been instilled into the bladder for the treatment and prophylaxis of superficial bladder tumors. The molecular weight of Mitomycin-C is 329. Myelosuppression, therefore, is rare as the absorption is low. As with Adriamycin, the most common side effect is chemical cystitis. An unusual side effect is a genital or systemic rash (Nissenkorn et al., 1981). Although uncommon, patients should wash their genitalia and hands following drug instillation and the first several voidings thereafter to avoid or reduce the incidence of contact of Mitomycin-C with their skin. This reduces the incidence of contact dermatitis, but an occasional systemic rash still occurs.

There are a number of studies which have demonstrated the efficacy of Mitomycin-C in a dose of 40 mg weekly for 8 weeks when used for the treatment of residual superficial bladder cancer. One of the few randomized trials was performed by the National Bladder Cancer Collaborative Group (Heney, 1985). Patients received either Thiotepa, 30 mg/30 ml or Mitomycin-C, 40 mg/40 ml. The complete response rate (negative cystoscopy, biopsy, and cytology) was 39% for Mitomycin-C and 26% for Thiotepa. This difference was significant, p=0.08. Local side effects were slightly higher for MMC, 43% versus 31%, respectively. Fourteen of the 71 who received Mitomycin had a local or systemic rash. Myelosuppression was low in both groups.

I have used intravesical Mitomycin-C for the treatment of residual tumor. Eighty patients received eight weekly instillations of Mitomycin-C beginning 7 to 14 days following incomplete transurethral biopsy or resection of stages Ta, CIS, or T1 bladder cancer. The dose was 40 mg in 40 ml sterile water with an instillation time of two hours. This was a select group of patients since they had a prior history of bladder cancer and most had multiple recurrences. 80% failed Thiotepa.

The first evaluation was at week 12. The criteria for a complete response included: no visible tumor at cysto-panendoscopy; biopsies from selected or random sites, including the location of the prior tumor, must contain no cancer; and no tumor cells in the bladder washing. I no longer use a partial response category (50% tumor decrease or positive cytology with negative cystoscopy) since we have shown that the long-term results of these partial responders are similar to those who do not respond, i.e., progression in stage, cystectomy, or radiation therapy (Cant et al., 1986). Some responders continued therapy at a dose of 40 mg monthly for nine months.

The 80 patients were divided by stage: Ta, 41 (51%); CIS, 21 (26%); and T1, 18 (23%). The avarage follow-up for the 80 patients is 40 months. 67% have been followed a minimum of three years and one third at least five years (range 12-109 months). 26% of the patients have had a cystectomy, however, only 15% developed a tumor which invaded the muscle. 9% died of bladder cancer. It must be stressed that Mitomycin-C was usually discontinued after one year. The figures for cystectomy, muscle invasion, or death from bladder cancer reflect events at any point in their follow-up.

37% (15/41) of those with initial Ta lesion, 33% of 21 patients with CIS, and 8 of 18 (44%) with an initial T1 lesion had a complete response. It was apparant in reviewing the subsequent events in these patients that those who had a complete response at 12 weeks were less likely to have a muscle invasive tumor (T2 or greater) or cystectomy than those who had biopsy or cytologic evidence of tumor after the eight weeks of Mitomycin-C (failure).

13% with an initial Ta tumor(s) who had a complete response later had a cystectomy compared to 23% of the 26 who failed. 7% of the complete responders and 15% of the failures developed a muscle invasive tumor. None of the complete responders died from bladder cancer, while 3 of 26 (11%) failures died of bladder cancer. Two of the eight cystectomies were for recurrence in the prostatic urethra or ducts.

Among the patients with initial multifocal carcinoma is situ who received Mitomycin-C, only one (14%) of the complete responders had a cystectomy compared to 8 of 14 (57%) non-responders. Only one complete responder and two failures progressed to muscle invasion. Only one patient died. This was an initial complete responders. The indication for cystectomy in two of the nine patients was for tumor in the prostatic ducts.

Only one of 8 (5%) T1 complete responders eventually had a cystectomy compared to 3 of 10 (30%) failures. None of the complete responders died of bladder cancer compared to 3 of the failures. Thus, only 4 of the 18 (22%) patients with an initial T1 tumor had a cystectomy. The pathology at the time of cystectomy was pT2 in two patients, CIS in one, and no tumor in one.

Since these were patients in which tumor was not resected prior to Mitomycin-C instillations, the results indicate that MMC is capable of eradicating residual superficial transitional cell carcinoma in 38%. Fewer of these complete responders had a change in treatment and this may be related to the successful therapy with MMC.

BACILLUS CALMETTE-GUÉRIN (BCG)

BCG is the only new intravesical agent introduced over the last five years. Repeated intravesical instillation of BCG organisms produces an inflammatory response which is responsible for or aids in eradication or prevention of superficial bladder tumors. Whether BCG induces a specific antitumor response is unclear and it has been the subject of some discussion.

There are several strains of BCG which have been used for intravesical therapy, e.g., the Pasteur, Tice, Connaught, and RIVM. Although the BCG organisms are attenuated, systemic infection can occur and anti-tuberculous therapy must be instituted promptly to prevent serious sequelae (Mirans and Bekirov, 1987; Rawls et al., 1988).

A number of trials have demonstrated that BCG is effective for preventing tumors following endoscopic resection, i.e. prophylaxis (Kavoussi et al., 1988). Other studies have demonstrated its efficacy in the treatment of residual bladder cancer. Herr conducted one of the randomized comparative trials which evaluated BCG for treatment following endoscopic resection, comparing it to a contral (TUR only) group (Herr et al., 1985). Patients had carcinoma in situ and papillary tumors and the authors indicated that all areas of CIS were not resected. Patients received 120 mg in 50 ml of the the Montreal (Pasteur) strain weekly for six weeks with no maintenance treatment. All patients who received BCG had a reduction in the recurrence rate when compared to their pretreatment tumor frequency whereas only 27 of the 43 control patients had a decrease in their recurrence rate. The likelihood of having a cystectomy and the tumor free survical was better for those patients who received BCG (Herr et al., 1988).

Debruyne reported the initial results of a prospective randomized trial comparing BCG to Mitomycin-C following resection of superficial bladder tumors (Debruyne et al., 1988). This was a low risk population since only 4% of the patients had carcinoma in situ and 70% had primary tumors. The initial results indicated no significant difference in the recurrence rate.

Two trials explored the need for maintenance therapy and both indicated that there was not a significant difference in the tumor free interval between patients who did or did not receive maintenance therapy after an initial 6- or 12-week BCG instillations (Badalament et al., 1987; Hudson et al., 1987).

I analyzed my experience with BCG in 60 patients with stages Ta, TCIS, or T1 bladder cancer. All were in a high risk category for recurrence since they had prior bladder tumors and multifocal disease. They cannot be separated into a treatment and prophylaxis group, since a post resection cytology was not routinely performed. In most cases there was residual tumor either by cystoscopic examination or a positive cytology.

The Tice strain was used. One ampule dissolved in 60 ml was instilled weekly for six consecutive weeks. Treatment was initiated 7 to 14 days following biopsy or transurethral resection. No patient received dermal scarification. Re-evaluation for response was six weeks following the last dose and the criteria for response were the same as for Mitomycin-C.

Histologic sections from all blocks of the pre-BCG tumors were reviewed by Jordan and Murphy and the tumors graded according to a recent classification system (Jordan et al., 1987). Grade is probably the most important factor in prognosis and thus the rationale for analyzing response by grade (Torti et al., 1987). This grading system uses the terms TCC grade I and papilloma synonymously. Tumors are classified: papilloma (TCC grade I), TCC low grade (TCC grade II), or TCC high grade (TCC grade III). Papillomas were most easily recognized by the uniform spacing of their nuclei and relatively large size of their cells as well as nuclear features. TCC low grade had nuclear features similar to those of the papilloma/grade I but differed in nuclear density even in the presence of uniform nuclear spacing. TCC high grade cancers exhibited nuclear clustering and cellular as well as nuclear pleomorphism in addition to irregularly distrubuted, coarse chromatin and prominent nucleoli. In situations where the tumors manifested areas of more than one grade, the highest grade was recorded. When patients had either papillary high grade or papillary low grade tumor plus carcinoma in situ, they were listed according to the dominant feature, which was usually the papillary tumor. Patients in the carcinoma in situ category had multifocal carcinoma in situ without exophytic lesions. The tumors were graded without knowledge of clinical outcome, interval progression, or treatment.

There were 15 patients with a mean follow-up of 35.6 months (range 15-59) who had multiple papillary TCC I (Papilloma) tumors and received BCG. Twelve (80%) had no tumor at the first three-month interval. Half of these complete responders recurred after Mitomycin-C. Only one of these 15 patients has had a cystectomy or a muscle invasive carcinoma. None of the 15 patients died of bladder cancer.

Eight patients had low grade (grade II) TCC. Three (38%) had a complete response. With a mean follow-up of 30.6 months, none of the three have recurred. Two of the five failures have had a muscle invasive tumor and a cystectomy. One of the failures died of bladder cancer.

As expected, patients with a papillary high grade tumor (TCC grade III) were more likely to develop progression despite BCG. 43% of 21 patients had a complete response. Only one of nine complete responders failed prior Mitomycin-C compared to 5 of 12 (42%) failures. Thus, a failure to Mitomycin-C was less likely to have a complete response to BCG. The likelihood of progression to muscle invasion was not much different between the complete responders and failures, 1 of 9 (11%) versus 2 of 12 (17%). The percentage of patients having a cystectomy, however, was quite different, 1 of 9 (11%) versus 6 of 12 (50%). One of the complete responders and two of those who did not respond died of bladder cancer. The mean follow-up for this group is 23 months.

The 21 patients with high grade TCC were divided according to invasion of the basement membrane, i.e., Ta or T1. The likelihood of being tumor-free at three months did not differ, 3 of 6 (50%) Ta versus 6 of 15 (40%) T1. None of those with Ta progressed and only one had a cystectomy compared to three T1s with subsequent muscle invasion and 6 of the 15 had a cystectomy.

The primary lesion was multifocal carcinoma in situ in 16 patients. Half of this group were free of tumor at three months (complete response) and once again, the likelihood of a complete response was higher if they did not fail Mitomycin-C. Two of the eight complete responders failed Mitomycin-C compared to 4 of the 8 who failed. Two of the complete responders and two of the failures have had a cystectomy (mean follow-up of 34 months). The only two who progressed to muscle invasion had an initial complete response. One of the 16 (6%) patients died of bladder cancer.

An examination of the five (8%) patients who died of bladder cancer after being treated with BCG indicates that only one had an initial low grade lesion and there was invasion of the lamina propria and positive lymph nodes at the time of cystectomy. Three patients had papillary high grade tumor, one of which was Ta. Interestingly, the patient with a high grade Ta lesion did not have invasion at cystectomy but nonetheless died of liver metastases three years after the cystectomy. One of the two with high grade T1 disease refused treatment; the second had positive lymph nodes. The only patients with multifocal carcinoma in situ who died had involvement of the prostatic substance. Despite radiation therapy, he died of metastatic disease.

Thus, there were 60 patients who received BCG. 53% had a complete response. 38% of the complete responders have required tumor resection for recurrence compared to 86% of the failures. Thus, 14% of the failures have only had a positive cytology but have not developed a visible tumor requiring therapy.

23% of the 60 patients have had a cystectomy, and 13% progressed with muscle invasion. 8% died of bladder cancer. The likelihood of having a cystectomy was three times greater for those who did not have an initial complete response. The incidence of progression and death from bladder cancer is almost identical to those reported by Kavoussi on the use of BCG in 104 patients (Kavoussi et al., 1988).

An effort was made to compare the response of patients who received Mitomycin-C and those who received BCG. Only those patients who had their pretreatment slides available for review by grade were analyzed. Patients who received Mitomycin-C prior to BCG were excluded as well as any who had BCG prior to MMC. Using these criteria, there were 65 patients who received Mitomycin-C for treatment of superficial bladder cancer. Thirty-one had a complete response (48%) at the first three-month interval. The complete response rate ranged from a low of 30% for those with papillary low grade (II) TCC to 56% for those with papillomas (TCC grade I). The initial complete response rate for 35 patients who received BCG as "first-line" therapy was 60%.

The likelihood of developing a muscle invasive tumor was 18% for the 65 patients receiving Mitomycin-C and 14% for the BCG group. 28% of the 65 patients who received Mitomycin-C subsequently had a cystectomy compared to 17% of those who received BCG. 15% of the patients who received Mitomycin-C eventually died of bladder cancer, compared to 8% (3/35) of those who received BCG. An accurate comparison is not possible since the follow-up interval was approximately twice as long for those who received Mitomycin-C.

SUMMARY

1. A thorough evaluation of the urinary tract is an integral part of the initial management of a patient with transitional cell carcinoma. The site of all urothelial abnormalities must be determined and adequate histologic material obtained and reviewed. The urothelium not involved by obvious tumor should also be evaluated by either cytology or mucosal biopsies. All patients with high grade tumor should have a biopsy from the prostatic urethra.

2. The clinician should determine the risk of progression by evaluating the tumor grade, stage, and the presence or absence of carcinoma in situ.

3. The likelihood of a recurrence following endoscopic resection of a superficial bladder tumor ranges from 20% for a solitary low grade tumor to over 90% for a patient with multifocal high grade cancer.

4. The reasons for the high incidence of a subsequent tumor include new occurrences related to the continued contact of carcinogens with the susceptible urothelium, failure to completely resect all tumor, and possibly the implantation of tumor cells on the altered urothelial surface following endoscopic resection.

5. Intravesical instillation of antineoplastic agents is capable of reducing the incidence of a subsequent tumor when used for prophylaxis. These agents are also capable of eradicating residual tumor.

6. The clinician should determine whether intravesical therapy is being used for treatment or prophylaxis.

7. Thiotepa is a relatively inexpensive and safe intravesical chemotherapeutic agent which, when used for treatment of existing tumor, will provide a complete response rate of from 35 to 45%. There is a suggestion that it is more effective in low grade than high grade tumors. Prospective randomized trials indicate that patients receiving Thiotepa are less likely to develop a subsequent tumor in a given period of time than patients who do not receive intravesical therapy.

8. Mitomycin-C will provide a complete response rate in high risk patients from 35 to 50% when used for treatment of existing tumor. Approximately 15% of such patients will progress to muscle invasion if followed for approximately three years. There are few randomized trials using Mitomycin-C to determine its efficacy for prophylaxis.

9. BCG has been used for treatment and prophylaxis of superficial bladder cancer. It is relatively inexpensive. The side effects vary with the strain. Several strains have been used but they have not been compared in randomized trials. When used for treatment, the complete response rate ranges from 50 to 65%. Approximately 10 to 15% of patients develop muscle invasion despite treatment with BCG.

10. Patients who receive Mitomycin-C or BCG and who are tumor-free at the first three-month interval are less likely to have tumor progression, require a cystectomy, or die from bladder cancer than patients who have endoscopically visible tumor or a positive cytology at the first three-month interval. If a desired antitumor response is not achieved in three to six months, a change in treatment should be seriously considered if the recurrent tumor is high grade, invasive or involves the prostate. This may be an alternative intravesical agent or cystectomy.

11. All trials do not indicate that intravesical therapy reduces the subsequent incidence of tumor. More prospective randomized trials are necessary to determine the most appropriate drugs, the role of combination intravesical therapy, and to gain a better understanding concerning the pharmacokinetics and tissue penetration of the various intravesical agents.

REFERENCES

Albarran J, Imbert L (1903). "Les Tumeurs de Rein." Paris: Masson et Cie, pp 452-459.
Anderstrom C, Johansson S, Nilsson S (1980). The significance of lamina propria invasion on the prognosis of patients with bladder tumors. J Urol 124: 23-26.
Ausfeld R, Beer M, Muhlethaler JP (1987). Adjuvant intravesical chemotherapy of superficial bladder cancer with monthly Doxorubicin or intensive Mitomycin. Eur Urol 13: 10-14.

Badalament RA, Herr HW, Wong GY, Gnecco G, Pinsky CM, Whitmore Jr WF, Fair WR, Oettgen HF (1987). A prospective randomized trial of maintenance versus non-maintenance intravesical Bacillus Calmette-Guérin therapy of superficial bladder cancer. J Clin Oncol 5: 441.

Boyd PJ, Bernand KG (1974). Site of bladder tumor recurrence. Lancet 2: 1290-1291.

Burnand KG, Boyd PJR, Mayo ME, Shuttleworth KED, Lloyd-Davies RW (1976). Single dose intravesical Thiotepa as an adjuvant to cystodiathermy in the treatment of transitional cell bladder carcinoma. Brit J Urol 48: 55-60.

Cant JD, Murphy WM, Soloway MS (1986). Prognostic significance of urine cytology on initial follow-up after intravesical Mitomycin-C for superficial bladder cancer. Cancer 57: 2119-2122.

Crawford ED, Lamm DL, Montie JE, Scardino PT, Grossman B, Stanis IK, Smith JA, Sullivan JW (1985). Intravesical Adriamycin for recurrent superficial bladder cancer: a Southwest Oncology Group protocol. J Urol 133: 213A

Debruyne FMJ, van der Meijden APM, Geboers ADH, Franssen MPH, van Leeuwen MJW, Steerenberg PA, de Jong WH, Ruitenberg EJ (1988). BCG (RIVM) versus Mitomycin intravesical therapy in patients with superficial bladder cancer. Urology (suppl.) 31: 20-25.

Eisenberg RB, Roth RB, Schwiensberg MH (1960). Bladder tumors and associated proliferative mucosal lesions. J Urol 84: 544-550.

Farrow GM, Utz DC, Rife CC (1976). Morphological and clinical observations of patients with early bladder cancer treated with local cystectomy. Cancer Res 36: 2495-3002.

Friedell G, Soloway MS, Hilgar AG, Farrow G (1986). Summary of workshop on carcinoma in situ of the bladder. J Urol 136: 1047-1048.

Greene LF, Yalowitz PA (1972). The advisability of concomitant transurethral excision of vesical neoplasm and prostatic hyperplasia. J Urol 107: 445-451.

Heney N, Ahmed S, Flanagan MJ, Frable W, Corder MP, Hafermann MD, Hawkins IR for National Bladder Cancer Collaborative Group A (1983). Superficial bladder cancer: progression and recurrence. J Urol 130: 1083-1086.

Heney NM (1985). First line chemotherapy of superficial bladder cancer: Mitomycin-C versus Thiotepa. Urology (suppl) 26: 27-29.

Herr HW, Pinsky CM, Whitmore Jr WF, Sogani PC, Oettgen HF, Melamed MR (1985). Experience with intravesical Bacillus Calmette-Guérin therapy of superficial bladder tumors.

Urology 25: 119-123.

Herr HW, Laudone VP, Whitmore Jr WF (1987). An overview of intravesical therapy for superficial bladder tumors. J Urol 138: 1363-1386.

Herr HW, Laudone VP, Badalament RA, Friedman BD, Whitmore Jr WF (1988). Bacillus Calmette-Guérin therapy alters progression of superficial bladder cancer. J Urol 139: 299A.

Hinman Jr F (1956). Recurrence of bladder tumors by surgical implantation. J Urol 75: 695-697.

Hudson MA, Ratliff TL, Gillen DP, Haaff EO, Dresner SM, Catalona WJ (1987). Single course versus maintenance Bacillus Calmette-Guérin therapy for superficial bladder tumor: a prospective randomised trial. J Urol 138: 295-298.

Jordan AM, Weingarten J, Murphy WM (1987). Transitional cell neoplasms of the urinary bladder - can biologic potential be predicted from histologic grading? cancer 60: 2766-2774.

Kavoussi LR, Torrence RJ, Gillen DP, Hudson MA, Haaff EO, Dresner SM, Ratliff TL, Catalona WJ (1988). Results of 6 weekly intravesical Bacillus Calmette-Guérin instillations on treatment of superficial bladder tumors. J Urol 139: 935.

Kiefer JH (1953). Bladder tumor recurrence in the urethra: a warning. J Urol 69: 652-655.

Koontz WW, Prout GR, Smith W, Frable WJ, Minnis JE (1981). The use of intravesical thiotepa in the management of non-invasive carcinoma of the bladder. J Urol 125: 307.

Mahadevia PS, Koss LG, Tar IJ (1986). Prostatic involvement in bladder cancer - prostate mapping in 20 cysto-prostatectomy specimens. Cancer 58: 2096-2102.

Mirans HY, Bekirov HM (1987). Granulomatous hepatitis following intravesical Bacillus Calmette-Guérin therapy for bladder carcinoma. J Urol 137: 11-112.

Monti J, Mersky H, Levin HS (1986). Transitonal cell carcinoma of the prostate in a series of cystectomies: incidence and staging problems. J Urol 135: 243A.

Nissenkorn I, Herrod H, Soloway MS (1981). Side effects associated with intravesical Mitomycin-C. J Urol 126: 596-597.

Page BH, Levison VB, Curwen MP (1978). The site of recurrence of non-infiltrating bladder tumors. Brit J Urol 50: 237-244.

Prout GR, Koontz WW Jr, Coombs LJ, Hawkins IR, Friedell GH for National Bladder Cancer Collaborative Group A (1983).

Long term fate of 90 patients with superficial bladder cancer randomly assigned to receive or not to receive Thiotepa. J Urol 130: 677-680.

Rawls WH, Lamm DL, Eyolfson MF (1988). Septic complications in the use of Bacillus Calmette-Guérin for non-invasive transitional cell carcinoma. J Urol 139: 300A.

Schade ROK, Swinney J (1983). The association of urothelial abnormalities with neoplasia: a ten-year follow-up. J Urol 129: 1125-1126.

Silverberg JM, Zarrabi MH (1987). Acute non-lymphocytic leukemia after Thiotepa instillation into the bladder: report of two cases and review of the literature. J Urol 138: 402-403.

Soloway MS, Murphy WM, Rao MK, Cox CE (1978). Serial multiple-site biopsies in patients with bladder cancer. J Urol. 120: 57-59.

Soloway M (1980). Rational for intensive intravesical chemotherapy for superficial bladder cancer. J Urol 123: 461.

Soloway MS, Masters S (1980). Urothelial susceptibility to tumor cell implantation. Cancer 46: 1158-1163.

Soloway MS, Ford KS (1983). Subsequent tumor analysis of 36 patients who have received intravesical Mitomycin-C for superficial bladder cancer. J Urol 130: 74.

Soloway MS (1988). An optical dilator to obviate blind urethral dilatation prior to endoscopic resection. Urology 31: 427-428.

Soto EA, Friedell GH, Tiltman AJ (1977). Bladder cancer as seen in giant histologic sections. Cancer 39: 447-455.

Torti FM, Lum DL, Aston D, MacKenzie N, Faysel M, Shortliffe LD, Freiha F (1987). Superficial bladder cancer: the primacy of grade in the development of invasive disease. J Clin Oncol 5: 125-130.

Weldon TE, Soloway MS (1975). Susceptibility of urothelium to neoplastic cellular implantation. Urology 5: 824-827.

EORTC Genitourinary Group Monograph 6:
BCG in Superficial Bladder Cancer, pages 237–252
© 1989 Alan R. Liss, Inc.

INTRAVESICAL THERAPY COMPARING BCG, ADRIAMYCIN, AND THIO-
TEPA IN 200 PATIENTS WITH SUPERFICIAL BLADDER CANCER: A
RANDOMIZED PROSPECTIVE STUDY

J.A. Martinez-Pineiro, J. Jimenez León, L. Martinez-
Pineiro Jr., L. Fiter, J.A. Mosteiro, J. Navarro,
M.J. García Matres, P., Cárcamo
Service of Urology, La Paz Hospital, Faculty of
Medicine, Universidad Autónoma, Madrid, Spain

INTRODUCTION

Since the initial report by Morales, the efficacy of
intravesical Bacillus Calmette-Guérin (BCG) for the treatment and prophylaxis of recurrence of superficial bladder
cancer has been shown in a number of non-randomized phase
II studies (Morales et al., 1976). An investigation started
in 1975 by our group showed that, of three possible routes
of administration (intralesional, intradermal, and intravesical), intravesical instillations was the most safe and
effective, and it yielded a significant reduction in number
of recurrences and a significant prolongation of the time
to recurrence (Martínez-Pineiro and Muntañola, 1977;
Martínez-Pineiro, 1980, Martínez-Pineiro, 1984).

In 1980, Lamm and Camacho reported the first randomized prospective studies that confirmed the value of intravesical plus percutaneous BCG in reducing bladder tumor
recurrences, compared with transurethral resection (TUR)
alone (Camacho et al., 1980; Lamm et al., 1980). In 1981,
Rodrigues Netto showed that BCG administered orally was
superior to either Thiotepa (TTPA) or TUR (Rodrigues Netto
and Caserta, 1981). Later, another two randomized trials
documented the superiority of adjuvant intravesical BCG to
either TTPA or Doxorubicin (ADM) (Brosman, 1982; Lamm et
al, 1985). Before the publication of those two papers, our
group had begun a trial to compare BCG, TTPA, and ADM; our
first preliminary results were reported in 1985 (Martínez-
Pineiro et al., 1985). We present here the second interim

report of our randomized prospective study, in which the final number of 202 patients has been recruited.

MATERIAL AND METHODS

Since 1980, 202 patients with histologically proven Ta or T1 transitional cell carcinoma (TCC) of the bladder have been enrolled in a randomized prospective trial to compare the prophylactic effects of intravesical instillations of BCG, TTPA, or ADM. The main criterion for exclusion was previous treatment with any of the substances to be tested in the trial. A total of 176 patients are now evaluable, with a median follow-up of 3 years.

After complete TUR of existing tumors, patients were assigned randomly to receive either BCG-Pasteur (Institute Pasteur, Paris) (150 mg in 2 ampules of 75 mg each), TTPA (50 mg) or ADM (50 mg). Each drug was instilled into the bladder in 50 ml of sterile saline solution and kept in the bladder for 1 hour. Instillations were given first within 14 days after TUR, and then every week for the first 4 weeks and once every month for 11 months thereafter (for a total of 15 treatments). If recurrence was histologically confirmed before the end of the treatment, the regimen was restarted (weekly for 4 weeks, and then monthly), but the total duration was limited to a year after the first TUR. If recurrence followed after completion of the treatment, the patient was removed from the study. Similarly, progression of the disease with muscle invasion (T2) or severe toxicity was cause for removal from the study.

The end points used were recurrence rate, time to first recurrence, and progression rate.

Patients were followed with cystoscopy and urinary cytologic studies every 3 months for the first year; if necessary, random biopsies or TUR of suspicious areas took place. Recurrent tumors were resected transurethrally and examined histologically. After the first year, evaluations were performed every 6 months.

Patients were stratified according to stage and grade, size, and number of tumors. The characteristics of the three treatment groups are summarized in Tables 1 and 2. Among the three patient populations, there were no significant differences with regard to age, sex, number, or size and grade of the papillary tumors. However, with regard to Ta category, there was an excess of patients in the TTPA group, although it was not significant (p = 0.07).

TABLE 1. Characteristics of patient groups

Characteristic	ADM	TTPA	BCG	TOTAL
No. patients evaluable	53	56	67	176
Median age (range), years	62 (34-87)	64 (41-82)	65 (30-87)	63.6 (30-87)
Sex:				
Male	47	47	55	149
Female	6	9	12	27
No. tumors:				
Single	31	32	41	104
Multiple	22	24	26	72
Tumor size:				
≤2 cm	19	26	27	72
>2 cm	34	30	40	104
Median folow-up (range), months	40 (5-97)	34 (6-78)	34 (3-92)	36 (3-97)

TABLE 2. Tumor Characteristics

Category	ADM	TTPA	BCG	TOTAL
Ta	6 (2)	14 (5)	8 (2)	28 (9)
T1	47 (17)	42 (17)	59 (23)	148 (57)
G1	33	32	41	106
G2	13	20	20	53
G3	7	4	6	17
Associated CIS	0	1	3	4

Only 28 of the 176 patients (15.9%) had Ta tumors and 148 patients (84.1%) had T1 tumors. Thus, the majority had tumors at high risk for recurrence or progression, and intravesical therapy held the greatest promise of benefit for them. Nine patients had recurrent tumors, owing to the small number, they have been excluded from this analysis, because a comparison with 193 primary tumors would be meaningless. The reason for such a low recruitment of patients with recurrent tumors was the exclusion of patients previously treated with any of the three agents tested.

RESULTS

The overall results after a median follow-up of 3 years (range, 3-97 months) are shown in Tables 3 and 4. The proportion of patients with recurrence was significantly lower in the BCG group, as was the number of new tumors detected per cystoscopy during the follow-up time (Ri/c = no. new tumors/no. cystoscopies) and the number or evaluations with new tumors per month of follow-up (Rec. index 100 pts. months = no. of new tumors x100/months of follow-up). The differences were significant between BCG and ADM and between BCG and TTPA (BCG vs. ADM, p = 0.007; BCG vs. TTPA, p = 0.001; TTPA vs. ADM, not significantly different).

The interval free of disease and the mean time between recurrences were in general very similar for the three therapeutic groups (Table 4).

Four (7.5%) of the 53 patients treated with ADM progressed. One patient developed invasive tumor in the prostatic urethra, one patient developed associated CIS. One progressed to muscle invasion, and one developed distant metastases.

The intervals to progression were 11, 17, 31, and 13 months respectively. Two patients were treated with radical cystectomy; both are alive without disease. Two patients were treated with systemic chemotherapy (MVAC) of whom one has died of metastatic disease. This is the single death of urothelial cancer sofar in this series.

TABLE 3. Effect of intravesical treatment on recurrences in patients followed for a median of 3 years (range, 3-97 months)

Characteristic	ADM (N=53)	TTPA (N=56)	BCG (N=67)	TOTAL (N=176)
No. patients with recurrences (%)	23 (43.4)	20 (35.7)	9 (13.4)	52 (29.5)
No. recurrences (recurrence/patient)	36 (1.57)	30 (1.5)	12 (1.3)	78 (1.5)

TABLE 4. Effect of intravesical treatment on recurrence index and other outcomes

Characteristic	ADM (N=53)	TTPA (N=56)	BCG (N=67)	TOTAL (N=176)
Time to recurrence (range), months	31 (3-45)	28.5 (3-40)	31.3 (3-70)	30.3 (3-70)
Mean time between recurrence, months	34	27	31.6	30.8
Recurrence index/ cystoscopy	0.21	0.16	0.04	0.13
Recurrence index/ 100 patients months	5	3	1	3
No. patients with:				
Progression (%)	4 (7.5)	2 (3.6)	1 (1.5)	7 (4.0)
Cystectomy (%)	2*(3.6)	0 (0)	1[a](1.5)	3 (1.7)
Metastatic disease (%)	1 (1.9)	0 (0)	0 (0)	1 (0.57)
No. non-cancer deaths (%)	0 (0)	1 (1.8)	0 (0)	1 (0.57)

* local progression   [a] contracted bladder

Two (3.6%) of the 56 patients receiving TTPA progressed. One had local urothelial progression from Ta G1 to
T1 G1 tumor at 12 months, which has recurred twice in 36
months; the other had a progression into the muscle from
T1 G1 to T2 G2 at 28 months, after 2 Ta recurrences. He was
treated with TUR and is now receiving BCG instillations.

One (1.5%) of the 67 patients treated with BCG progressed from T1 G2 to T2 G1 at 23 months; he underwent a
repeated TUR and is free of disease after 46 months of
follow-up.

The disease-free-survival according to Kaplan-Meier's
method was significantly better for the BCG group than for
the TTPA group ($p < 0.01$) or the ADM group ($p < 0.001$)
(Fig. 1).

Analysis of the diverse stratifications revealed an
advantage for BCG in most subgroups (Table 5). Particularly
noteworthy are the statistically significant differences in
the disease-free-survival curves of T1 tumors (Fig. 2), G3
tumors (Fig. 3), and multiple tumors (Fig. 4) subgroups,
considered as populations at high risk of recurrence.
Tables 6 and 7 indicate the respective recurrence rates of
single and multiple tumors.

Complications of therapy are outlined in Table 8. The
toxicity of intravesical BCG was notably higher than that
of the other drugs, but side effects generally were mild
and transient, and limited to bladder irritability for 2-3
days. In 16.4% of the patients, cystitis was severe, but
its intensity diminished with the administration of
Isoniazid and non-steroidal anti-inflammatory agents. No
patient had to stop treatment because of cystitis.

One patient in the BCG group with a T1m G2 tumor
developed a contracted bladder at 15 months after having
had three recurrences that were treated with TUR and
additional TTPA instillations for 4 months. He underwent a
cystectomy, and the pathologic examination revealed no
tumor (pT0 pNo), but only fibrosis.

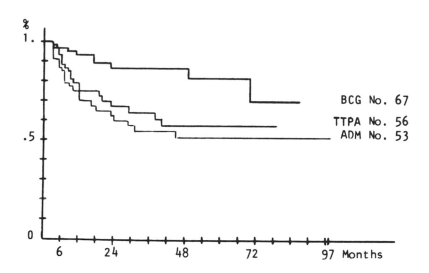

Figure 1. Overall disease-free-survival curves according to Kaplan-Meier. BCG/TTPA p < 0.01; BCG/ADM p < 0.01; TTPA/ADM not significant.

TABLE 5. Overall tumor recurrences according to stage and grade

| | \multicolumn{8}{c}{No. patients with recurrence (%)} |
	ADM		TTPA		BCG		TOTAL	
Ta	0/6	(0.0)	6/14	(42.0)	0/8	(0.0)	6/28	(21.4)
T1	23/47	(48.9)	14/42	(33.3)	9/59	(15.2)	46/148	(31.0)
G1	12/33	(36.3)	14/32	(43.7)	4/41	(9.7)	30/106	(28.3)
G2	6/13	(46.1)	5/20	(25.0)	5/20	(25.0)	16/53	(30.2)
G3	5/7	(71.4)	1/3	(25.0)	0/6	(0.0)	6/17	(35.3)

Statistical significance of differences for T1 tumors: TTPA vs. ADM, not significant; BCG vs. ADM, p = 0.002; BCG vs. TTPA, p = 0.0327.

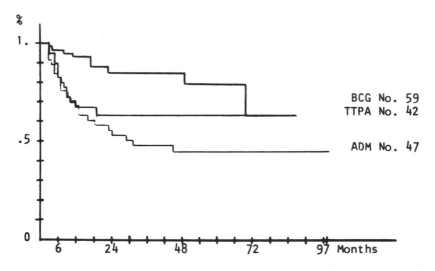

Figure 2. Disease-free-survival curves of patients with T1 tumors. BCG/TTPA p < 0.05; BCG/ADM p < 0.001; TTPA/ADM not significant.

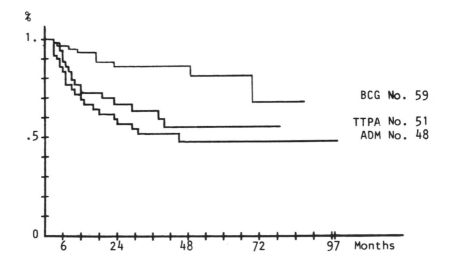

Figure 3. Disease-free-survival curves of patients with G2 tumors. BCG/TTPA p < 0.02; BCG/ADM p < 0.01.

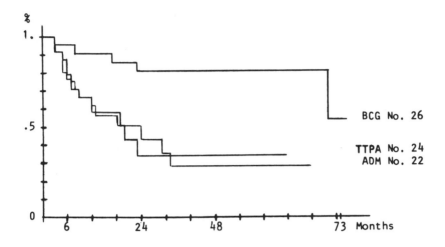

Figure 4. Disease-free-survival curves of patients with multiple tumors. BCG/TTPA p < 0.01; BCG/ADM p < 0.01; TTPA/ADM not significant.

TABLE 6. Recurrences according to stage and multiplicity

| | No. patients with recurrence | | | |
	ADM	TTPA	BCG	TOTAL
Ta Single	0/4 (0.0)	3/9 (33.3)	0/6 (0.0)	3/19 (15.8)
Ta Multiple	0/2 (0.0)	3/5 (60.0)	0/2 (0.0)	3/9 (33.3)
T1 Single	11/30 (36.7)	4/25 (16.0)	4/36 (11.1)	19/91 (20.9)
T1 Multiple	12/17 (70.5)	10/17 (58.8)	5/23 (21.7)	27/57 (47.4)

Statistical significance of difference: T1 Single: TTPA vs. ADM, not significant; BCG vs. ADM, p = 0.013; BCG vs. TTPA, not significant. T1 multiple: TTPA vs. ADM, not significant; BCG vs. ADM, p = 0.002; BCG vs. TTPA, p = 0.016.

TABLE 7. Recurrences of T1 tumors according to grade and multiplicity

| Tumors | No. patients with recurrence | | | |
	ADM	TTPA	BCG	TOTAL
T1 single				
G1	7/14 (41.2)	2/13 (15.4)	3/23 (13.0)	12/53 (22.6)
G2+G3	4/13 (30.8)	2/12 (16.7)	1/13 (7.7)	7/38 (18.4)
T1 multiple				
G1	5/10 (50.0)	7/9 (77.7)	1/11 (9.1)	13/30 (43.3)
G2+G3	7/7 (100)	3/8 (37.5)	4/12 (33.3)	14/27 (51.9)
Associated with CIS	--	1/1 (100)	1/3 (33.3)	2/4 (50.0)

Statistical significance of difference: Single G1: TTPA vs. ADM, not significant; BCG vs. ADM, p = 0.035; BCG vs. TTPA, not significant. Single G2+G3: not significant. Multiple G1: TTPA vs. ADM, not significant; BCG vs. ADM, p = 0.055; BCG vs. TTPA, p = 0.007. Multiple G2+G3: TTPA vs. ADM, p = 0.018; BCG vs. ADM, p = 0.0065; BCG vs. TTPA, not significant.

TABLE 8. Complications of therapy

| Complication | No. patients with recurrence (%) | | |
	ADM	TTPA	BCG
Bladder irritability	7 (13.2)	8 (14.3)	28 (41.8)
Severe cystitis	0 (0.0)	0 (0.0)	11 (16.4)
Epididymitis	0 (0.0)	0 (0.0)	1 (1.5)
Fever	0 (0.0)	0 (0.0)	5 (7.5)
Leukopenia	0 (0.0)	3 (5.4)	0 (0.0)
Thrombopenia	0 (0.0)	1 (1.8)	0 (0.0)
Contracted bladder	0 (0.0)	0 (0.0)	1 (1.5)

DISCUSSION

Our preliminary analysis of the data seems to confirm our previous experience that intravesical BCG can reduce the rate of recurrence of superficial bladder carcinomas treated with TUR (Martínez-Pineiro, 1980; Martínez-Pineiro, 1984) and seems to confirm results of other studies that indicated that BCG is more effective than Thiotepa and Doxorubicin (Brosman, 1982; Lamm, 1985; Rodrigues Netto and Caserta, 1981). Our study has compared BCG simultaneously with ADM and with TTPA -- the latter two among the most widely used drugs for intravesical prophyxis -- at the most commonly used schedules: 50 mg a week for the first month and then monthly for 11 months (Allona et al., 1984; Herr et al, 1987; Kurth et al., 1984; Schulman et al., 1982). We used BCG-Pasteur at the same dose and dilution as in our previous studies (150 mg BCG in 50 ml saline).

After a median follow-up of 36 months (range, 3-97), the rate of patients with recurrence was 43.3% (23/53) in the ADM group, 35.7% (20/56) in the TTPA group, and 13.4% (9/67) in the BCG group (BCG vs. ADM, p = 0.0002; BCG vs. TTPA, p = 0.0037). The recurrence index per 100 patient-months was also significantly lower for BCG than for TTPA and ADM (BCG vs. ADM, p = 0.007; BCG vs. TTPA, p = 0.001). BCG was superior in preventing recurrences of high-grade (G2+G3) tumors and T1 multiple tumors the groups at highest risk for recurrence (Allona et al., 1984; Herr et al., 1987). Considering that recurrence rates within the first year vary from 30% in patients with solitary T1 tumors to more than 90% in patients with multiple tumors (Allona et al., 1984; England et al., 1981; Herr et al., 1987; Lutzeyer et al., 1982), the benefit of using BCG is clear; ADM was much less efficacious, and TTPA was in between the two in efficacy.

Progression, either local progression resistant to TUR and intravesical therapy or muscle invasion with or without metastasis, was also notably prevented by BCG (1.5%) and by TTPA to a lesser degree (3.6%). Without prophylaxis, around 5-30% of all patients with superficial tumor exhibit progression of the disease; and in the particular case of T1 G3 tumors, 45-50% progress to muscle invasion within 3 years (England et al., 1981; Lutzeyer et al., 1982).

The 1.5% progression rate yielded by BCG in the 67 patients in our study, followed for a median of 31.3 months, is comparable to the 3% overall progression rate found by Lamm and associates in a series of 64 patients treated with shorter courses and followed for a median of 27 months (Reynold et al., 1985).

Considering the recurrence and progression rates of patients with the most dangerous tumors -- T1 associated with carcinoma in situ, which usually recur and progress in up to 80% (Althausen et al., 1976; Utz and Farrow, 1980) -- we found two recurrences in four cases. One tumor recurred at 3 months in a patients treated with TTPA, and another at 70 months among three patients treated with BCG. Both patients are still free of disease. The other two patients had never recurrences and are in complete remission at 17 and 24 months after entry into the study.

The most important objective of intravesical therapy for superficial bladder tumors is prevention of tumor progression from a non-invasive tumor to muscle-infiltrating cancer (Herr et al., 1987). We feel that our study documents the value of BCG in retarding that event, at least after 3 years of follow-up. We hope that the final analysis, at 5 years, will confirm the preliminary data.

The second most important objective, reduction of the rate of recurrence, seems also to have been achieved with BCG and TTPA; BCG was superior. That finding accords with the results of a review of randomized clinical trials by Herr, who reported an overall potential benefit for chemotherapy of 16%, compared with 52% for BCG (Herr et al., 1987).

Toxicity in our study has been modest, despite the long duration of treatment (1 year). The most important complication was bladder contraction in one patient among the 67 patients treated with BCG, which occurred after the end of treatment. In another 11 cases (16.4%), granulomatous cystitis developed and needed treatment with Isoniazid. No patient had to interrupt treatment because of toxicity.

Although repeated administration of intravesical therapy, in particular with BCG, admittedly increased the duration and severity of cystitis (Lamm et al., 1986), without additional therapeutic benefit over short courses (Badalament et al., 1987), the controversy of short-term versus long-term prophylaxis is still open to discussion.

In conclusion, our preliminary results show that at the dose, schedule, and duration used in our study, BCG is superior to ADM or TTPA in retarding progression and reducing recurrence of superficial bladder cancer.

SUMMARY

This report presents the second interim analysis of data from a randomized prospective trial that compares the prophylactic effect of 15 intravesical instillations of 50 mg Doxorubicin (ADM), 50 mg of Thiotepa (TTPA), or 150 mg of Bacillus Calmette-Guérin (BCG) against recurrence and progression of superficial transitional cell bladder cancer. Of 202 enrolled patients, 176 patients are currently evaluable after a mean follow-up of 3 years (range, 3-97 months).

The number of patients with recurrence was significantly lower in the BCG group (9/67) than in the ADM group (23/53, $p = 0.002$) or the TTPA group (20/56, $p = 0.003$). The overall recurrence index per 100 patient-months was also significantly lower for the BCG group (BCG vs. ADM, $p = 0.07$; BCG vs. TTPA, $p = 0.001$; TTPA vs. ADM, not significant).

BCG was superior in preventing recurrence and progression of high risk tumors (T1, G2-3, multiple growth, and tumors associated with carcinoma in situ) The recurrence in this group of high risk tumors was for ADM treated patients 12/17, for TTPA treated patients 10/17 and for BCG treated patients 5/23 (BCG vs. ADM, $p = 0.002$; BCG vs. TTPA, $p = 0.016$; TTPA vs. ADM, not significant).

Toxicity of intravesical BCG was higher than that of the other drugs, but not limiting the treatment. Bladder irritability occurred in 42% of the patients, granulomatous cystitis in 16.4%, and bladder contraction in 1.5% of the patients.

Two patients of the ADM group (2/53 = 3.8%) underwent radical cystectomy for local urothelial progression. One

patient (1.9%) in the same group died of distant
metastases.

The preliminary results suggest that BCG is significantly superior to the chemotherapeutic agents ADM and TTPA
when used as an adjuvant intravesical therapy in superficial bladder cancer.

ACKNOWLEDGMENT

We wish to thank Rosario Madero Jarabo of the
Biostatistics Unit of La Paz Hospital for her help and
advice in the statistical analysis.

REFERENCES

Allona A, Santos I, Polo G, Diza R, Gonzalez M, Zuloaga A,
    Martinez JL, Rodrigues J, Duarte J, Megino JF, Gomez F,
    Martinez-Pineiro JA (1984). Resultados preliminares de un
    estudio randomizado entre ADM y Thiotepa intravesical en
    el tratamiento de los tumores superficialis de vejiga.
    Arch Esp Urol 37: 113.
Althausen AF, Prout GRJ, Daly JJ (1976). Non-invasive
    papillary carcinoma of the bladder associated with
    carcinoma in situ. J Urol 116: 575.
Badalament RA, Herr HW, Wong GY, Gnecco C, Pinsky CM,
    Whitmore Jr WF, Fair WR, Oettgen HF (1987). A prospective
    randomized trial of maintenance vs non-maintenance intra-
    vesical BCG therapy for superficial bladder cancer.
    J Clin Oncol 5: 441.
Brosman SA (1982). Experience with Bacillus Calmette-Guérin
    in patients with superficial bladder carcinoma. J Urol
    128: 27.
Camacho FJ, Pinsky CM, Kerr D, Whitmore Jr WF, Oettgen HF
    (1980). Treatment of superficial bladder cancer with
    intravesical BCG. Proc Amer Ass Cancer Res and Amer Soc
    Clin Oncol 21: 359.
England HR, Paris AMI, Blandy JP (1981). The correlation of
    T1 bladder tumor history with prognoses and follow-up
    requirements. Br J Urol 53: 593-597.
Herr HW, Laudone VP, Whitmore Jr WF (1987). An overview of
    intravesical therapy for superficial bladder tumors. J
    Urol 138: 1363-1386.
Kurth KH, Schröder FH, Tunn UAR, Pavone Macaluso M,

Debruyne F, de Pauw M, Dalesio O, ten Kate F, and members of the EORTC GU Co-operative Group (1984). Adjuvant chemotherapy of superficial transitional cell bladder carcinoma: preliminary results of an EORTC randomized trial comparing Doxorubicin hydrochloride, ethoglucid and transurethral resection alone. J Urol 132: 258.

Lamm DL, Thor DE, Harris SC, Reyna JA, Stogdill VD, Radwin HM (1980). Bacillus Calmette-Guérin immunotherapy of superficial bladder cancer. J Urol 124: 38-43.

Lamm DL, Crawford ED, Montie JE, Scardino PT, Stanisic TH, Grossman HB, Sullivan JW (1985). BCG versus Adriamycin in the treatment of transitional cell carcinoma in situ: A Southwest Oncology Group Study. J Urol 133: 184A.

Lamm DL, Stogdill VD, Stogdill BJ, Crispen RG (1986). Complications of Bacillus Calmette-Guérin immunotherapy in 1278 patients with bladder cancer. J Urol 135: 272.

Lutzeyer W, Rubben H, Dahm H (1982). Prognostic parameters in superficial bladder cancer: an analysis of 315 cases. J Urol 127: 250-252.

Martinez-Pineiro JA, Muntanola P (1977). Non-specific immunotherapy with BCG vaccine in bladder tumors. A Preliminary report. Eur Urol 3: 11.

Martinez-Pineiro JA (1980). BCG vaccine in the treatment of non-infiltrating papillary tumors of the bladder. In Pavone Macaluso M, Smith PH, Edsmyr F (eds.): "Bladder tumors and other topics in Urological Oncology," New York: Plenum Press, pp 175.

Martinez-Pineiro JA (1984). BCG vaccine in superficial bladder tumors: eight years later. Eur Urol 10. 93.

Martinez-Pinoiro JA, de la Pena J, Hidalyu L, Cisneros J, Jiménez Léon J, Machuca J, Perdices C (1985). Tumores vesicales superficiales. Resultados preliminares de un estudio prospectivo comparando BCG, Adriamicina y Thiotepa endovesical. Arch Esp Urol 38: 545.

Morales A, Eidinger D, Bruce AW (1976). Intracavitary Bacillus Calmette-Guérin in the treatment of superficial bladder tumors. J Urol 116: 18.

Reynold RH, Stogdill VD, Lamm DL (1985). Disease progression in BCG treated patients with transitional cell carcinoma of the bladder. J Urol 133: 211A.

Rodriguez Netto Jr N, Caserta F (1981). Estudio comparativo del tratamiento en el carcinoma vesical. RTU, THIO, BCG. Arch Esp Urol 34: 369.

Schulman CC, Robinson M, Denis L, Smith P, Viggiano G, de Pauw M, Dalesio O, Sylvester R (1982). Prophylactic chemotherapy of superficial transitional cell bladder carcinoma: an EORTC randomized trial comparing Thio-tepa, VM-26 and TUR alone. Eur Urol 8: 207.

Utz DC, Farrow GM (1980). Management of carcinoma in situ of the bladder: the case for surgical management. Urol Clin N Amer 7: 533.

EORTC Genitourinary Group Monograph 6:
BCG in Superficial Bladder Cancer, pages 253–261
© 1989 Alan R. Liss, Inc.

LOW-DOSE BCG-PASTEUR STRAIN IN THE TREATMENT OF SUPERFICIAL BLADDER CANCER: PRELIMINARY RESULTS

Francesco Pagano, Pierfrancesco Bassi, Claudio Milani, Agostino Meneghini, Giuseppe Tuccitto, Antonio Garbeglio, Stefano Guazzieri
Department of Urology, University of Padova, Padova, Italy

INTRODUCTION

Since the 1976 pilot study of Morales the therapeutic and prophylactic effects of intravesical Bacillus Calmette-Guérin (BCG) on superficial bladder cancer have been definitively confirmed (Brosman, 1985; Debruyne and van der Meijden, 1987; Herr et al., 1986; Kavoussi et al., 1988; Kelley et al., 1985; Lamm, 1985, 1987; Martinez Pineiro, 1984; Morales et al., 1976; Steg et al., 1986). Besides its documented effect in reducing tumor recurrence rates and the need for radical surgery, many aspects of the treatment remain unclear (Lamm, 1987): the mechanism of action is unknown, and various frequencies and durations of administration, doses, and strains are used.

The main purpose of our study was to evaluate the efficacy and relative toxicity of a low-dose (75 mg) BCG-Pasteur regimen in the treatment and prevention of superficial bladder cancer. We report here the preliminary results of our randomized study, which continues.

MATERIALS AND METHODS

Patients selection

Patients eligible for BCG treatment were divided in two groups: prophylaxis (prevention of papillary recurrences after transurethral resection) and therapy (treatment of carcinoma in situ).

Multiple papillary tumors

Since February 1986, we have randomized 108 patients with multiple papillary superficial bladder tumors (at least three tumors at stage Ta, T1a, or T1b) to receive either transurethral resection (TUR) alone (50 patients, the control group) or TUR plus BCG (58 patients, the prophylaxis group). All visible lesions were removed by TUR. Multiple biopsies of abnormal- and normal-looking bladder mucosa and bladder washing cytologic tests after TUR were carried out regularly. In the prophylaxis group, 17 (29%) patients were treated with intravesical chemotherapy (Mitomycin or Adriamycin) before entering the study.

Carcinoma in situ

In the same period, 42 patients (therapy group) with carcinoma in situ (CIS), with or without concomitant multi-focal papillary tumors, were treated with intravesical BCG. Bladder-washing cytologic tests, multiple biopsies on abnormal- and normal-looking mucosa, and TUR of papillary lesions (when associated) were performed in all patients. No randomization was done, because of the high progression potential and the difficulty of controlling CIS with TUR alone). In this group, 12 (29%) patients were unsuccess-fully treated with intravesical chemotherapy (Mitomycin or Adriamycin) before entering the trial.

Follow-up

Follow-up of patients in both groups has been 6–30 months (mean, 14.3 months).

BCG therapy

The induction course consisted of 75 mg (5×10^8 colony froming units (CFU)) of BCG-Pasteur (Institute Pasteur-Paris, France) given intravesically in 50 cc of saline solution and patients kept the BCG in their bladder for 2 hours. The treatment was initiated within 3 weeks after TUR. BCG was administered weekly for 6 consecutive weeks. No intradermal inoculations of the vaccine were given. When tumor was not demonstrated at cystoscopy after the 6 week induction course, maintenance therapy was started and was administered monthly by instillation for the first year and thereafter every 3 months for the second year. An additional 6-weeks course of therapy was given when tumor recurrence or persistence without progression was observed after the induction course. Colony-forming units of BCG-Pasteur lots were counted periodically to confirm the vaccine viability. We performed serial endoscopic evaluations with bladder-washing cytologic tests and multiple biopsies in abnormal- and normal-looking bladder mucosa in all patients after treatment. If papillary tumors were present they were removed by TUR. All posttreatment clinical evaluations were carried out 30-40 days after the last BCG instillation. PPD skin tests were not performed.

Response criteria

Results were classified as complete response or no response; partial responses were not considered. The criteria for complete response in both prophylaxis and therapy groups were absence of tumor recurrence and negative cytologic findings. Histologic evidence alone or positive cytologic findings alone were considered as no response. In the prophylaxis group, the recurrence rate was estimated as follows:

$$\text{Recurrence rate} = \frac{\text{No. of positive cystoscopic findings}}{\text{Overall follow-up in months}} \times 100$$

RESULTS

We report here the preliminary results in patients with 12 months follow-up (30 patients in the papillary control group, 33 patients in the prophylaxis group, and 27 patients in the CIS therapy group) and with 18 months follow-up (15 patients in the papillary control group, 19 patients in the prophylaxis group, and 12 patients in the CIS therapy group). Toxicity related to the treatment was eveluated in all 98 BCG-treated (58 papillary tumors and 40 CIS) patients.

BCG in multiple papillary tumors

In the prophylaxis group (TUR plus BCG), 85% (28/33) of evaluable patients showed complete response at 12 months, compared with 17% (5/30) in the control group (TUR alone). After 18 months, the percentages were 89% (17/19) and 13% (2/15) respectively. A complete response was obtained after induction therapy in 21 (63%) patients. The recurrence rates observed in prophylaxis and control groups were 3.3% and 12.4%, respectively. The small number of patients prevents attaching statistical significance to the correlation between stage or grade and tumor progression or recurrence.

With regard to the previous endovesical chemotherapy (ADM or MMC), a complete response at 12 months was obtained in 87.5% (14/16) of the previously untreated patients and in 76% (13/17) of those previously treated. No significant statistical differences were demonstrated.

Recurrence was reported in two patients 18 months after initial complete response to BCG therapy; no tumor progression was seen after initial response. Tumor progression during BCG therapy was observed in 5.2% (3/58) of all patients with multiple papillary tumors in the trial, compared with 20% (10/50) in the control group. In two of three BCG treated patients who experienced progression, squamous or glandular metaplasia had been evident before therapy.

BCG in carcinoma in situ

A complete response was observed after 12 months in 78% (21/27) of patients with BCG therapy and after 18 months in 83% (10/12). After the induction course 52% (14/27) were complete responders; 54% (7/13) of patients who had an additional course of BCG therapy showed complete response at 12 months. Of 12 patients (44%) previously treated with endovesical chemotherapy (MMC or ADM), 92% (11) had complete response after 12 months, compared with 67% (10/15) of untreated patients. No statistical significance was evident, because of the small number of patients. Of all 42 patients, 10% (4) experienced tumor progression during BCG therapy and underwent radical cystectomy. One patient who discontinued therapy because of toxicity during the additional course and two non-responders underwent the same treatment. Interesting histologic findings came from the patients who experienced tumor progression: glandular, or squamous metaplasia (three patients) was evident before immunotherapy was initiated.

TABLE 1. Complete response at 12 and 18 months of follow-up

Group	Complete response	
	12 month follow-up	18 month follow-up
Papillary control	5/30 (17%)	2/15 (13%)
Prophylaxis	28/33 (85%)	17/19 (89%)
Therapy (CIS)	21/27 (78%)	10/12 (83%)

TABLE 2. Evidence of complications (%) according to dose and "substrain" of BCG-Pasteur

	Cystitis			Fever
	overall	slight	severe	
"Paris" Pasteur-BCG 75 mg - current series (N= 98)	26	22	4	16
"Paris" Pasteur-BCG 150 mg - Steg et al., 1986 (N= 89)	"frequently"	--	--	8
- Martinez-Pineiro, 1984 (N= 33)	54	48	6	75
BCG-Armand Frappier (Pasteur) 120 mg - Lamm et al., 1986 (N= 127)	91	--	--	28
- Kavoussi et al., 1988 (N= 104)	91	--	--	39
- Morales et al., 1986 (N= 82)	--	--	10	70
- Herr et al., 1985 (N= 88)	51	--	--	44

Toxicity

The overall incidence of cystitis in our series (Table 2) was 26% -- slight cystitis (irritative disturbances lasting no more than 24 hours) in 22% and severe cystitis (irritative disturbances lasting for more than 24 hours and leading to request for a symptomatic treatment) in 4%. Persistent hematuria (more than 24 hours), prostatitis, and orchi-epididymitis were observed in 3%, 2%, and 2% of patients, respectively. One patient had a contracted bladder early after the induction course; no systemic BCG-itis, hepatic or pulmonary granulomatosis, death, or urethral obstruction was reported in our series. Associated toxicity, however, was severe enough to interrupt treatment in two cases and to delay instillation in two. No patient in the maintenance group required a dose reduction.

DISCUSSION

The preliminary results of this randomized study demonstrate the effectiveness of a low-dose BCG regimen in the prevention of papillary tumor recurrence and in the therapy of carcinoma in situ of the bladder.

Percentage of complete response (89% in the prophylaxis group and 83% in the therapy group at 18 months of follow-up) are similar to those reported in previous studies with different strains (Tice, Frappier, Connaught) and schedules of BCG administration. Comparison of results is therefore difficult. Comparison of our data with those reported by Steg and Martinez-Pineiro, who used BCG-Pasteur in similar patient populations, confirm the value of a low-dose regimen (Martinez-Pineiro, 1984; Steg et al., 1986). Steg, who used 150 mg of BCG weekly for 6 weeks plus a maintenance course, reported complete response rates of 79% and 75% in patients with carcinoma in situ and papillary tumors respectively. Martinez-Pineiro, in a longer follow-up experience with combined intravesical BCG therapy (150 mg BCG-Pasteur a week for a month plus a maintenance course) and intradermal BCG therapy, reported complete response in 49%.

In our experience, previous unsuccessful endovesical chemotherapy did not seem to affect the clinial response to BCG treatment; the data appear similar to those reported by others (Brosman, 1982; Soloway et al., 1986).

No definitive conclusions could be drawn in regards to the predictive value of grade and stage, because of the small number of patients. The value of an additional course of therapy after initial failure was confirmed in our series.

Tumor progression was more frequent in the control group (20%) than in the CIS and papillary tumor groups (10% and 5%, respectively). The benefit of BCG therapy in reducing tumor progression or improving patient survival has not been established. Preliminary and limited data suggest that BCG therapy will reduce tumor progression (Lamm, 1987). No conclusion can be drawn on the basis of our series, because of the short period of follow-up. The predictive role of squamous and grandular metaplasia before BCG therapy in patients who did not respond to treatment and who experienced tumor progression has to be confirmed in a larger series of patients. If confirmed, this finding could be considered to be related to a poor prognosis and could suggest early alternative therapeutic choices.

The low-dose regimen achieved significant therapeutic results with decreased toxicity. Toxicity is the most threatening side effect of BCG therapy: its incidence and importance explain the frequency of treatment interruption and delays. In our series (Table 2), slight and severe cystitis (total, 26%), fever (16%), and hematuria (3%) were less frequent than in previous reports (Herr, 1985; Kavoussi et al., 1988; Lamm et al., 1986; Morales, 1986). In a review of 1,274 BCG treated patients Lamm reported that 91% had cystitis, 28% fever of 102°F or higher and 48% hematuria (Lamm et al., 1986). Comparison of our data with those reported by others, who used "Paris" BCG-Pasteur, confirms a significant reduction in the incidence of the side effects (Martinez-Pineiro, 1984; Steg et al., 1986). Similar data were reported by Debruyne and van der Meijden, who used BCG-RIVM (Debruyne and van der Meijden, 1987). The incidence of major complications appeared insignificant in our series. Our data definitively confirmed the correlation between dose and toxicity.

CONCLUSIONS

Low doses (75 mg) of BCG-Pasteur were effective in the treatment of superficial papillary tumors and carcinoma in situ of the bladder.

Incidence of complete response, recurrence, and progression are similar to those reported elsewhere.

Toxicity related to this treatment regimen appears to be of a lower incidence than that observed when a higher dose was administered.

Previous intravescial chemotherapy does not seem to affect response rate.

Our date must be replicated in a larger series of patients with a longer follow-up. It appears, however, justified to propose low-dose treatment with BCG for superficial bladder cancer. Definitive success of BCG therapy -- greater benefits with minimal toxicity -- should be established if greater efforts are directed toward the improvement of prediction of response to the treatment and adjustment of the BCG regimen according to tumor behavior. Earlier determination of the number of viable bacilli required for the highest success rate of BCG immunotherapy with low toxicity would be successful. Eventually, manufacturers must guarantee with substantial reliability the number of viable bacilli per ampule, if researchers are to determine the optimal number of viable bacilli required for successful BCG immunotherapy.

ACKNOWLEDGMENT

We thank Marina Calore for her editorial assistance in the preparation of this manuscript.

REFERENCES

Brosman SA (1982). Experience with Bacillus Calmette-Guérin in patients with superficial bladder carcinoma. J Urol 128: 27.

Brosman SA (1985). The use of Bacillus Calmette-Guérin in the therapy of bladder carcinoma in situ. J Urol 134: 36.

Debruyne FMJ, van der Meijden APM (1987). BCG vs Mitomycin-C intravesical therapy in patients with superficial bladder cancer: first results of a randomized prospective trial. J Urol 137: 179.

Herr HW, Pinsky CM, Whitmore Jr WF, Sogani PC, Oettgen HF, Melamed MR (1985). Experience with intravesical Bacillus

Calmette-Guérin of superficial bladder tumors. Urology 25: 119.

Herr HW, Pinsky CM, Whitmore Jr WF, Sogani PC, Oettgen HF, Melamed MR (1986). Long-term effect of intravesical Bacillus Calmette-Guérin on flat carcinoma in situ of the bladder. J Urol 135: 265.

Kavoussi LR, Torrence RJ, Gillen DP, Hudson MA, Haaff EO, Dresner SM, Ratliff TL, Catalona WJ (1988). Results of 6 weekly intravesical Bacillus Calmette-Guérin instillations on treatment of superficial bladder tumors. J Urol 139: 935.

Kelley DR, Ratliff TL, Catalona WJ, Shapiro A, Lage JM, Bauer WC, Haaff EO, Dresner SM (1985). Intravesical Bacillus Calmette-Guérin therapy for superficial bladder cancer: effect of Bacillus Calmette-Guérin viability on treatment results. J Urol 134: 4.

Lamm DL (1985) Bacillus Calmette-Guérin immunotherapy for bladder cancer. J Urol 134: 40.

Lamm DL, Stogdill VD, Stogdill BJ, Crispen RG (1986). Complications of Bacillus Calmette-Guérin immunotherapy in 1278 patients with bladder cancer. J Urol 135: 272.

Lamm DL (1987). BCG immunotherapy for superficial bladder cancer. In Ratliff TL, Catalona WJ (eds): "Genitourinary cancer," Boston: Martinus Nijhoff Publishers, pp 205-224.

Martinez-Pineiro JA (1984). BCG vaccine in superficial bladder tumors: eight years later. Eur Urol 10: 93.

Morales A, Eidinger D, Bruce AW (1976). Intracavitary Bacillus Calmette-Guérin in the treatment of superficial bladder tumors. J Urol 116: 10.

Morales A, Nickel JG (1986). Immunotherapy of superficial bladder cancer with BCG. World J Urol. 3: 209.

Soloway MS, Murphy WM, Perry A (1986). BCG treatment for Thiotepa of Mitomycin-C failures. J Urol 135: 184A.

Steg A, Leleu C, Boccon-Gibod L, Debre B (1986). Traitement des tumeurs superficielles et des carcinomes in situ de vessie par la BCG thérapie intra-vésicale. Ann Urol 20: 26.

EORTC Genitourinary Group Monograph 6:
BCG in Superficial Bladder Cancer, pages 263–270
© 1989 Alan R. Liss, Inc.

ADRIAMYCIN VERSUS BCG IN SUPERFICIAL BLADDER CANCER: A SOUTHWEST ONCOLOGY GROUP STUDY

D.L. Lamm, J Crissmann, B. Blumenstein, E.D. Crawford, J. Montie, P. Scardino, H.B. Grossman, T. Stanisic, J. Smith, J. Sullivan, M. Sarosdy
Department of Urology, West Virginia University, Morgantown, USA

INTRODUCTION

The classic approach to the prevention of recurrence and progression in patients with superficial transitional cell carcinoma of the bladder has been the intravesical instillation of chemotherapeutic agents. This approach dates to 1955 when Thiotepa was first instilled intravesically. Since that time, intravesical Thiotepa has become the standard for comparison of treatments. Newer chemotherapies, including Epodyl, Adriamycin, and Mitomycin-C, have held promise of increased efficacy. Complete response rates in the treatment of residual bladder cancer suggest that these agents are more effective: while the complete response for Thiotepa is 29%, complete response is reported in 55% of patients treated with Epodyl, 38% of those treated with Adriamycin, and 49% of those treated with Mitomycin-C (Kowalkowski and Lamm, 1988). Controlled trials, however, have generally failed to demonstrate superiority of any of the newer chemotherapies over Thiotepa. While controlled studies still need to be completed, Adriamycin has historically had the highest response in the treatment of carcinoma in situ of the bladder. Reported complete response rates are as high as 88% and average 49% in 88 patients (Kowalkowski and Lamm, 1988).

Following Morales' report of a 12 fold reduction in tumor recurrence in patients given intravesical and percutaneous BCG and the confirmation of the efficacy of BCG in randomized prospectively controlled studies (Brosman, 1982; Camacho et al., 1982; Lamm, 1985), BCG immunotherapy has become an increasingly popular treatment modality. Complete response rates with BCG are reported to be 59% in 124 patients in combined series (Kowalkowski and Lamm, 1988). Two controlled studies have suggested that BCG is superior to intravesical Thiotepa, and in 177 reported patients with carcinoma in situ complete response occurred in 86%. To confirm the high efficacy of BCG in the treatment of superficial and in situ carcinoma of the bladder and compare its efficacy with ADM, a randomized prospective multicenter trial was initiated by the Southwest Oncology Group.

METHODS

Beginning in January, 1983, 285 patients with transitional cell carcinoma of the bladder with 2 recurrences in the most recent 12 months and/or carcinoma in situ were enrolled from 46 separate institutions. Patients were stratified by the presence or absence of carcinoma in situ and the presence or absence of previous chemotherapy treatment and then randomized by central computer to receive Adriamycin (ADM) or Connaught substrain BCG. Of the 285 patients registered 44 (15 ADM, 29 BCG) were later considered to be ineligible: 12 due to incomplete resection of papillary tumor, 9 due to pathologic review showing muscle invasive tumor, 8 due to inadequate histology, 4 due to the presence of additional non-transitional tumors of the bladder, and 3 due to only 1 recurrence in the most recent 12 months. Two hundred twenty-seven patients (115 ADM, 112 BCG) were considered to be evaluable for toxicity and 228 (119 ADR, 109 BCG) were considered to be evaluable for response. One hundred six of these patients (55 ADM, 51 BCG) had carcinoma in situ and 122 (64 ADM, 58 BCG) had papillary grade 1-4, stage Ta or T1 transitional cell carcinoma.

Patients in both groups were similar with respect to age (66.8 in both groups, range 24 to 95), sex (81% male ADM, 76% male BCG), and race (80% caucasian ADM, 90% BCG). Stage Ta tumors were present in 57% of ADM treated patients and 43% of BCG treated patients, and stage T1 tumors in 43% and 57% respectively. Tumor grade was similarly distributed among groups: grade 1 tumors comprised 12% of patients in the ADM group and 10% of the BCG group; grade II tumors 45% and 44% respectively; and grade III tumors 43% and 46% respectively.

RESULTS

Toxicity

No significant difference in overall toxicity was observed between groups. Moderate cystitis was seen in 20% of patients treated with ADM and 29% of patients treated with BCG. Fever was seen in the BCG group only, and affected 13% of the patients. Malaise was seen in both groups, but was more common in the BCG group (12%) than in the ADM group (2%). Arthralgia, which has been previously associated with BCG treatment occurred in 2% of the BCG-treated patients. Arthralgia has not been formerly associated with ADM instillation but was seen in 1% of our patients. Mucositis (1%) and leukopenia (1%) were limited to the ADM group.

Severe toxicity was also seen with equal frequency in both groups. Four patients in the ADM group and 3 patients in the BCG group withdrew from the protocol because of toxicity. Major bleeding after treatment occurred in 7% of patients in both groups. Cystitis graded as severe occurred in 6% (ADM) and 4% (BCG) respectively. High fever with chills occurred in 3% of the BCG group and one patient (1%) developed ureteral obstruction.

Tumor recurrence

In patients with stage Ta and T1 tumors the primary end point for comparison of treatment efficacy was time to first tumor recurrence. Illustrated in Figure 1 is the Kaplan Meier time to recurrence curves for each group. Mean time to recurrence for the ADM group was 10 months; mean time to recurrence for the BCG group was 22 months. This prolongation of disease free interval was statistically significant, by 2 tailed log rank testing, at the $p = 0.006$ level. The curves clearly illustrate the relative advantage of BCG treatment. In this relatively high-risk group of patients with previously confirmed rapidly recurring disease or co-existing carcinoma in situ 79% of patients treated with ADM had tumor recurrence versus 57% of patients treated with BCG.

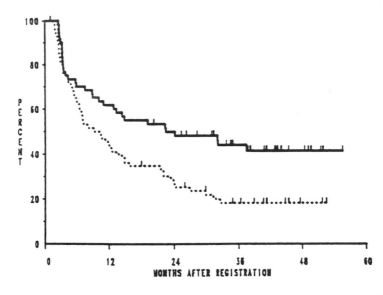

Figure 1. Illustrated is the highly significant (p = 0.006), log rank prolongation of time to recurrence with BCG (solid line) compared to Adriamycin (dotted line).

Tumor recurrence was further compared in patients who had previously been treated with and subsequently failed intravesical chemotherapy with Thiotepa or Mitomycin-C. Of the 127 patients with stage Ta or T1 transitional cell carcinoma, 78 (61%) had been previously treated with intravesical chemotherapy. Forty one of these patients randomized to ADM treatment, of whom 36 (88%) had tumor recurrence. Thirty seven randomized to BCG treatment and 23 of these (62%) had tumor recurrence. In patients who had not had previous chemotherapy, 17 of 26 patients (65%) randomized to ADM had tumor recurrence compared with 11 of 23 patients (48%) who randomized to BCG treatment. The time to recurrence curves for these 4 groups of patients is illustrated in Figure 2. Both of the BCG treatment subgroups had rates of tumor recurrence which were less than the ADM groups. Mean time to recurrence for the ADM group with and without previous chemotherapy treatment were 7 and 13 months respectively. Mean time to recurrence for the BCG treatment groups with and without previous chemotherapy treatment were in excess of 50 months (not yet reached) and 22 months.

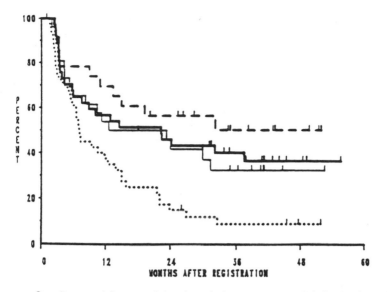

Figure 2. Separating patients into groups which had prior chemotherapy and those which had no prior chemotherapy reveals a consistent advantage for patients receiving BCG. Prolongation of time to recurrence was longest (>50 months) for the BCG treated patients who had not received prior chemotherapy (dashed line), followed by the BCG treated patients who had received prior chemotherapy (22 months, thick solid line), followed by Adriamycin treated patients without previous chemotherapy (13 months, thin solid line), and finally Adriamycin treated patients with previous chemotherapy (7 months, dotted line).

Carcinoma in situ

Unlike patients with papillary or solid tumors who were evaluable for prophylaxis against tumor recurrence, patients with carcinoma in situ were considered to be evaluable for response to therapy. Patients with previous Ta and T1 tumors in addition to carcinoma in situ were also included in this evaluation. Only complete response to treatment, defined as biopsy confirmation of no residual carcinoma in situ as well as no recurrence of papillary or solid transitional cell carcinoma, was considered. One hundred and nine patients had carcinoma in situ, of whom 57 randomized to ADM and 52 randomized to BCG. Complete response was seen in 27 patients (47%) treated with ADM and 37 patients (71%) treated with BCG. Increasing extent of disease was found in 37% of patients in the ADM group and 15% of patients in the BCG group.

In patients with prior chemotherapy, complete resolution of carcinoma in situ was seen in 60% in the ADM group and 79% in the BCG group. In the absence of prior chemotherapy, surprisingly, only 33% of patients had complete response to Adriamycin and 64% had complete response to BCG.

Survival

No significant difference in survival between treatment groups or disease categories were noted. Overall, 198 of 240 patients (82.5%) survived with a median follow-up of 3 years. In the ADM group, 102 of 126 patients (81%) are alive and in the BCG group 96 of 114 patients (84%) are alive. In patients with carcinoma in situ 97 of 114 patients (86%) evaluable for survival are alive, 8 of 59 (86%) in the ADM group and 8 of 54 (85%) in the BCG group. In patients with Ta or T1 tumors, 112 of 127 patients (88%) survived, including 52 of 67 patients (78%) treated with ADM and 50 of 60 patients (83%) treated with BCG.

DISCUSSION

The efficacy of BCG has been confirmed in multiple studies, but its relative efficacy and toxicity in comparison to intravesical chemotherapy has been less certain. Historical reviews provide limited data regarding both efficacy and toxicity since criteria for treatment, disease status, and criteria for determination of both response to treatment and degree of toxicity vary with each investigator and each protocol. A randomized protocol therefore is far superior and can provide statistically as well as clinically significant comparisons.

BCG has been considered to be the most toxic of currently-employed intravesical therapies. While recent reports support this concept in that severe and even fatal septic complications of BCG can occur (Rawls et al, 1988; Steg et al, 1988), the current study suggests that the majority of patients tolerate BCG as well as ADM.

In the prevention of tumor recurrence, historical series suggest BCG is among the best of agents currently available. Clearly relative efficacy, however, cannot be calculated on the basis of historical comparisons of patients with different characteristics treated with varying protocols. Our data confirm that BCG provides improved protection against tumor recurrence when compared with ADM. This observation is supported, as well, by controlled series which have compared BCG and ADM respectively with control patients treated with transurethral resection (TUR) alone. In two ADM studies, only one reported ADM to be significantly superior to TUR alone, and ADM reduced tumor recurrence by only 13% relative to controls (Lamm, in press). By comparison, three BCG studies have found treatment to be significantly better than no treatment with an average reduction in tumor recurrence of 47%.

Our results in the treatment of carcinoma in situ are remarkably consistent with historical series reported in literature. The average complete response rate to ADM treatment is 49% (Kowalkowski and Lamm, 1988) in the literature and 47% in our randomized study. Similarly, our response rate of 71% with BCG treatement is remarkably similar to recently reported series. These observations further support the increased efficacy of BCG over ADM in the treatment of carcinoma in situ.

While increasing disease, defined as tumor recurrence in patients with carcinoma in situ or increasing stage or extent of disease, was found in 37% of patients treated with ADM and only 15% of patients treated with BCG, this beneficial response has not resulted, to date, in any significant improvement in survival. A statistically significant improvement in survival in patients has recently been reported in a randomized prospective comparison of BCG with TUR alone (Herr et al., 1988). In that report, despite the earlier use of cystectomy in controls, progression was significantly reduced and mortality from bladder cancer reduced from 37% in controls to 14% with BCG treatment. To date, no controlled trial of chemotherapy has demonstrated that treatment significantly reduces disease progression or improves survival. Our failure to demonstrate a survival advantage for the BCG group may mean that no advantage exists when compared to ADM, or, more likely, that our relatively short follow and crossover design precluded the demonstration of such advantage.

Our date from 46 different institutions in the United States confirm that BCG can be given by multiple investigators. While recent severe toxic reactions have raised concern about the toxicity of BCG, in this study of 285 patients BCG was found to be have no more toxicity than ADM. It is noteworthy that the superiority of BCG in multiple single institution trials has now been confirmed by a multigroup study. While BCG is clearly superior to ADM in the prevention of recurrence of Ta and T1 tumors and the treatment of carcinoma in situ, ADM and the other intravesical chemotherapeutic drugs in use will continue to play an important role in the management of these patients. With the confirmed efficacy of both immunotherapy and chemotherapy in the future holds even greater promise for the development of new agents which will be more effective and less toxic than those currently available.

REFERENCES

Brosman SA (1982). Experience with Bacillus Calmette-Guérin in patients with superficial bladder carcinoma. J Urol 128: 27.

Camacho FJ, Pinsky CM, Kerr D (1982). Treatment of superficial bladder cancer with intravesical BCG. In Terry WT, Rosenberg SA (eds): "Immunotherapy of Human Cancer," New York: Elsevier North Holland, pp 309.

Herr HW, Laudone VP, Badalament RA, Freedman BD, Whitmore Jr WF (1988). Bacillus Calmette-Guérin (BCG) therapy alters progressions of superficial bladder cancer. J Urol 139: 299A.

Kowalkowski TS, Lamm DL (1988). Intravesical therapy of superficial bladder cancer. In Resnick MI (ed): "Current Trends in Urology," Baltimore: The Williams and Wilkens Co., pp 89-107.

Lamm DL (1985). BCG immunotherapy in bladder cancer. J Urol 134: 40.

Lamm DL. Immunotherapy versus chemotherapy in the treatment of superficial bladder cancer. In Bloom HJG, Hanham IWF (eds): "Urological Oncology: Dilemmas and Developments," Chichester: John Wiley & Sons Ltd., in press.

Rawls WH, Lamm DL, Eyolfson MF (1988). Septic complications in the use of Bacillus Calmette-Guérin for non-invasive transitional cell carcinoma. J Urol 139: 300A.

Steg A, Leleu C, Debre B, Boccon-Gibod L (1988). Systemic Bacillus Calmette-Guérin infection in patients treated by intravesical Bacillus Calmette-Guérin therapy for bladder cancer. J Urol 139: 300A.

EORTC Genitourinary Group Monograph 6:
BCG in Superficial Bladder Cancer, pages 271–274
© 1989 Alan R. Liss, Inc.

MITOMYCIN-C AND BCG IN INTRAVESICAL CHEMOTHERAPY AND
IMMUNOTHERAPY OF SUPERFICIAL BLADDER CANCER

Erkki Rintala, Kari Jauhiainen, Olof Alfthan and the
Finnbladder Research Group, Helsinki University,
Urological Unit, Second Department of Surgery,
Helsinki, E.R. and O.A) and Mikkeli Central Hospital,
Department of Surgery, (K.J.), Mikkeli, Finland

The efficacy of intravesical chemotherapy and immunotherapy of frequently recurrent superficial bladder cancer
has been confirmed. There have been few randomized studies
of Mitomycin-C (MMC) versus Bacillus Calmette-Guérin (BCG).
We describe two of them here: Finnbladder I and Finnbladder
II. Finnbladder I was a randomized multicenter study of
clinical efficacy and drawbacks of MMC and BCG. Finnbladder
II uses two patterns of treatment: MMC and MMC with alternating BCG.

MATERIALS AND METHODS

Finnbladder I

The first study, in 1984–1988, included 116 patients,
24 with carcinoma in situ (CIS) and 92 with tumors stage
Ta–T1. Randomization was based on date of birth. The
criterion for randomization was histologically evident
malignancy, three consecutive cytologic tests showing
papillary cancer at least twice in 1.5 years for the Ta–T1
group. Instillation therapy started 2 weeks after transurethral resection (TUR) and was repeated weekly for the
first month and thereafter monthly for 2 years. The dose of
MMC was 20–40 mg diluted with phosphate buffer, according
to bladder capacity. For BCG therapy we used 75 mg immune
BCG-Pasteur strain in 50 ml of saline solution. This is
half of the dose normally used in most protocols. As the
end point for CIS, we used complete response (CR) and

progression of disease (PD); for the Ta-T1 group, we used recurrence rate (RR = number of recurrences/100 months) and recurrence index (RI = number of recurrent tumors/100 months). The mean follow-up time was 21 months (range, 1-36) in CIS patients and 26 months in Ta-T1 patients. Prerandomization characteristics were identical in both treatment groups.

Finnbladder II

The second study started July 1987. By August 1988, 69 patients had entered the trial. The patients were randomized in two groups. In both groups, instillation of MMC started postoperatively and continued once a week for 5 weeks. Thereafter, patients in one group received MMC monthly, as in the first study; patients in the other group received MMC and BCG alternating each month (doses as in the first study). Before treatment, every patient had a PPD skin test. Eight PPD-negative patients were changed to the MMC-only group.

RESULTS

Finbladder I

Carcinoma in situ. In 14 CIS patients treated with MMC, the CR was 39% and the PD, 7%. In 10 CIS patients treated by BCG the CR was 40% and PD 20% respectively.

Stage Ta-T1. Each patient served as his own control when the results before therapy were compared with those during therapy. The number of recurrences of Ta-T1 tumors during the chemotherapy or immunotherapy (MMC or BCG) was significantly lower than that before therapy, especially in patients with multifocal frequently recurrent cancer. As evaluated by RR (Table 1) and by RI/m (Table 2), the efficacy of BCG was significantly better than that of MMC ($p < 0.0001$). The disease-free interval was also significantly longer in patients treated with BCG ($p < 0.01$). There was only one progression in the two groups. Because of local side effects of BCG (hematuria and dysuria), treatment had to be stopped in 19.2%; because of side effects of MMC (chemical cystitis, skin reactions and allergy) treatment had to be stopped in 6.6%. No severe side effects, such as BCG-itis, were seen in this study.

TABEL 1. RR (recurrence rate) in Ta-T1 patients

	MMC	BCG
RR before treatment	18.4	17.4
RR during treatment	9.1*	2.5*
Adjusted RR difference	- 7.8	- 14.6*
Number of patients	40	36

* p < 0.001

TABEL 2. RI/m (recurrence index/month) in Ta-T1 patients

	MMC	BCG
RI/m before treatment	0.52	0.66
RI/m during treatment	0.18*	0.03*
Adjusted RI/m difference	- 0.40	- 0.56*
Number of patients	40	36

* p < 0.001

Finbladder II

Up to August 1988, the mean follow-up period in 53 patients was 6 months. Preliminary results were evaluated according to CR and PD. In the CIS patients treated with MMC, the CR was 6/9, and in those treated with alternating MMC and BCG, it was 4/5. In the Ta-T1 patients treated with MMC, the CR was 16/25 (64%), and in those patients treated with the alternating therapy, it was 13/14 (93%). There were no progressions.

Because of side effects, treatment was stopped once in the MCC group (allergy). One patient in the other group refused BCG instillation, because of dysuria. On the basis of comparison with corresponding figures from the 6 month follow-up in Finnbladder I, it seems that the alternating treatment yields better results and fewer side effects.

COMMENTS

1. Chemotherapy and immunotherapy with MMC and BCG alternating are effective, especially in frequently recurrent multifocal cancers.

2. MMC seems to be better than BCG in the long-term treatment of carcinoma in situ with less progression. However, the number of patients is too small for definitive conclusions.

3. BCG was significantly more effective than MMC in the prophylaxis of Ta-T1 cancer, in spite of small doses of BCG-Pasteur. Our results are similar to those reported using a two-fold dose.

4. MMC was better tolerated than BCG. There were no systemic complications (such as BCG-itis) in the treatment groups.

5. An alternating treatment with MMC and BCG seems to be a new, exciting pattern of treatment, but more data are necessary.

EORTC Genitourinary Group Monograph 6:
BCG in Superficial Bladder Cancer, pages 275–283
© 1989 Alan R. Liss, Inc.

BCG VERSUS THIOTEPA IN NON-CIS, STAGE Ta, T1 BLADDER
CANCER: RATIONALE AND DESIGN OF ECOG TRIAL

Hugh A.F. Fisher

Department of Urologic Oncology, Albany medical
College, Albany, New York, USA

The majority of bladder tumors (80%) are superficial
and papillary when first detected and involve the mucosa
(Stage Ta) and/or the lamina propria (T1). Following
complete transurethral resection or fulguration new tumor
occurrences are found in 40-80% of patients within 36
months (Gilbert ct al., 1978; Lerman et al., 1970; Williams
et al., 1977). Factors predicting both the new occurrence
of tumor and progression to muscle invasion or metastases
have been defined in longitudinal studies and allow definition of high and low risk groups for these events (Dalesio
et al., 1983; England et al., 1981; Heney et al., 1983;
Lutzeyer et al., 1982). Intravesical chemotherapy with a
variety of agents and immunotherapy with BCG have proven
efficacy in reducing recurrence rates and prolonging the
time to recurrence when compared with control groups
treated by transurethral resection alone. However, sizable
randomized prospective trials with appropriate patient
entry, stratification and response criteria which compare
effective agents are few. In this hctcrogeneous population
of patients only direct comparison of agents will enable
determination of the best single agent or agents for treatment of bladder cancer Stages CIS, Ta, T1. Also, many
questions regarding timing, dose and treatment schedules of
intravesical agents remain unanswered, and the possibility
that "low risk" groups may not need the same intensity of
treatment as "high risk" groups needs to be explored. Such
meaningful comparative trials can be performed most quickly
in a well organized co-operative group setting.

This paper will review past and present Eastern Co-operative Oncology Group initiatives with use of BCG in superficial bladder cancer.

INITIAL STUDY - PC-881

From January to September 1982 in a pilot study involving four ECOG institutions, 37 patients with completely resected Stage Ta or T1 low grade (I-II) papillary transitional cell carcinoma were treated with six weekly bladder instillations of 120 mg Pasteur strain BCG. Patients were required to have two recurrences in the preceding 18 months or greater tumors at presentation. All visible disease was removed from the bladder and carcinoma in situ was ruled out by random bladder biopsy. It was not required that urine cytology be negative post resection prior to BCG treatment. Dwell time was two hours. Intradermal BCG was not given. Patients were treated 2-4 weeks after definitive resection or fulguration.

Following BCG instillation, all patients underwent cystoscopy at three montly intervals for two years, every six months in years three and four and yearly thereafter. Primary end point for the study was a visible recurrent tumor within the bladder. Patients were then followed for later progression and long term survival. Subsequent treatment was at the discretion of the treating urologist.

Average age was 65.7 years. There were 22 males and 14 females. 17 Patients had been treated with prior thiotepa and one patient with additional Mitomycin. 19 Patients had received no prior chemotherapy. Of the previously treated patients, eight were judged to have had a partial or complete response in the past.

RESULTS

One patient with CIS was removed from study. Mean follow-up was 61.2 months for all patients and 69.2 months for surviving patients. 27 Of 36 evaluable patients (75%) had recurrent visible tumor within the bladder during the course of the study. Mean time to recurrence was 11.7 months. Median time to recurrence was 6.0 months. 82% Of patients were disease free at three months, 56% at six months, 44% at nine months, 42% at 10-18 months, 36% at 19-24 months, 28% at 25-36 months and 25% at 37-48 months. Nine of the 36 (25%) had no recurrence during the entire study. 15 Of 17 (88%) patients with prior Thiotepa therapy relapsed compared with 12 of 19 (64%) patients who had not received prior Thiotepa.

Three patients (8.3%) had muscle invasive disease or distant metastases. Two underwent cystectomy 17 and 28 months post therapy. There was one bladder cancer death in the patient not undergoing cystectomy. There were seven non bladder cancer deaths, mainly from cardiovascular or pulmonary disease.

TOXICITY

All patients completed six weeks of treatment. Ten patients had no side effects. Mild to moderate frequency and dysuria occurred in 16 patients (43%), mild hematuria in 10 patients (27%), fever in 4 patients (11%). Other side effects included: nausea in two patients (5%), fatigue in two patients (5%), urinary retention or chills in one patient (2%). No serious toxicity was observed.

These data indicate a relatively high incidence of early tumor recurrence at three-six months post therapy. However, several patients in the early failure group had fewer tumors and a longer interval to recurrence than prior to therapy, implying a delayed salutary effect of BCG on rate of recurrence. These data are presently being analyzed to compare the rate of tumor formation pre and post BCG. Such analyses in other studies have indicated clear BCG efficacy (Pinsky et al., 1985).

EST 4884 - BCG VERSUS THIOTEPA

A phase III randomized study comparing BCG with intravesical chemotherapy was designed. Review of the few available direct comparative trials for prophylaxis revealed no clear advantage for Mitomycin, Adriamycin or Thiotepa, although early results indicated a favorable response to BCG when compared with Adriamycin and Thiotepa (Table 1). Only two studies compare Thiotepa with BCG, both with small numbers of patients. Brosman (1982) compared 19 evaluable Thiotepa treated patients with 25 BCG treated patients with recurrence rates of 40% and 0% respectively. Cytology was not used as an exclusion or response criterion. BCG (one ampule of Tice strain) and Thiotepa (60 mg) were administered weekly for six weeks, every two weeks for three months and monthly until a total treatment period of 24 months had elapsed. Although recurrences were not seen in the BCG group, 11 patients (28%) experienced significant toxicity. Six patients required Isonazid therapy. Four patients required hospitalization and triple drug therapy with evidence of abnormal liver function studies and evidence of pulmonary infection. In contrast, seven patients treated with Thiotepa had bladder irritability with cessation of therapy in one patient.

TABLE 1. Comparative prophylactic studies.

Author	Study	Result
Zincke et al. 1983	Thiotepa vs. Doxorubicin	No difference
Denis et al. 1985	Thiotepa vs. Doxorubicin	No difference
Llopis et al. 1985	Thiotepa vs. Doxorubicin	No difference
Zincke et al. 1984	Thiotepa vs. Mitomycin	No difference
Flanigan et al. 1986	Thiotepa vs. Mitomycin	No difference
Brosman 1982	Thiotepa vs. BCG (Tice)	BCG superior
Netto and Lemos 1983	Thiotepa vs. BCG (Moreau)	BCG superior
Lamm and Crawford 1985	Doxorubicin vs. BCG (Connaught)	BCG superior

The second randomized trial by Netto and Lemos (1983) comparing BCG with Thiotepa used oral BCG of the Moreau strain with patients treated over an 11 year period. There were 14 patients in the Thiotepa group and 16 in the BCG treated group. Thiotepa dose was 60 mg daily for seven days beginning 24 hours post resection, every month for three months for one year, every three months for one year, every six months for two years and yearly for two years with retreatment at recurrence. With mean follow-up of 30 months 6 of 14 (42.9%) Thiotepa treated patients recurred compared with 1/16 (6.2%) BCG treated patients. There has been no other published experience with this strain of BCG administered orally, although Tice strain seems to be ineffective. These two studies indicate superiority of BCG, although in the Brosman study the toxicity of the BCG was unacceptably high and in the Netto and Lemos study oral BCG was used.

Thiotepa continues to be a widely used and effective first line agent for prophylaxis of superficial transitional cell carcinoma (Koontz et al., 1981; Schulmann et al., 1982). A variety of treatment schedules have proved to be effective. Toxicity has been acceptable (Soloway and Ford, 1983). 30 mg and 60 mg are equivalent in terms of therapeutic response, with less toxicity with the 30 mg dose (Koontz et al.m 1981). It is a relatively inexpensive agent. Long term tumor free intervals have been observed in patients who have had a complete response to 6-8 weeks of induction therapy for residual disease (Prout et al., 1982). Maintenance prophylaxis has added additional protection against recurrence (Prout et al., 1982). However, data regarding response to re-induction with Thiotepa at first recurrence are lacking and it is possible that rather than changing to another chemotherapeutic agent or BCG that a second induction with Thiotepa might produce additonal response. In a long term follow-up study, Prout (1983) noted that the longest tumor free intervals occurred in patients with low grade tumors. Thiotepa has been considered less effective for treatment of carcinoma in situ, although it has been inadequately studied in this disease. BCG on the other hand has been a very effective agent for treatment of carcinoma in situ (Brosman, 1985; Herr et al., 1986).

EST 4884 (see Fig. 1) is a randomized trial, comparing BCG with Thiotepa as first line prophylaxis in non CIS patients with recurrent or multiple ($\geq$ 3) completely resected stage Ta, T1 tumors with negative cytology post resection. This patient population is one with a high probability of local recurrence in the bladder if treatment failed, but a low probability of progression to muscle invasion, extravesical failure or distant metastases and therefore could be retreated at recurrence without the fear that progressive disease would occur during the retreatment. Such a study population will allow long term surveillance for determination of recurrence rates and the tumor free interval for these patients. One ampule of Tice strain BCG (5-8 times 10^8 culturable particles) is administered weekly for six weeks within four weeks after complete tumor resection or fulguration. Thiotepa dose is 30 mg in 30 cc sterile water administered weekly for six weeks. Dwell time is two hours for both. Patients are then followed at three monthly intervals. If a new tumor occurrence is seen at any time during the study, the tumor is completely resected, a cytology is obtained and patient is retreated with the original agent for an additional six weeks. At second recurrence the patients is removed from the study.

220 Patients are required. End points for this study will be the percent of patients with recurrence, time to first recurrence, recurrence rate (number of tumors per 100 months follow-up or number of cystoscopies at which tumors were seen) and response to retreatment. Secondary end points are the progression rate to muscle invasion or metastases and bladder cancer death rate, although it is expected that these events will be infrequent in this non CIS study population.

The first patient was entered in February 1988. 11 Patients have been accrued. No results are currently available.

Within ECOG institutions, patients with prior intravesical chemotherapy or those failing in the Thiotepa arm of EST 4884 or who have concomitant CIS will be entered into an Intergroup study with the Southwest oncology group comparing BCG (Tice) with Mitomycin-C. This study will begin shortly.

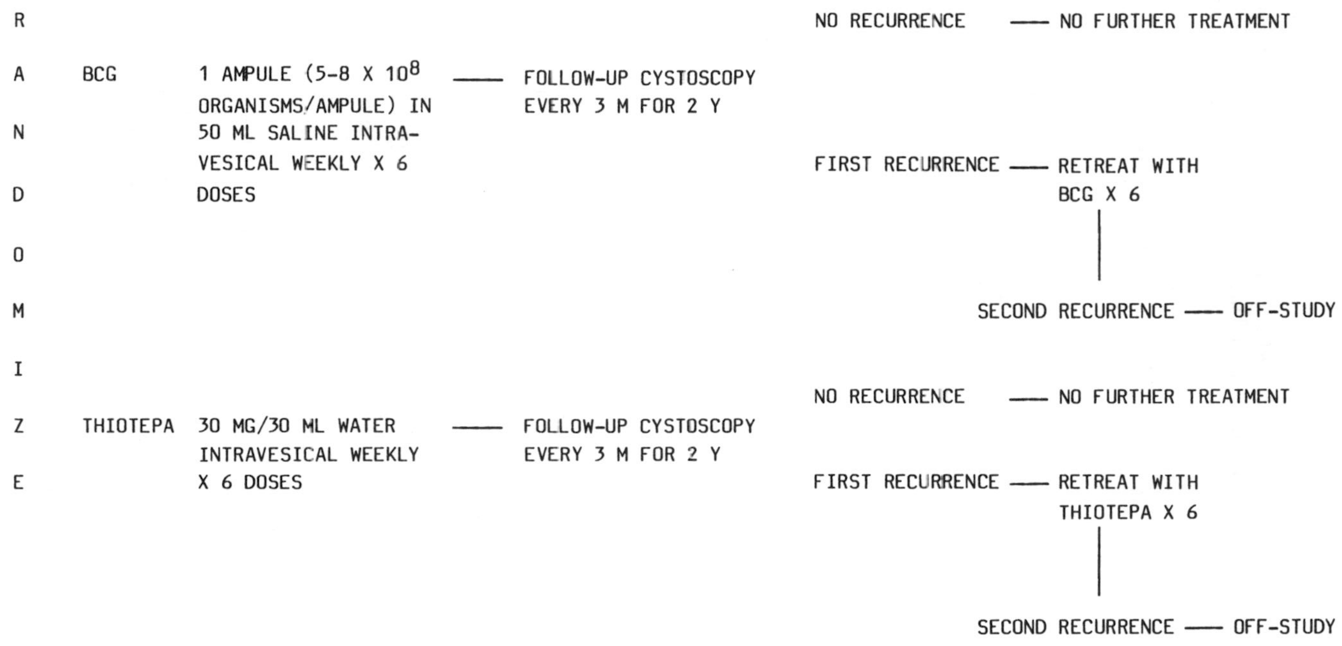

```
R          NO RECURRENCE ——— NO FURTHER TREATMENT

A    BCG    1 AMPULE (5-8 X 10^8    ——— FOLLOW-UP CYSTOSCOPY
            ORGANISMS/AMPULE) IN         EVERY 3 M FOR 2 Y
N           50 ML SALINE INTRA-
            VESICAL WEEKLY X 6     FIRST RECURRENCE ——— RETREAT WITH
D           DOSES                                       BCG X 6

O
                                          SECOND RECURRENCE ——— OFF-STUDY
M

I          NO RECURRENCE ——— NO FURTHER TREATMENT

Z    THIOTEPA  30 MG/30 ML WATER   ——— FOLLOW-UP CYSTOSCOPY
               INTRAVESICAL WEEKLY      EVERY 3 M FOR 2 Y
E              X 6 DOSES
                                   FIRST RECURRENCE ——— RETREAT WITH
                                                        THIOTEPA X 6


                                          SECOND RECURRENCE ——— OFF-STUDY
```

Figure 1. Schema EST 4884

REFERENCES

Brosman SA (1982). Experience with Bacillus-Calmette-Guérin in patients with superficial bladder cancer. J Urol 128: 27-30.

Brosman SA (1985). The use of Bacillus-Calmette-Guérin in the therapy of bladder carcinoma in situ. J Urol 134: 36-39.

Dalesio O, Schulman CC, Sylvester R, de Pauw M, Robinson M, Denis L, Smith P, Viggiano G (1983). Prognostic factors in superficial bladder tumors, a study of the European Organisation for Research on Treatment of Cancer: Genito-urinary Group. J Urol 129: 730-733.

Denis LJ, Viggiano G, Oosterlinck W, Bouffioux C, Sylvester R, de Pauw MM, Schröder FH and Members of the EORTC Urological Group (1985). Phase 3 chemotherapy with Thiotepa, Adriamycin and Cisplatinum for recurrent superficial bladder tumors. J Urol 133: 185A.

England HR, Paris AMI, Blandy JP (1981). The correlation of T1 bladder tumor history with prognoses and follow-up requirements. Br J Urol 53: 593-597.

Flanigan RC, Ellison MF, Butler KM, Mc Roberts JW (1986). Adjuvant intravesical thiotepa versus Mitomycin-C in recurrent or multiple stage 0 and A transitional cell cancers. J Urol 136: 35-37.

Gilbert HA, Logan JL, Kagan AR, Friedman HH, Cove JK, Muldoon TM, Lonni YW, Rowe JH, Cooper JF, Nussbaum H, Chan P, Rao A, Starr A (1978). The natural history of papillary transitional cell carcinoma of the bladder and its treatment in an unselected population on the basis of histologic grading. J Urol 119: 488-492.

Heney N, Ahmed S, Flanigan MJ, Frable W, Corder MP, Hafermann MD, Hawkins IR for National Bladder Cancer Collaborative Group A (1983). Superficial bladder cancer: progression and recurrence. J Urol 130: 1083-1086.

Herr WH, Pinsky CM, Whitmore Jr WF, Sogani C, Oettgen HF, Melamed MF (1986). Long term effect of intravesical Bacillus-Calmette-Guérin (BCG) on carcinoma in situ of the bladder. J Urol 135: 265-267.

Koontz WW Jr, Prout GR Jr, Smith W, Frable WJ, Minnis JE (1981). The use of intravesical Thiotepa in the management of non invasive carcinoma of the bladder. J Urol 125: 307-312.

Lamm DL, Crawford ED (1985). BCG versus Adriamycin in bladder cancer: A Southwest Oncology Group Study. Proc. ASCO.

Lerman IL, Hutter RVP, Whitmore WF Jr (1970). Papilloma of the urinary bladder. Cancer 25: 333-342.

Llopis B, Gallego J, Mompo JA (1985). Thiotepa versus Adriamycin verus Cisplatinum in the intravesical prophylaxis of superficial bladder tumors. Eur Urol 11: 73-78.

Lutzeyer W, Rubben H, Dahm H (1982). Prognostic parameters in superficial bladder cancer: an analysis of 315 cases. J Urol 127: 250-252.

Netto Jr NR, Lemos GC (1983). A comparison of treatment methods for the prophylaxis of recurrent superficial bladder tumors. J Urol 129: 33-34.

Pinsky CM, Camacho FJ, Kerr D (1985). Intravesical administration of Bacillus Calmette-Guérin in patients with recurrent superficial carcinoma of the urinary bladder: Report of a prospective, randomized trial. Cancer Treat Rep 69: 47-53.

Prout GR, Koontz WW Jr, Coombs LJ, Hawkins IR, Friedell GH for National Bladder Cancer Collaborative Group A (1983). Long term fate of 90 patients with superficial bladder cancer randomly assigned to receive or not to receive Thiotepa. J Urol 130: 677-680.

Schulmann CC, Robinson M, Denis L, Smith P, Viggiano G, de Pauw M, Dalesio O, Sylvester R, and Members of the EORTC Genito-Urinary Tract Cancer Group (1982). Prophylactic chemotherapy in superficial transitional cell bladder carcinoma: An EORTC randomized trial comparing Thiotepa and Podophyllotoxin (VM26) and TUR alone. Eur Urol 8: 207-212.

Soloway MS, Ford KS (1983). Thiotepa induced myelosuppression: review of 670 bladder instillation. J Urol 130: 889-891.

Williams JL, Hammond JC, Saunders N (1977). T1 bladder tumors. Br J Urol 49: 663-668.

Zincke H, Benson Sr RC, Fleming TR. Tumor recurrence after intravesical instillation of Thiotepa and Mitomycin at time of transurethral resection of bladder cancer Ta, T1, CIS and postoperatively. J Urol.

Zincke H, Utz DC, Taylor WF, Meyers RP, Leary FJ (1983). Influence of Thiotepa and Doxorubicin instillations at time of transurethral surgical treatment of bladder cancer on tumor recurrence: a prospective, randomized, double blind, controlled trial. J Urol 129: 505-509.

EORTC Genitourinary Group Monograph 6:
BCG in Superficial Bladder Cancer, pages 285–298
© 1989 Alan R. Liss, Inc.

BCG-RIVM VERSUS BCG-TICE VERSUS MITOMYCIN-C IN SUPERFICIAL
BLADDER CANCER. RATIONALE AND DESIGN OF THE TRIAL OF THE
SOUTHEAST CO-OPERATIVE UROLOGICAL GROUP, THE NETHERLANDS

Ad P.M. van der Meijden, Frans M.J. Debruyne, Peter
A. Steerenberg, Wim H. de Jong, Wim Doesburg.
Departments of Urology (A.P.M.v.d.M., F.M.J.D.) and
Statistical Consultation (W.D.), University of
Nijmegen and National Institute of Public Health and
Environmental Protection (P.A.S., W.H.d.J.),
Bilthoven, The Netherlands

INTRODUCTION

In 1976 a new approach to adjuvant therapy for superficial bladder cancer was developed by Morales and
co-workers (Morales, 1976). They were the first to use
Bacillus Calmette-Guérin (BCG), an attenuated strain of
mycobacterium bovis, the bovine tubercle bacillus for non-
specific active immunotherapy. BCG was administered intravesically and intradermally. The preliminary results were
promising. Morales deducted this new avenue to treat superficial bladder cancer from a linkage between the observations made by Coe and Feldman and the results of experiments performed by the reseach group of Zbar and Rapp (Coe
and Feldman, 1966; Zbar et al., 1972).

Coe and Feldman demonstrated that the bladder is a
suitable organ for the development of delayed hypersensitivity reactions. Zbar and Rapp showed that optimum results
with BCG were obtained if certain basic principles were
fulfilled.
1. Tumor burden must be small.
2. Direct contact between tumor cells and BCG is essential.
3. Dose of immunizing agent must be adequate.
4. Tumors respond better, when confined to the parent organ
   or in case of metastases, when spread is limited to the
   regional lymph nodes.

Superficial bladder cancer appears to be ideally
suited for non-specific active immunotherapy with BCG after
endoscopic surgery, which remains the initial and most

effective treatment, only a small tumor burden or no tumor at all is left in the bladder. Intensive contact between possible residual tumor cells and BCG is guaranteed by intravesical instillation of BCG.

Also from another point of view immunotherapy seems to be indicated for transitional cell carcinoma of the bladder, as tumor associated antigens were demonstrated, and these antigens can be recognized by the host (Bubenik et al., 1970). In addition patients with advanced disease show impaired immunologic respons (Catalona and Chretien, 1973). So there seems to be an interaction between the immune system and bladder cancer.

Because of the encouraging preliminary results obtained by Morales, 2 prospective randomized trials were conducted in the USA (Camacho et al., 1980; Lamm et al., 1981). In these trials patients were treated either with transurethral resection only, or with additional intra-vesical BCG, according to the regimen Morales had used. The results were significantly better in the BCG treated patients. Brosman conducted a prospective randomized trial comparing intravesical BCG with intravesical chemotherapy using Thiotepa (Brosman, 1982). Here a more intensive dose schedule was used. BCG was instilled weekly for 6 conse-cutive weeks, every 2 weeks for 3 months and thereafter monthly for 2 years. This long term therapy with repeated instillations is called maintenance therapy. No intradermal injections of BCG were given. It was demonstrated that intravesical instillations without intradermal injection were capable to induce systemic sensitization to BCG in nearly all patients after 3 months.

Recent data suggest that a single 6-week course of BCG instillations is suboptimal (Haaff et al., 1986). Haaff and co-workers observed a considerable cumulative response rate after a second 6-week course of intravesical BCG in those patients who failed to respond to the initial 6-week course. Although most investigators are convinced that a single 6-week course of intravesical BCG is a suboptimal therapy, Badalament, however, in a prospective randomized study comparing maintenance versus non-maintenance therapy could not demonstrate a significant difference between the two groups. Patients receiving maintenance therapy had similar recurrence and progression rates as those who were treated with a single 6-week course (Badalament et al., 1987).

Intravesical instillation of BCG has also been successful in the treatment of carcinoma in situ of the bladder (Brosman, 1982; Herr et al., 1983). Without any surgical treatment, complete cure was obtained in a marked number of patients. Several investigators consider BCG as one of the best available treatments for carcinoma in situ (Herr et al., 1986; Morales, 1980).

In the Netherlands a BCG-strain is produced at the Rijksinstituut voor Volksgezondheid en Milieuhygiëne (RIVM) (National Institute of Public Health and Environmental Protection, Bilthoven). In contrast to most other BCG-preparations, such as BCG-Tice, the Dutch BCG-RIVM is produced as a homogeneously dispersed culture. Although differences in immunostimulating properties may be present between BCG-preparations cultured as a surface pellicle or homogeneously dispersed, similar antitumor activity was exerted by these products in experimental tumors (Ruitenberg et al., 1981). The antitumor potency of BCG-RIVM conclusively was established in different animal tumor systems e.g. murine fibrosarcoma (Ruitenberg et al., 1981), line 10 hepatocellular carcinoma in the guinea pig (de Jong et al., 1986), bovine ocular squamous cell carcinoma (Klein et al., 1982) and equine sarcoid (Klein et al., 1986).

In a prospective randomized joint study of the EORTC GU-Group and IKO-IKZ (the Netherlands) BCG-RIVM was compared with Mitomycin-C as an adjuvant therapy after transurethral resection for superficial bladder cancer. The immediate toxicity of BCG-RIVM instillation therapy is known, as the accrual for this joint study was closed on October the first 1986. From the literature it is known that long term toxicity has to be established in the future but it is not likely to expect long term toxicity, if immediate toxicity not is encountered (Lamm et al., 1986; Morales and Nickel, 1986). It is clear that BCG-RIVM is a safe strain and that this strain seems to have less side effects compared with other strains e.g. Tice strain. On the other hand BCG-RIVM, administered intravesically without percutaneous support was able to induce a systemic immunologic reaction as a conversion of the PPD skin reaction was observed in the guinea pig (van der Meijden et al., 1987) and in man (van der Meijden, unpublished observations).

RESULTS

A total number of 337 patients took part in this study, which was closed October 1st, 1986. The toxicity data from 165 patients entered by the Dutch Southeast Co-operative Group (enrolled by 14 Institutions) were analyzed in January 1987.

Stratification for CIS, and stages Ta and T1, as well as for G-category, number of tumors, primary and recurrent tumors was similar in both treatment arms (Tables 1-4). Local and systemic toxicity and comparison of the occurrence of bacterial and drug-induced, or chemical, cystitis by both number of patients and number of instillations are shown in Table 5. Drug-induced cystitis was observed in 13 (16.7%) of 78 BCG treated patients and in 12 (13.8%) of 87 MMC treated patients. In the same group, bacterial cystitis occurred in 17 (21.8%) patients and in 16 (18.4%) patients, respectively. No significant difference between the two treatment groups was observed. Severe systemic toxicity was absent in both treatment arms. The number of occurrences of allergic reactions is shown in Table 5. Allergic reactions, requiring cessation of the therapy, was seen in 1 (1.3%) of 78 BCG treated patients and in 6 (6.9%) of 87 patients of the MMC group. This analysis shows more frequent allergic reactions in the MMC arm. With regard to recurrence, the results are presented for 308 patients after a follow-up period of twelve months (Table 6). In the BCG-treated group (N=148), 44 (29.8%) patients had recurrent tumors, while in the Mitomycin group (N=160) 40 (25%) patients had a recurrence (Table 6). The recurrence rate for BCG-treated patients was 0.33. For MMC-treated patients, the rate was 0.29 (p = 0.560, not significant).

TABLE 1. Protocol 30845: pT-category

| Therapy | No. of Patients | | | Total No. |
	pTis	pTa	pT1	Pts. (%)
BCG RIVM	5	106	59	170 (50.4)
MMC	5	107	55	167 (49.6)
Total	10	213	114	337 (100)

TABLE 2. Protocol 30845: G-category

| Therapy | G0 | No. of Patients | | | | Total No. |
		GI	GII	GIII	GX	Pts. (%)
BCG RIVM	3	48	90	27	2	170 (50.4)
MMC	0	60	79	24	4	167 (49.6)
Total	3	108	169	51	6	337 (100)

TABLE 3. Protocol 30845: Number of tumors

| Therapy | 0 | No. of Patients | | | Total No. |
		1	2-3	4-10	Pts. (%)
BCG RIVM	1	89	44	36	170 (50.4)
MMC	1	89	41	36	167 (49.6)
Total	2	178	85	72	337 (100)

TABLE 4. Protocol 30845: Primary/recurrent bladder cancer

| Therapy | No. of Patients | | Total No. |
	Primary (%)	Recurrent (%)	Pts. (%)
BCG RIVM	117	53	170 (50.4)
MMC	118	49	167 (49.6)
Total	235 (69.7)	102 (30.3)	337 (100)

TABLE 5. Protocol 30845: Occurrences of chemical cystitis and bacterial cystitis and allergic reactions

	BCG No. (%)	MMC No. (%)
Chemical cystitis		
Total patients	78	87
Occurrences	13 (16.7%)	12 (13.8%)
Instillations	510	727
Occurrences	32 (6.3%)	28 (3.9%)
Bacterial cystitis		
Total patients	78	87
Occurrences	17 (21.8%)	16 (18.4%)
Instillations	510	727
Occurrences	29 (5.7%)	23 (3.2%)
Allergic reactions		
Total patients	78	87
Occurrences	1 (1.3%)	6 (6.9%)
Instillations	510	727
Occurrences	2 (0.4%)	14 (1.9%)

TABLE 6. Protocol 30845: Available follow-up until August, 1987

	BCG RIVM	MMC
Patients with follow-up	148	160
Mean follow-up (months)	11.63	11.78
Mean no. of cystoscopies	4	4
Total number of recurrences	47	45
Recurrence rate	0.33	0.29

These preliminary results demonstrate no statistically significant difference between the two therapeutic regimens.

In conclusion, there remains a need to establish the exact value of non-specific active immunotherapy, with BCG in superficial bladder cancer. Further prospective randomized trials are demanded in which BCG is compared with potent chemotherapeutic agents with proven antitumor activity. Since BCG is a biological product, variations in immunostimulation and antitumor effect can be expected. Therefore it is necessary to standardize and select active BCG-preparations. On the other hand the local and systemic side effects must be limited to a minimum.

Therefore this protocol is proposed, in which two different BCG-strains are compared with a standard intravesical chemotherapeutic agent. One BCG-strain (Tice) has proved its efficacy but side effects can not be ignored. The second BCG-strain (RIVM) also has proved antitumor activity. The side effects of this therapy, however, are less frequent, compared with other strains. In this protocol intravesical instillation of Mitomycin-C is compared with intravesical instillation of BCG-Tice and with intravesical instillation of BCG-RIVM in primary and recurrent Ta, T1 papillary carcinoma and primary carcinoma in situ of the urinary bladder.

For the proposed trial selected batches of BCG-RIVM and BCG-Tice have been reserved. Repeated quality controls revealed that each vial of the two strains (Tice and RIVM) contain at least 5×10^8 lyophilized bacilli per ampule. This means, that with regard to the dosage, the two preparations are comparable.

Summarizing, it is expected that this study will bring two important answers:
1. What is the efficacy of a well known BCG-preparation (BCG-Tice) compared to the efficacy of one of the most potent cytotoxic drugs (Mitomycin-C) in superficial bladder cancer.
2. Is the antitumor activity of BCG-RIVM, known as a safe strain with minor toxicity, comparable to BCG-Tice and/ or Mitomycin-C.

OBJECTIVES OF THE STUDY

This randomized trial is designed to compare the effect of intravesically administered BCG-Tice, BCG-RIVM and Mitomycin-C (MMC) in patients with primary and recurrent superficial bladder cancer including CIS on:
* recurrence rate,
* the duration of disease-free interval,

* the rate of progression to a higher stage (T-category) of the disease,
* the incidence and severity of side effects,
* the number, size and localisation of the primary or recurrent tumor(s).

THERAPEUTIC REGIMEN

The therapeutic scheme is depicted in Fig. 1.

PRELIMINARY RESULTS ON TOXICITY

A first analysis of 165 patients entered in the protocol was performed in January 1989. The stratification for CIS and the stages Ta and T1 as well for the G-category, primary versus recurrent tumors, number of tumors was comparable in the three treatment arms (Table 7-10).

TABLE 7. Distribution of patients after T-category

	pTis	pTa	pT1	TOTAL
MMC	1	34	20	55
BCG-RIVM	2	32	22	56
BCG-TICE	3	33	18	54
TOTAL	6	99	60	165

TABLE 8. Distribution of patients after G-category

	G1	G2	G3	Gx	TOTAL
MMC	18	28	8	1	55
BCG-RIVM	16	25	13	2	56
BCG-TICE	16	24	11	3	54
TOTAL	50	77	32	6	165

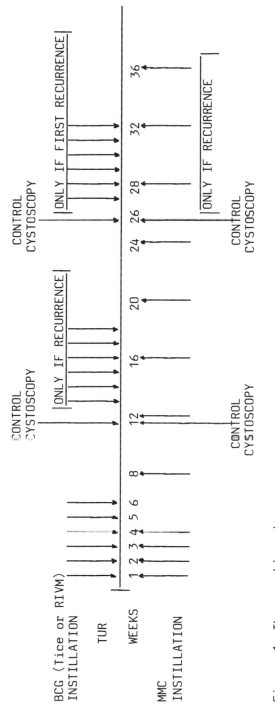

Figure 1. Therapeutic scheme

TABLE 9. Distribution of patients after primary/recurrent bladder cancer

	PRIMARY	RECURRENT	TOTAL
MMC	38	17	55
BCG-RIVM	39	17	56
BCG-TICE	38	16	54
TOTAL	115	50	165

TABLE 10. Distribution of patients after number of tumors

	NUMBER OF TUMORS				TOTAL
	0	1	2-3	4-9	
MMC	0	30	12	13	55
BCG-RIVM	2	23	14	17	56
BCG-TICE	1	22	17	14	54
TOTAL	3	75	43	44	165

The side effects were divided into 4 categories: drug induced cystitis, bacterial cystitis, allergic reactions and other side effects (Table 11-15). A total of 144 patients was evaluable for toxicity.

TABLE 11. Side effects: drug induced cystitis

	MMC	BCG-RIVM	BCG-TICE
PATIENTS	44	51	49
OCCURRENCES	8	21	17
PERCENTAGE	18.2	41.2	34.7

TABLE 12. Side effects: bacterial cystitis

	MMC	BCG-RIVM	BCG-TICE
PATIENTS	44	51	49
OCCURRENCES	10	9	14
PERCENTAGE	22.7	17.6	28.6

TABLE 13. Side effects: allergic reactions

	MMC	BCG-RIVM	BCG-TICE
PATIENTS	44	51	49
OCCURRENCES	1	0	0
PERCENTAGE	2.3	0.0	0.0

TABLE 14. Side effects: local side effects

	MMC	BCG-RIVM	BCG-TICE
PATIENTS	44	51	49
OCCURRENCES	2	6	6
PERCENTAGE	4.5	11.8	12.2

TABLE 15. Side effects: systemic side effects

	MMC	BCG-RIVM	BCG-TICE
PATIENTS	44	51	49
OCCURRENCES	2	14	14
PERCENTAGE	4.5	27.5	28.6

Although no definitive conclusions can be made it seems that Mitomycin-C has the least toxicity. The importance of comparing toxicity in a prospective way is clearly shown when one considers the data from the two BCG-strains. We expected from our earlier experiences with BCG-RIVM and from reports by other investigators, who reported on the toxicity of BCG-Tice that we would find differences in toxicity in favor for BCG-RIVM. These preliminary results, however, show drug induced cystitis in 21 (41.2%) of 51 BCG-RIVM treated patients and in 17 (34.7%) of 49 BCG-Tice treated patients. Bacterial cystitis was observed in 9 (17.6%) and in 14 (28.6%) respectively in the same groups. Allergic reactions were not observed in the BCG groups and in 1 (2.3%) of the MMC group. It also shows clearly that toxicity should be defined more precisely, so that standardization of scoring the side effects is performed by each investigator in the same way.

Other systemic side effects e.g. fever, malaise, myalgia were present in 14 (27.5%) of the BCG-RIVM treated patients and in 14 (28.6%) of the patients who received BCG-Tice.

It must be stated, however, that non of these side effects was severe, requiring anti-tuberculous drugs. Severe side effects were not encountered sofar in this ongoing study.

REFERENCES

Badalament RA, Herr HW, Wong GY, Gnecco G, Pinsky CM, Whitmore Jr WF, Fair WR, Oettgen HF (1987). A prospective randomized trial of maintenance versus non-maintenance intravesical Bacillus Calmette-Guérin therapy of super-ficial bladder cancer. J Clin Oncol 5: 441.
Brosman SA (1982). Experience with Bacillus Calmette-Guérin in patients with superficial bladder carcinoma. J Urol 128: 27.
Bubenik J, Peremann P, Helmstein K (1970). Cellular and humoral immune responses to human urinary bladder carci-nomas. Int J Cancer 5: 310.
Camacho F, Pinsky C, Herr D, Whitmore W, Oettgen H (1980). Treatment of superficial bladder cancer with intravesical BCG. Abstract C-160, Proc Amer Ass Cancer Res and Amer Soc Clin Oncol 21: 359, 1980.
Catalona WJ, Chretien PB (1973). Correlation among host im-munocompetence and tumor stage, tumor grade and vascular

premedation in transitional carcinoma. J Urol 110: 526.

Coe JE, Feldman JD (1966). Extracutaneous delayed hypersensitivity, particularly in the guinea pig bladder. Immunology 10: 127.

Haaff EO, Dresner SM, Ratliff TL, Catalona WJ (1986). Two courses of intravesical Bacillus Calmette-Guérin for transitional cell carcinoma of the bladder. J Urol 136: 820.

Herr HW, Pinsky CM, Whitmore Jr WF, Oettgen HF, Melamed MR (1983). Effect of intravesical BCG on carcinoma in situ of the bladder. Cancer 51: 1323.

Herr HW, Pinsky CM, Whitmore Jr WF, Sogani PC, Oettgen HF, Melamed MR (1986). Long-term effect of intravesical Bacillus Calmette-Guérin on flat carcinoma in situ of the bladder. J Urol 135: 265.

de Jong WH, Teppema JS, Wagenaar SS, Paques M, Steerenberg PA, Ruitenberg EJ (1986). Histological evaluation of immunologically mediated tumor regression of the line 10 guinea pig hepatocarcinoma. Virchows Arch (Cell Pathol) 50: 249.

Klein WR, Ruitenberg EJ, Steerenberg PA, de Jong WH, Kruizinga W, Misdorp W, Bier J, Tiesjema RH, Kreeftenberg JG, Teppema JS, Rapp HJ (1982). Immunotherapy by intravesical injection of BCG cell walls or live BCG in bovine ocular squamous cell carcinoma: a preliminary report. J Natl Cancer Institute 69: 1095.

Klein WR, Bras GE, Misdorp W, Steerenberg PA, de Jong WH, Tiesjema RH, Kersjes AW, Ruitenberg EJ (1986). Equine sarcoid: BCG immunotherapy compared to cryosurgery in a prospective randomized clinical trial. Cancer Imm Immunoth 21: 133.

Lamm DL, Thor DE, Winters WD, Stogdill VD, Radwin HM (1981). BCG immunotherapy of bladder cancer: inhibition of tumor recurrence and associated immune responses. Cancer 48: 82.

Lamm DL, Stogdill VD, Stogdill BJ, Crispen RG (1986). Complications of Bacillus Calmette-Guérin immunotherapy in 1278 patients with bladder cancer. J Urol 135: 272.

van der Meijden APM, de Jong WH, Steerenberg PA, Geerse E, de Boer EG, Ruitenberg EJ (1987). Histological changes and immunological response after intravesical immunotherapy with BCG-RIVM in the guinea pig. J Urol 137: 165A.

van der Meijden APM. Unpublished observations.

Morales A, Eidinger D, Bruce AW (1976). Intracavitary Bacillus Calmette-Guérin in the treatment of superficial bladder tumors. J Urol 116: 180.

Morales A (1980). Treatment of carcinoma in situ of the bladder with BCG. A phase II trial. Cancer Immunol Immunother 9: 69.

Morales A, Nickel JC (1986). Immunotherapy of superficial bladder cancer with BCG. World J Urol 3: 209.

Ruitenberg EJ, de Jong WH, Kreeftenberg PA, Kruizenga W, van Noorle Jansen LM (1981). BCG preparations, cultured homogeneously dispersed or as surface pellicle, elicit different immunopotentiating effects but have similar antitumor activity in a murine fibrosarcoma. Cancer Immunol Immunoth 11: 45.

Zbar B, Bernstein ID, Bartlett GL, Hanna MG, Rapp HJ (1972). Immunotherapy of cancer: regression of intra-dermal tumors and prevention of growth of lymph node metastases after intralesional injection of living Myco-bacterium bovis. J Natl Cancer Inst 49: 119.

PART IV. CONTROVERSIES AND FUTURE GUIDELINES ON BCG-IMMUNOTHERAPY FOR SUPERFICIAL BLADDER CANCER

EORTC Genitourinary Group Monograph 6:
BCG in Superficial Bladder Cancer, pages 301–310
© 1989 Alan R. Liss, Inc.

PERCUTANEOUS, ORAL, OR INTRAVESICAL BCG ADMINISTRATION:
WHAT IS THE OPTIMAL ROUTE?

Donald L. Lamm, Michael S. Sarodosy, Jean I. DeHaven

Department of Urology, West Virginia University,
Morgantown, USA

BCG immunotherapy for recurrent superficial bladder cancer is perhaps the most successful form of immunotherapy for human malignancy. As illustrated in this volume, current data suggest that BCG is the most effective intravesical treatment of carcinoma in situ (CIS) and the most effective prophylaxis for the prevention of recurrence of transitional cell carcinoma (TCC).

Multiple investigators have confirmed the efficacy of BCG in the prevention of bladder tumor recurrence and the treatment of residual TCC and CIS of the bladder. Two studies comparing BCG with Thiotepa intravesical chemotherapy have found BCG to significantly further improve tumor prophylaxis (Brosman, 1982; Netto and Lemos, 1983), and the multicenter study conducted by the Southwest Oncology Group presented earlier in this volume provides convincing evidence that BCG immunotherapy is superior to Doxorubicin chemotherapy of superficial bladder cancer.

Although the optimal protocol for BCG immunotherapy remains undefined, the experience of multiple investigators has provided extensive information from which reasonable though tentative conclusions can be drawn. Substrains which have been demonstrated by clinical trials to be effective intravesically include Armand Frappier, RIVM, Connaught, Pasteur, Japanese, and Tice. The optimal dose of vaccine has not been established since treatments have been given empirically. Commonly used and effective intravesical doses of these vaccines are 120 mg for Armand-Frappier, RIVM, Connaught, and Pasteur preparations, 50 mg for Tice, and

40 mg for Japanese BCG. Table 1 lists BCG doses and the common treatment schedules used.

TABLE 1. Treatment schedules/Effective vaccines/doses

Effective Schedules

Morales (1986) : weekly x 6

Brosman (1982) : weekly x 6 (-24)
                     then monthly

Catalona (1987):weekly x 6,
                   repeat with weekly x 6 if recurrence

Lamm (1985)   : weekly x 6,
                     every other week x 3, at 6 months,
                     and then every 6 months

Effective Vaccines/Doses

Armand-Frappier:	120 mg	
RIVM	:	1×10^9 CFU
Connaught	:	120 mg
Pasteur	:	120 mg
Tice	:	50 mg
Japanese	:	40 mg
Glaxo/Evans	:	1×10^9 CFU*

---

* This is not the preparation commercially available in the USA.

Patients have been treated empirically at weekly intervals for six weeks. It has not been firmly established that longer courses are better or that shorter courses are equally effective. The necessity of maintenance BCG immuno-therapy remains debatable. In theory, since it is known that the immune stimulation induced by BCG wanes with time and the proclivity of the urothelium to tumor formation persists, periodic retreatment with BCG should improve long term results. Long term protection from a single course of BCG would suggest the correction of an immune deficit, the induction of specific antitumor immunity, or the elimination or reversal of malignant transformation in the urothelium. In our experience with previously randomized patients followed for at least one year or until tumor recurrence, maintenance BCG immunotherapy reduced the rate of tumor recurrence four-fold, from 1.9 to 0.49 tumors per 100 patient months (Lamm, 1985).

In a randomized study of 42 evaluable patients, Hudson found no difference in tumor recurrence in patients receiving a 6 week course of intravesical BCG and those receiving an additional BCG treatment every three months (Hudson et al., 1987). Similarly, Badalament reported equal recurrence in 93 patients randomized to non-maintenance or maintenance BCG at monthly intervals beginning at 3 months (Badalament, 1987).

These randomized studies document the remarkable effectiveness of a single 6 week course of BCG and cast serious doubt on the benefit of maintenance therapy. However, maintenance therapy is, by definition, designed to sustain complete response after optimal induction therapy. Both of these studies used a single 6 week induction, and did not initiate maintenance until the third month. Since a single 6 week course of BCG is highly effective and our controlled animal model studies have demonstrated that the protective effect of BCG is long term, that is, persists for at least 8 months in mice without further BCG administration, it is likely that more patients followed for longer periods of time will be needed to determine whether maintenance BCG therapy will further improve clinical results.

While Stober and Peters have clearly demonstrated in a randomized prospective study that percutaneous BCG alone has no antitumor activity, the added value of percutaneous BCG has been controversial (Stober and Peters, 1980). Clearly excellent results can be obtained with high-dose intravesical BCG alone (Brosman, 1985). My early experience with Armand-Frappier BCG given only intravesically was disappointing: 40% of patients developed tumor recurrence, and no patient converted from skin test negative to positive with 6 weekly intravesical instillations. Subsequently, with the addition of percutaneous BCG and additional course of intravesical therapy, patients both converted skin test reactivity and reduced the rate of tumor recurrence. While percutaneous administration may enhance the systemic immunity conferred by intravesical BCG treatment and perhaps decrease the need of high dose intravescial BCG to achieve a response, adequate comparison studies had not been performed. To evaluate the added benefit, if any, of percutaneous BCG, we conducted a randomized prospective comparison.

Even more controversial has been the use of oral rather than intravescial BCG in the treatment and prophylaxis of bladder cancer. Our animal data (Reichert and Lamm, 1984), and that of multiple investigators (Bast and Bast, 1976), has demonstrated that juxtaposition of BCG and tumor antigens provides the best antitumor response. The reported dramatic reduction in tumor recurrence with oral BCG, as reported by Netto and Lemos, and the subsequent report of regression of muscle invasive disease with oral therapy were therefore surprising (Netto and Lemos, 1983; 1984). Oral BCG therapy has been reported by many to be virtually without side effects, but the widely proven efficacy of intravesical BCG and the potential expense of the massive doses of oral BCG diminish enthusiasm for this approach. Why then, should oral BCG therapy be investigated? For two reasons: first, animal data from 2 independent laboratories have in fact confirmed that high-dose systemic BCG does inhibit peripheral transitional cell carcinoma (Drago and Sipio, 1985; Pang and Morales, 1982), and second, if BCG given orally inhibits TCC in the bladder it might be equally effective in inhibiting TCC in the lung or pelvic lymph nodes. Such therapy could thus provide the effective adjuvant to cystectomy that has thus far eluded us. To evaluate the potential role of oral BCG immunotherapy a randomized prospective comparison with standard intravesical therapy was performed.

METHODS

Percutaneous BCG

Consenting patients with biopsy-confirmed TCC of the bladder were stratified by tumor recurrence (1 versus 2 or more in the most recent year) and tumor grade (1 versus 2 or more) and then randomized to receive intravesical BCG-Tice, 50 mg in 50 cc saline each week for 6 weeks, at 8, 10, and 12 weeks, at 6 months and every 6 months with or without simultaneous percutaneous BCG administered by the multiple puncture technique. Patients were followed with cystoscopy at 3 month intervals with biospy of suspicious lesions and cytology.

Oral BCG

Consenting patients with biopsy-confirmed TCC of the bladder were stratified by tumor recurrence (1 versus 2 or more in the most recent year) and tumor grade (1 versus 2 or more) and then randomized to receive oral or intravesical plus percutaneous BCG. Because of a shortage in vaccine, the original one to one randomization had to be modified to a 1 oral to 3 intravesical randomization mid way through the study, resulting in an increased number of patients in the standard BCG treatment arm. Intravesical and percutaneous BCG-Tice was given as described above. Oral BCG consisted of 200 mg BCG-Tice given on Monday, Wednesday, and Friday of each week. Patients were instructed to rinse their mouths with apple juice after taking oral BCG.

RESULTS

Percutaneous BCG

Seventy eight patients with superficial transitional cell carcinoma of the bladder were enrolled. Sixty-six completed therapy and had sufficient follow-up (3 to 25 months) to be considered evaluable. Mean follow-up for the intravesical only group (IVES) was 12 months; mean follow-up for the intravesical plus percutaneous group (IVPRC) was 11 months. Mean comparable with respect to sex distribution with 70% and 80% male in IVES and IVPRC groups respectively. Fifty-nine percent of the IVES group had more than 2 recurrences in the most recent year compared with 54% of the IVPRC group. Of the 30 evaluable patients randomized to receive intravesical only BCG, 13 (43%) had biopsy-confirmed tumor recurrence at a mean of 7 months. Of the 36 patients who received intravesical plus percutaneous BCG, 15 (42%) had tumor recurrence at a mean of 5 months. As illustrated in Figure 1, the time at which recurrence occurred was virtually identical in the 2 groups.

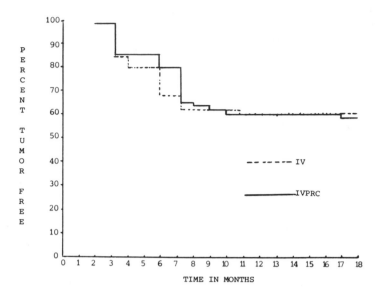

Figure 1. Illustrated is the time to recurrence for intravesical (IV) and intravesical plus percutaneous (IVPRC)
groups. No difference in recurrence was observed.

Oral BCG
    Minimal side effects confirmed the safety of oral BCG.
An occasional patient noted mild transient gastro-
intestinal upset or diarrhea, but serious toxicity was not
observed. No elevation of liver function tests occurred.
The toxicity of intravesical and percutaneous BCG has been
well documented and no unexpected complications occurred in
these patients.

    Tumor recurrence was documented in 21 of the 33
patients (64%) treated with oral BCG and 18 of the 55
patients (33%) treated with intravesical BCG (p < 0.001,
chisquared). The time to recurrence curves for the two
groups are illustrated in Figure 2.

    Twelve patients with CIS of the bladder were studied,
4 in the oral group and 8 in the intravesical group. Resolution of CIS documented by biopsy and cytology occurred in
1 patient (25%) in the oral group and 6 patients (75%) in
the intravesical group.

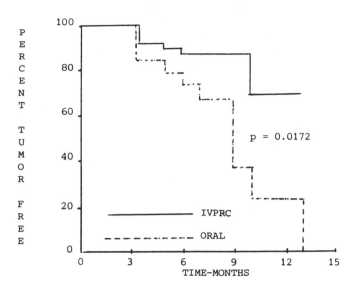

Figure 2. Illustrated is the time to recurrence for the intravesical plus percutaneous group (IVPRC) and the oral BCG group. The advantage for intravesical plus percutaneous BCG was highly significant.

DISCUSSION

BCG immunotherapy in superficial bladder cancer has been remarkably successful and has exceeded the expectations of even the most optimistic researchers and clinicians. In treating superficial disease, exclusive of CIS, 58% of 118 reported cases have responded with complete resolution of all tumor (Lamm, 1987). Efforts to improve the efficacy of BCG immunotherapy continue. Our initial experience suggested that percutaneous BCG enhanced the efficacy of 6 weekly intravesical therapy. However, no evidence of enhanced efficacy (reduced tumor recurrence) was observed in our randomized prospective comparison in patients treated with maintenance BCG. Although our numbers are relatively small and our length of follow-up averages only one year, it is highly unlikely that percutaneous BCG has any impact on immunotherapy results in patients who receive more than 6 weekly treatments. Whether percutaneous BCG has a role in less intensive treatment regimens has not been tested.

    Despite the proven efficacy of intravesical BCG immunotherapy, many patients, particularly those with extensive disease or disease invading the prostatic urethra or involving the ureters, will fail. Even more problematic is the patient who undergoes radical cystectomy for invasive bladder cancer, who has no clinical evidence of metastatic disease, and yet has more than a 50% probability of dying of metastatic disease. Unfortunately, even though combination chemotherapy with agents such as Cisplatinum, Cyclophosphamide, and Doxorubicin (CISCA); Cisplatinum, Methotrexate, and vincristine (CMV); and Methotrexate, Vinblastine, Doxorubicin, and Cisplatinum (MVAC) have demonstrated complete responses in as high as 50% of patients, to date adjuvant chemotherapy has not proven to be superior to radical cystectomy alone in controlled trials. Therefore, it is unlikely that post-operative chemotherapy with drugs currently available will significantly impact on survival of patients undergoing cystectomy. Moreover, chemotherapy with these drugs in the population at risk is highly toxic and would inflict significant morbidity to one half of these patients without benefit. An ideal adjuvant would effectibely remove occult metastatic disease without imposing significant risk or morbidity. The reported efficacy of high-dose oral BCG in preventing tumor recurrence and inducing regression of muscle-invasive disease suggested that such treatment could provide an ideal adjuvant to cystectomy. It could also be an effective modality in patients with disease that could not be reached by topical intravesical instillation. This goal prompted our evaluation of oral BCG and the comparison oral and intravesical routes of administration.

    Our results confirm the efficacy of intravesical and percutaneous BCG-Tice in the prevention of bladder tumor recurrence and the treatment of CIS, and demonstrate its marked superiority over oral BCG. In fact, we were unable to demonstrate any antitumor activity of oral BCG with the dose and substrain utilized. Unfortunately, the exact protocol of Netto and Lemos was not used in this study so the efficacy of that technique remains to be confirmed or refuted. Animal data clearly suggest that systemic BCG is effective only when given in high doses. Soloway found no antitumor effect using low-dose intraperitoneal BCG in a mouse model (Soloway, 1977). However, Pang and Morales in the same model and Drago and Sipio in the Nb rat bladder tumor model clearly demonstrated that high-dose systemic (intraperitoneal) BCG could effectively inhibit the growth of peripherally transplanted TCC (Drago and Sipio, 1985; Pang and Morales, 1982). In our study, BCG-Tice rather than BCG-Moreau R.J. was utilized in an average dose of 200 mg three times each week rather than 400 mg. These protocol modifications were imposed by the availability of vaccine and the advantage of using the same preparation. The dosage of BCG was reduced because of reported increased potency of the Tice preparation, but considerations was not given to the fact that the Moreau preparation was used fresh while Tice is supplied as a lyophylized vaccine. Lyophilization results in a ten-fold loss of viability when compared with the fresh vaccine, and therefore the effective dose employed in this experiment may have been only one fiftieth of that used by Netto and Lemos. While our results clearly confirm that intravesical and percutaneous BCG-Tice is superior to oral BCG-Tice in doses of 200 mg thrice weekly, we cannot say that higher doses or other strains may not be as effective as topically administered BCG.

CONCLUSIONS

BCG immunotherapy has significantly improved the management of superficial bladder cancer, and, as such, holds the promise that immunotherapy may eventually play a role in the management of invasive or metastatic disease. Our data suggest that the addition of percutaneous BCG does not materially improve the efficacy of intravescial administration given on a maintenance schedule. Effective cytomic immunity should improve local control and reduce metastasis of TCC. The addition of systemic percutaneous BCG does not appear to enhance such immunity. The confirmed animal data and preliminary clinical experience which suggested that systemic BCG administration can cause regression of localized tumor implies that BCG might have a role as an adjuvant to cystectomy. Out inability to confirm the efficacy of oral BCG precludes such trials at the present time, but should not diminish the intensity of our search for other systemically effective immunotherapies.

REFERENCES

Badalament RA, Herr HW, Wong GY, Gnecco C, Pinsky CM, Whitmore Jr WF, Fair WR, Oettgen HF (1987). A prospective randomized trial of maintenance vs non-maintenance intra-vesical BCG therapy for superficial bladder cancer. J Clin Oncol 5: 441.

Bast RC, Bast BS (1976) Critical review of previously reported animal studies of tumor immunotherapy with non-specific immunostimulants. Ann NY Acad Sci 277: 60-93.

Brosman SA (1982). Experience with Bacillus Calmette-Guérin in patients with superficial bladder carcinoma. J Urol 128: 27-30.

Brosman SA (1985). The use of Bacillus Calmette-Guérin in the therapy of bladder carcinoma in situ. J Urol 134: 36.

Catalona WJ, Hudson, M'Liss A, Gillen DP, Andriole GL, Ratliff TL (1987). Risk and benefits of repeated courses of intravesical Bacillus Calmette-Guerin therapy for superficial bladder cancer. J Urol 137: 220.

Drago JR, Sipio J (1985). Characterization of the Nb rat bladder cancer model. Surg Forum 36: 645.

Hudson MA, Ratliff TL, Gillen DP, Haaff EO, Dresner SM, Catalona WJ (1987). Single course versus maintenance Bacillus Calmette-Guérin therapy for superficial bladder tumors. A prospective randomized trial. J Urol 138: 295-298.

Lamm DL (1985). BCG immunotherapy in bladder cancer. J Urol 134: 40.

Lamm DL (1987). BCG immunotherapy in bladder cancer. In Rouse SN (ed): "Urology Annual," Los Altos: Appleton and Lange, pp 67.

Morales A, Nickel JG (1986). Immunotherapy of superficial bladder cancer with BCG. World J Urol 3: 209.

Netto Jr NR, Lemos CG (1983). A comparison of treatment methods for prophylaxis of recurrent superficial bladder tumors. J Urol 129: 33.

Netto Jr NR, Lemos CG (1984). Bacillus Calmette-Guérin immunotherapy of infiltrating bladder cancer. J Urol 132: 675.

Pang AS, Morales A (1982). Immunoprophylaxis of a murine bladder cancer with high dose BCG immunization. J Urol 127: 1006.

Reichert DF, Lamm DL (1984). Long term protection in bladder cancer following intralesional immunotherapy. J Urol 132: 570.

Soloway MS (1987). Intravesical and systemic chemotherapy of murine bladder cancer. Cancer Res 37: 2918.

Stober U, Peters HH (1980). BCG-Immunotherapie zur Rezidiv-prophylaxe beim Harnblasenkarzinom. Therapiewoche 30: 6067.

EORTC Genitourinary Group Monograph 6:
BCG in Superficial Bladder Cancer, pages 311–323
© 1989 Alan R. Liss, Inc.

A PRACTICAL GUIDE TO THE USE OF INTRAVESICAL BCG FOR THE MANAGEMENT OF STAGE Ta, T1, CIS, TRANSITIONAL CELL CANCER

Stanley A. Brosman, Donald L. Lamm, Ad. P.M. van der Meijden, Frans M.J. Debruyne
Kaiser Permanente Medical Center (S.A.B.), Los Angeles, USA, University School of Medicine (D.L.L.), Morgantown, USA, University Hospital Nijmegen, (A.P.M.v.d.M, F.M.J.), Nijmegen, The Netherlands

The increasing use of BCG in the treatment of patients with low-stage bladder cancer will inevitably bring attention to problems of proper usage and toxicity. There is a need to identify patients who are most likely to benefit from this therapy and a need to identify patients who may be at risk for serious complications.

As the use of intravesical BCG for the management of transitional cell carcinoma increases, the number of problems and complications associated with its usage is likely to increase. Although BCG instillations have been shown to be effective and well tolerated by the majority of patients, there are situations where potentially serious problems might arise. Careful selections and management of the patients can reduce and prevent serious complication. Our experience in treating 1,254 patients over the past 15 years has taught us how to avoid some of the problems which can be associated with BCG instillation. During this time we have observed or consulted on almost every complication or adverse effect which has been reported. There have been 2 deaths from confirmed BCG sepsis in outside hospitals in patients treated on our protocols and several patients in our early experience nearly died as a result of sepsis.

This experience taught us how to recognize the early warning signs of a potentially serious problem and institute therapy to prevent complications. We now recognize that there are situations when BCG should not be administered and other times when BCG therapy should be halted or delayed.

Tice strain BCG was used in the majority of the patients. A small number were treated with the Connaught, Armand Frappier, and Glaxo strains while in the Netherlands the RIVM strain was used. The Connaught strain seems to be equivalent to Tice in terms of tumor response and toxicity but there have been no comparative studies done to prove this impression. A comparative study between Tice and RIVM strain is ongoing in the Netherlands. The Glaxo strain was ineffective in the situations where it was used.

WHO IS ELIGIBLE FOR BCG THERAPY

Prophylaxis

Potential candidates for BCG instillations can be divided into three categories. The prophylaxis group consists of patients who have a high risk of developing a tumor recurrence and an attempt to reduce this probability is warranted. Most patients with stage pTa and pT1 TCC which has been completely resected are potential candidates if they have high grade and multiple tumors.

Of all patients with TCC of the bladder, 70-80% have stage pTa/pT1 disease. Since 50% to 70% of all patients with pTa/pT1 TCC are likely to develop a recurrence, the clinician has the dilemma of deciding which patient to treat. Those with stage pTa tumors comprise 60-70% of this category but in those who are treated only with TUR, less than 6% are likely to develop tumor progression, at the time of a subsequent recurrence (Cutler et al., 1982). Patients with stage T1 disease have a 30% to 46% probability of developing tumor progression and when this occurs it is most likely to do so within the first 12 months (Heney et al., 1983).

When tumor grade is analyzed, it has been shown that only 6% of grade 1 lesions become invasive and rarely metastasize, whereas 52% of grade 2 and 82% of grade 3 tumors become invasive and are likely to become metastatic (Gilbert et al., 1978; Pauwels et al., 1988). Only 5% of patients whose original tumor was grade 1 will die of their disease (Van der Meijden, 1988), but 16% of those with grade 2 and 60% of those with grade 3 eventually die of their tumors (Cutler et al., 1982; Gilbert et al., 1978;

Heney et al., 1983). Recurrence rates within 3 years for Ta G1 are 25%, Ta G2 53%, Ta G3 60%, T1 G2 59%, and T1 G3 80% respectively.

Other risk factors for recurrence include tumor multiplicity (> 3), a history of previous TCC and, to a lesser extent tumor size greater than 5 cm. In a study by Cutler, patients with single tumors had a 67% chance of recurrence compared to a 90% probability for multiple tumors (Cutler et al., 1982). Others have suggested that the number of tumors at the time of original diagnosis is the single most important factor influencing tumor recurrence (Dalesio et al., 1983). After an analysis of the data it would seem reasonable to conclude that patients with their first episode of bladder cancer which is stage pTa, grade 1, and is a solitary lesion less than 3 cm, do not need to receive intravesical instillation of chemotherapeutic agents or BCG. Fortunately, a substantial number of patients fall into this category.

Residual tumor

The second group of patients who may benefit from therapy are those who are known to have residual papillary tumors in the bladder or develop a recurrence but are not good candidates for surgery (Brosman, 1982; Lamm et al., 1981; Lamm, 1985). Since one of the caveats for successful BCG therapy states that the tumor burden should be small, tumors that are greater than 2 cm are less likely to respond favorably. The number of tumors seems of no consequence as long as they are small and accessible to the action of BCG. One of the problems in assigning patients to the proper treatment protocol, has been the finding of a tumor at the first cystoscopy following BCG induction phase. Whether or not the tumor represents a recurrence or a tumor which was previously unidentified cannot be ascertained. Therefore, it is difficult to decide whether the BCG prophylaxis therapy was ineffective or the patient should have been assigned to the proper protocol for eliminating existing tumor. One method to obviate this situation is to obtain a post TUR urine cytology and to perform a cystoscopy before initiating therapy.

Carcinoma in situ

The third group of patients who are candidates for BCG instillations either have carcinoma in situ as a primary disease or have residual CIS following resection of a papillary or sessile TCC (Herr et al., 1986; Morales and Nickel, 1986). CIS has a variable form of presentation and the diffuse form is associated with the most rapid development of invasive disease and is associated with the highest mortality.

WHO SHOULD NOT BE TREATED

Because BCG must be in contact with the epithelial surface containing the CIS, intravesical instillations are inadequate to treat disease in the ureters. Patients with CIS growing into the prostatic ducts or cancer which has invaded the bladder muscle are not likely to benefit from this type of therapy. If the CIS is confined to the bladder epithelial surface, the treatment is likely to be effective.

The largest group of patients who do not need therapy are those with their first episode of pTa G1 tumors which are solitary and less than 3 cm in size. Since these tumors rarely progress, it is safe to await a recurrence before beginning prophylaxis therapy of any type.

Patients who are immunocompromised may be unable to mount a local inflammatory response. They may be unable to control the systemic spread of the live organisms. Fortunately, most patients with stage Ta G1 bladder cancer do not fall into this category. We have instilled BCG into the bladder of a patient who we later learned was HIV positive. He had no adverse effect but neither did have a beneficial response. In general it may be unwise to use BCG in HIV positive individuals or individuals who have other malignant tumors which are progressing. There has been concern about BCG overwhelming the immune system and enhancing the growth of a second cancer. While our controlled comparison of BCG and Adriamycin intravesical therapy showed no increase in second malignant tumors of other origin in either group. Caution should be exercised in patients who have other malignancies.

WHEN TO START TREATMENT

Therapy can begin several days to two weeks following the TUR for individuals who are in the prophylaxis protocol. There may be some advantage to beginning treatment a few days following the TUR while the bladder is still inflamed and the mucosa has not healed completely but this issue has not yet been resolved. A fresh, bleeding wound in the urethra or bladder can be the place where living BCG bacilli may penetrate into the circulation with the consequent danger of sepsis.We prefer to start treatment when the patients had a negative urine culture, a negative cytology, a cystoscopy showing no residual tumor and when there is no gross hematuria or bladder irritability.

Patients with existing tumor can begin therapy when the bladder has been carefully mapped, the tumor(s) size noted (e.g. photographically) and the urine culture is negative. The same is true for patients with CIS.

PREPARING AND INSTILLING THE BCG

The BCG comes in a lyophilized form which should be reconstituted with saline rather than water. The preparation of the solution should be done using sterile technique and the individual responsible for mixing the solution may wear gloves and a mask to avoid inadvertent exposure of open sores or inhalation of live organisms. The suspension, consists of one ampule of BCG gently swirled and mixed with 50 cc of preservative and antibiotic-free saline, can be instilled shortly after it is ready, or within the next several hours. The swirling prevents clumping of the bacteria. It is usually wise to wait until the patient has arrived in the office before preparing the solution because it cannot be used the following day.

Although it is unnecessary to state that the catheterization should be as atraumatic as possible, there are some special considerations when BCG is being instilled. We have found that the number of severe reactions is much higher when the patient has had a traumatic catheterization or instrumentation. Therefore there are situation where the instillation should be postponed. Although we have instilled BCG at the time of cystoscopy, the patients often report that the reaction is more severe than that experienced after the usual instillation.

THERAPEUTIC PROTOCOL

The most effective protocol for administering BCG has not yet been found and in fact may never be found because there may be no protocol which is optimal for each patient. There is general agreement, that an initial or induction phase is necessary to establish an inflammatory response within the bladder epithelium. Most patients achieve this response within six weekly instillations but there are those who require fewer and some who need even more instillations before their bladders begin to show inflammatory reaction. Once the inflammation of the epithelium has developed, it is not clear whether or not there is a need for maintenance therapy. The purpose of maintenance therapy is to maintain the antitumor response or reactivate it in the hope of preventing a recurrence of the neoplasm. Because we are dealing with a biologic product with inherent variability in the dose and great variability in host response to the treatment, the plan for each patient may need to be individualized. The need for maintenance therapy has not been established and there is early data which indicates that it is of no benefit (Badalament et al., 1987). There are patients in the prophylaxis protocol whose risk for recurrence is low and who develop a potent inflammatory reaction to BCG during the induction phase. They would not benefit to a great extent from maintenance therapy. The decision to use maintenance therapy is likely to be made on an individual basis. If the urologist deems that maintenance therapy is beneficial then the question arises as to how long it should be given. Some earlier protocols suggested monthly instillations for 1-2 years. But this program was arbitrary and there are no data to indicate that if maintenance therapy is beneficial at all, there is an advantage to monthly instillations compared to every 3 months, or 6 months or at any interval. There are also no data to indicate how long maintenance therapy should be utilized.

When treating patients with CIS or those with existing tumor the exact number of instillations necessary to achieve an optimum response in the bladder is unknown (Catalona et al., 1987; Haaff et al., 1986). We have had successful responses in some patients who received only three instillations and others have had 24 instillations. Based upon our experience, we would judge that most patients who respond will do so with six to twelve instillations and maintenance therapy is arbitrary (unpublished observations).

Patients who fail to respond to therapy and who do not show an inflammatory response may be given additional treatment or a stronger dose. The failure to develop an in- flammatory reaction, not necessarily a granulomatous reac- tion, suggests that BCG may be defective, the individual is unable to mount an inflammatory reaction to the dosage schedule being utilized or there is some other mechanism at work about which we have no knowledge sofar. It must also be acknowledged that an occasional patient who failes to develop an inflammatory response in the bladder will remain tumor free for a prolonged period of time.

Patients whose tumor persists or recurs in spite of having histologic evidence of an inflammatory reaction represent true failures of this therapy. Although there is a systemic and local immunologic component to the BCG reaction, this is likely to be a weak antitumor effect to a poorly antigenic tumor, as suggested by the development of cancer at other sites in the urinary tract in patients whose bladder cancer was effectively eliminated and in whom a strong local inflammatory reaction developed.

ADVERSE REACTIONS AND THEIR MANAGEMENT

The majority of patients tolerate BCG instillations reasonably well but adverse effects can and do occur (Lamm et al., 1986). It is important that patients be advised that an infectious agent is being utilized and that any unusual reactions should be reported to the physician. Adverse reactions often are localized in the bladder but may be accompanied by systemic symptoms. The commonest local reactions relate to the inflammatory response in the bladder and can be experienced after the first instillation but more commonly are noted after the third administration. They begin 3-4 hours after the instillation and usually last 24-72 hours. These reactions consist of bladder irri- tability but there may be gross hematuria. The reactions can become progressively more severe after each instilla- tion and there are patients who have developed such severe reactions that their bladder capacity was permanently reduced.

Complications associated with intravesical BCG have been reviewed by Lamm who analyzed 1278 patients (Lamm et al., 1986). This author reported on 195 of his own patients and an additional 1083 patients reported by different investigators in the USA and Europe (Lamm et al., 1986). Lamm could find no difference in the incidence of side effects in patients treated with either the Pasteur (Armand Frappier), Tice, or Connaught preparations and found no difference in toxicity. Van der Meijden observed that patients treated with a Dutch BCG strain (BCG-RIVM) showed drug induced cycstitis in 16.7% of 78 patients (van der Meijden, 1988). In the same group no severe systemic complications were encountered. Recently, however, a patient developed a biopsy confirmed granulomatous pneumonitis. Frequency and dysuria occured to a variable degree in 90% of the patients. Pyuria was found in nearly every patient but urine cultures are rarely positive. Hematuria occurred in 43% of the patients and was severe in 0.5-1%.

Systemic side effects consist of a fever > 103°F in 28%, malaise in 24% and nausea in 8%. More serious side effects occur in 5% of all patients. A wide variety of systemic reactions have been reported and we have seen enough indications of the generalized spread of the organism to be very cautious about the continued use of treatment in patients who develop severe reactions. The commonest observation is the "flu-like syndrome" consisting of a modest temperature elevation, aching in the muscles and joints, and a feeling of malaise. Among the more serious reactions which we have seen, are prostatitis, orchitis, hepatitis, arthritis including one patient wiht Sjogren's syndrom, granulomatous changes in a vertebra, leukopenia from BCG-itis in the bone marrow, pulmonary changes and generalized septic reactions.

There have been three deaths associated with intravesical instillations of BCG in which patients developed sepsis with granulomas and inflammation developing almost everywhere in the body. In these patients the systemic reaction occurred after the fifth, sixth and eighth instillations. Other instances of sepsis have occurred after the third instillation and another patient developed sepsis six months after completing BCG therapy (Steg et al., 1988).

There is a recurring observation in the patients who develop sepsis or have severe systemic complications. These indivuduals usually show signs of an increasingly severe reaction with high temperatures or the reactions last longer. A common thread in all fatal cases and most septic cases is intravasation of intravesically instilled BCG. Steg reported that one patient had a fever of 104°F due to traumatic catheterization or absorption through inflamed, friable bleeding bladder urothelium. This followed the sixth BCG instillation and the patient became septic and died after the eighth instillation which was associated with a traumatic catheterization (Steg, 1988). Rawls and Lamm reported on the deaths of two patients which were brought to their attention (Rawls and Lamm, 1988). One was 66 years old and had Ta G2 tumor and CIS. After the fifth instilation there was a fever of 103°F. The patient was given INH but the patient became septic and died. The second death occured in a 63-year-old being treated for the prevention of disease in whom the original tumor was Ta G2. Two hours after the fifth dose the patient became hypotensive and was started on INH. The patient was given a sixth instillation a week later without INH. Four days later the patient became hypotensive and died with sepsis. Although the numbers are small, Lamm has observed that 2 of his patients with life threatening BCG sepsis have survived with the use of triple anti-tuberculous antibiotics including cycloserine, while none of the fatal cases received the benefit of this more rapidly acting antibiotic.

Our own observations on the development of sepsis in several patients indicate the need to know how to predict when this is likely to occur, how to prevent sepsis when possible, and how to manage sepsis when it is diagnosed. Our policy has been to start patients on oral INH when they report that they are having any systemic reaction which is associated with a fever of over 100°F (38°C) and which lasts longer than 24 hours. We feel that the risk associated with the potential hepatotoxicity of INH is less than that associated with a septic episode from BCG. Patients are instructed to take INH 300 mg daily beginning on the day of each instillation and continuing for the next two days. Liver function studies are obtained and if they are abnormal, therapy is withheld until they have become normal. Non-steroidal anti-inflammatory agents and antihistamines are beneficial in controlling some of the milder systemic symptoms. However, BCG therapy is stopped in patients who continue to have a febrile reaction, if there is a recurring evaluation of the liver function enzymes or the patient develops signs of prostatitis, orchitis etc. Experience over 8 years has shown that septic episodes and severe complications can be virtually eliminated if traumatic catheterization is avoided, BCG is withheld until symptoms of cystitis or signs and symptoms of systemic reaction have resolved, and INH coverage is provided. We have had patients who developed orchitis and prostatitis while they were using INH and some patients continued to have side effects severe enough to stop BCG treatment.

Concern has been raised regarding the possibility that INH might abrogate the antitumor effect of BCG. Animal studies have clearly demonstrated that this does not occur, and theoretical considerations strongly suggest that withholding INH in these circumstances is much more likely to reduce the antitumor effect. Data from our laboratory and others demonstrates that excess BCG administration reduces antitumor effect and can, on rare occasion, even result in enhancement of tumor growth. To withhold INH in a patient who has clearly demonstrated increased susceptability to BCG infections is to risk not only severe toxicity but also diminished antitumor efficacy.

Comparing our complications before and after beginning INH and learning when to withhold and stop therapy has greatly reduced the incidence and severity of adverse consequences of BCG. We experienced that it is not necessary to treat patients every week during the induction phase. Once a patient has a strong reaction to the BCG, the goal of the induction phase has been achieved and we consider it safer to wait one week or even two before giving the next dose allowing the patient to recover. If the patient has two successive adverse reactions such as severe bladder irritative symptoms and fever > 101°F in spite of taking the medications prescribed, therapy with BCG is stopped. Therapy is withheld if the patient reports that the inflammatory symptoms persisted for more than 5 days or when the patient has a viral infection.

Lamm has recommended that patients with reactions severe enough to produce sepsis be treated with triple drug anti-tuberculosis therapy which includes cycloserine (Lamm, 1988). The effect of anti-tuberculous antibiotics, with the exception of cycloserine, is not evident until 3 days after administration. The patient with fullminant BCG sepsis is at high risk of expiring within 3 days and therefore initial management should include cycloserine. BCG retains sensitivity to anti-tuberculous antibiotics. Recommended therapy for systemic BCG infection is INH 300 mg orally per day, Rifampicin 600 mg orally per day, and Ethambutol 1200 mg orally per day. In patients with life-threatening sepsis, cycloserine 250 to 500 mg is given orally twice daily for the first 3 days or until the acute crisis has resolved. The duration of therapy is uncertain but the minimum time should be 3-6 months.

Therapy should be withheld in patients with abnormal liver function tests until these have become normal. BCG can be restarted with the patient taking INH but should be stopped if the liver enzymes become abnormal again.

SUMMARY

Intravesical instillations of BCG are effective in preventing tumor recurrence, eliminating existing tumor and treating CIS in a substantial number of patients. As with any type of therapy, side effects can occur. Because a live organism is being used, care must be taken in the handling and administration of the product. Patients should be informed about the common types of reactions so that these may be reported to the urologist. In turn, the urologist must decide if the treatment plan needs to be modified or the patient started on medications which can prevent or reduce the severity of the side effects. At times a decision must be made regarding withholding or delaying treatment and there are situations when BCG should be stopped.

REFERENCES

Badalament RA, Herr HW, Wong GY, Gnecco C, Pinsky CM, Whitmore Jr WF, Fair WR, Oettgen HF (1987). A prospective randomized trial of maintenance vs non-maintenance intravesical BCG therapy for superficial bladder cancer. J Clin Oncol 5: 441.
Brosman SA (1982). Experience with Bacillus Calmette-Guérin in patients with superficial bladder carcinoma. J Urol 128: 27.
Catalona WJ, Hudson, M'Liss A, Gillen DP, Andriole GL, Ratliff TL (1987). Risk and benefits of repeated courses

of intravesical Bacillus Calmette-Guérin therapy for superficial bladder cancer. J Urol 137: 220.

Cutler SJ, Heney NM, Friedell GW (1982). Longitudinal study of patients with bladder cancer: factors associated with disease recurrence and progression. In Bonney Ww, Prout DR (eds.): "Bladder Cancer," AUA Monographs, Baltimore: Williams and Wilkings, pp 35-46.

Dalesio O, Schulman CC, Sylvester R, de Pauw M, Robinson M, Denis L, Smith P, Viggiano G (1983). Prognostic factors in superficial bladder tumors. A study of the European Organization for Research on treatment of cancer: Genito-Urinary Tract Cancer Co-operative Group. J Urol 129: 730-733.

Gilbert HA, Logan JL, Kagan AR (1978). The natural history of papillary transitional cell carcinoma of the bladder and its treatment in an unselected population on the basis of histologic grading. J Urol 119: 488-492.

Haaff EO, Dresner SM, Ratliff TL, Catalona WJ (1986). Two courses of intravesical Bacillus Calmette-Guérin for transitional cell carcinoma of the bladder. J Urol 136: 820.

Heney N, Ahmed S, Flanagan MJ, Frable W, Corder MP, Hafermann MD, Hawkins IR for National Bladder Cancer Collaborative Group A (1983). Superficial bladder cancer: progression and recurrence. J Urol 130: 1083-1086.

Herr HW, Pinsky CM, Whitmore Jr WF, Sogani PC, Oettgen HF, Melamed MR (1986). Long-term effect of intravesical Bacillus Calmette-Guérin on flat carcinoma in situ of the bladder. J Urol 135: 265.

Lamm DL, Thor DE, Winters WD, Stogdill VD, Radwin HM (1981). BCG immunotherapy of bladder cancer: inhibition of tumor recurrence and associated immune responses. Cancer 48: 82.

Lamm DL (1985). BCG immunotherapy in bladder cancer. J Urol 134: 40.

Lamm DL, Stogdill VD, Stogdill BJ, Crispen RG (1986). Complications of Bacillus Calmette-Guérin immunotherapy in 1278 patients with bladder cancer. J Urol 135: 272.

van der Meijden APM (1988). Non-specific immunotherapy with BCG-RIVM in superficial bladder cancer. Histological, imunological and therapeutic aspects. Thesis, University of Nijmegen, the Netherlands.

Morales A, Nickel JG (1986). Immunotherapy of superficial bladder cancer with BCG. World J Urol 3: 209.

Pauwels RBE, Scheepers RFM, Smeets AWGB (1988). Grading in superficial bladder cancer. Morphological criteria. Brit J Urol 61: 129-134.

Rawls WH, Lamm DL, Eyolfson MF (1988). Septic complications in the use of Bacillus Calmette-Guérin (BCG) for non-invasive transitional cell carcinoma. J Urol 139: 300A.
Steg A, Leleu C, Debré B, Boccon-Gibod L (1988). Systemic Bacillus Calmette-Guérin (BCG) infection in patients treated by intravesical BCG-therapy for bladder cancer. J Urol 139: 300A.

EORTC Genitourinary Group Monograph 6:
BCG in Superficial Bladder Cancer, pages 325–334
© 1989 Alan R. Liss, Inc.

SYSTEMIC BACILLUS CALMETTE-GUÉRIN INFECTION IN PATIENTS TREATED BY INTRAVESICAL BCG THERAPY FOR SUPERFICIAL BLADDER CANCER

Adolphe Steg, Christian Leleu, Bernard Debré, Laurent Boccon-Gibod, Didier Sicard.
Dept. of Urology (A.S., C.L, B.D.) and Medicine (D.S.), Hôpital Cochin, Dept. of Urology (L.B.G.), Hôpital Bichat, Paris, France

INTRODUCTION

Bacillus Calmette-Guérin (BCG) therapy in superficial bladder cancer often causes side effects (such as bladder irritation and hematuria) or local complications (such as epididymitis), but major complications are rare and self-limiting. Intravesical BCG therapy, however, can be followed by a severe life-threatening, disseminated BCG infection called BCG-itis.

We report here five cases of such BCG-itis that we have observed among 169 patients treated with intravesical BCG for superficial bladder tumors.

Treatment was started 3 weeks after transurethral resection (TUR). We instilled 150 mg BCG-Pasteur (Institute Pasteur, Paris) once a week for 6 consecutive weeks and every 2 weeks for the next 3 months. Some patients received montly maintenance therapy thereafter for the next 2 years.

CASE 1

A 66-year-old man presented with an 8-year history of four TURs for superficial transitional cell carcinoma of the bladder.

At admission, a grade 1 stage Ta tumor was resected. BCG treatment was started 3 weeks later.

The sixth instillation was followed by fever (temperature up to 39°C), which lasted for 48 hours and then subsided spontaneously. At the eighth instillation, introduction of the catheter was difficult, and there was urethral bleeding. The patient presented with chills and a temperature of 39°C 24 hours later. Ampicillin and Gentamicin had no effect, and the patient's temperature stayed at 40-41°C for 10 days.

The patient was then readmitted to the hospital. There was neither splenomegaly, nor hepatomegaly, but auscultation revealed cracking rales on the right lung. His sedimentation rate was 53/86, there was a moderate leukopenia (3,700 leukocytes with 35% lymphocytes), the gamma-GT was 66 UI/l (n = 20 UI/l), his alkaline phosphatase was 124 UI/l (n = 90 UI/l), his ALAT was 51 UI/l (n = 40 UI/l) and his ASAT was 34 UI/l (n = 40 UI/l). All blood cultures had negative results. No mycobacteria were found by gastric lavage or in the urine. The tuberculin test was negative.

The patient's chest X-ray showed basal lobar infiltration of the right lung (Fig. 1). Bronchofibroscopy with biopsy demonstrated active interstitial fibrosis, and lung lavage showed aveolar lymphocytosis (70% of 310,000 cells/mm^3). Hepatic biopsy revealed hepatic granulomatosis (Fig. 2).

Treatment with Isoniazid, Rifampicin, Prednisolone, was successful and was maintained for 3 months.

CASE 2

A 71-year-old man with a history of resections for a Grade III, stage Ta bladder tumor was treated intravesically with BCG for 2 years. The standard 6-weekly induction treatment was followed by monthly instillations. Treatment was completed in June 1985.

In December 1985, the patient presented with chills and flu-like symptoms, and a temperature of 39°C. A chest X-ray showed basal infiltration of the right lung. Hepatic biopsy showed granulomatous hepatitis.

Because there were leukopenia (3,800 leukocytes) thrombopenia (50,600 platelets) and anemia, we performed a medullary biopsy, which demonstrated intramedullary granulomatosis (Fig. 3). Treatment was successful.

CASES 3, 4 AND 5

Cases 3, 4, and 5 are presented schematically in Table 1.

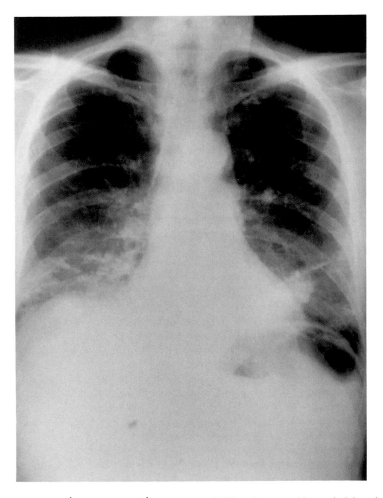

Figure 1. (Case No. 1) Lung infiltrate on the right side.

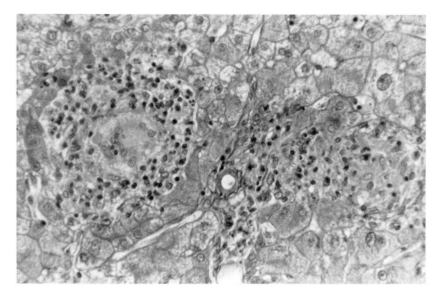

Figure 2. (Case No. 1) Typical granulomatous hepatitis.

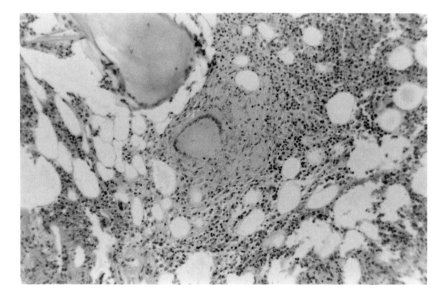

Figure 3. (Case No. 2) Intramedullar granulomatosis.

TABLE 1. Schematic presentation of 5 patients with systemic complications of intravesical BCG instillation

Case	Age of patients	Tumor stage and grade	No. of installations before onset of BCG-itis	Lung infiltration	Aleveolar lymphocytosis	Granulomatous hepatitis	Urethral trauma (catheterisation)
1	66	Ta, I	8th	+	+	+	+
2	71	T1, III	6 months after completion of 18 months maintenance therapy	+	lung lavage not performed	+	0
3	64	Ta, II	6th	+	lung lavage not performed	+	+
4	39	Ta, III	3rd	+	+	+	+
5	62	T1, III	6th	+	lung lavage not performed	hepatic biopsy not performed	0

TREATMENT

All five patients were treated with Isoniazid (300 mg daily), Rifampicin (600 mg daily), and Prednisolone (40 mg intravenously daily). Their temparature decreased slowly and became normal 10-15 days after treatment began. Treatment was maintained for 3 months.

All the patients are without symptoms with a follow-up for more than 2 years.

DISCUSSION

Systemic BCG complications were observed very rarely when BCG was used for vaccination against tuberculosis (Esterly et al., 1971, Matsaniotis, 1967). Among hundreds of millions of BCG vaccinations, about 30 deaths were reported (Matsaniotis and Economou-Mavrou, 1966; Sicevic, 1972; Watanabe et al., 1969).

Disseminated BCG disease was more frequently observed during the 1970s, when BCG was administered either by scarification (Ritch et al., 1978), by intradermal injection (Aungst et al., 1975), or by intralesional injection in immunotherapy for malignant tumors, especially melanomas (McKhan et al., 1975).

When BCG is used intravesically, systemic complications can occur, although they are rarely reported:
- three patients had pulmonary complications.
- four patients had abnormal liver-functions and evidence of pulmonary infection (Brosman, 1982, 1985).
- five patients had pneumonitis and hepatitis (Lamm, 1985, 1986).
- fewer than 2% of patients in one series had "systemic complications" (Morales, 1984).

We have shown that BCG-itis is not so rare, having observed it in five (3%) of our 169 patients.

In four of our cases, BCG-itis complicated the early stage of treatment. In three cases, BCG-itis followed a traumatic urethral catheterization with bleeding, which might have favored the BCG hematogenous dissemination. This hypothesis is supported by the report that Mycobacterium bovis introduced via intralesion injection was isolated from blood up to 30 minutes after injection (Pinsky et al., 1972).

Even pulmonary tuberculosis has been reported after hematogeneous spread of BCG (Jenkins et al., 1971). Furthermore, a biopsy specimen obtained from a patient with granulomatous hepatitis that complicated BCG immunotherapy yielded a growth of Mycobacterium bovis in culture (Flippin et al., 1980) which is evidence of a true infectious process.

Some authors have interpreted the BCG-itis as a possible hypersensitivity reaction (Hunt et al., 1973; McKahn et al., 1975; New England Journal of Medicine Case reports, 1975).

Hematogeneous spread of BCG during a traumatic instillation could contribute to the presensitization of a patient to BCG. Later spread of BCG could then represent a massive antigen load and lead to granuloma formation, as in some experimental models (Masih et al., 1979).

Case 2 is particularly interesting in that not only granulomatous hepatitis and a pulmonary lesion developed, but also intramedullar granulomatosis, while symptoms did not appear until 6 months after a 2-years treatment had been completed. Such a long interval between the last BCG instillation and the development of granulomatous hepatitis might represent a problem in the differential diagnosis. In fact, the fever and basal lung infiltration were first diagnosed as signs of pulmonary embolism.

In our cases, because there was a delay in diagnosis, specific treatment was generally initiated several days after fever had appeared. Earlier treatment might have prevented the disseminated localizations.

Because, simple uncomplicated febrile reactions to BCG cannot be distinguished from systemic BCG infection, we recommand, like Lamm, that patients with such conditions be treated with anti-tuberculous therapy (Lamm et al., 1986).

CONCLUSIONS

1. Intravesical BCG therapy may be complicated by disseminated disease with pulmonary involvement, granulomatous hepatitis and even intramedullary granulomatosis.

2. Although BCG-itis usually develops during treatment it may also occur after treatment has been completed.

3. Urethral trauma might favor BCG dissemination.

4. Treatment includes the association of Isoniazid, Rifampicin and Prednisolone and has to be maintained for 3 months.

5. We suggest that any patient with a febrile response ($>38°C$) should be treated with anti-tuberculous drugs for 3 days.

ABSTRACT

Among 169 patients treated for superficial bladder tumors with intravesical instillations of 150 mg BCG-Pasteur, five developed BCG-itis -- a severe systemic infection with bronchopulmonary lesions and granulomatous hepatitis. In four cases, the complication appeared early during treatment (after three, six, six and eight instillations respectively).

In one case, BCG-itis appeared 6 months after completion of 2 years monthly maintenance therapy. In addition to pulmonary basal infiltration and granulomatous hepatitis, intramedullary granulomatosis was observed.

In three patients, the role of trauma has to be considered, as BCG-itis appreared after a traumatic instillation with bleeding.

All patients were cured by combined treatment with Rifampicin, Isoniazid and Prednisolone.

REFERENCES

Aungst CW, Sokal JE, Jager BV (1975). Complications of BCG vaccination in neoplastic disease. Ann Intern Med 82: 666-669.

Brosman SA (1982). Experience with Bacillus Calmette-Guérin in patients with superficial bladder cancer. J Urol 128: 27-29.

Brosman SA (1985) The use of Bacillus Camette-Guérin in the therapy of bladder carcinoma in situ. J Urol 134: 36.

Case reports of the Massachusetts General Hospital (1975). N Engl J Med 293: 443-448.

Esterly JR, Sturner WQ, Esterly NB, Windhorst DB (1971). Disseminated BCG in twin boys with presumed chronic granulomatous disease of childhood. Pediatrics 48: 141-144.

Flippin T, Mukherji B, Dayal Y (1980). Granulomatous hepatitis as a late complication of BCG immunotherapy. Cancer 46: 1759-1762.

Hunt JS, Silverstein MJ, Sparks FC, Haskell EM, Pilch YH, Morton DL (1973). Granulomatous hepatitis: a complication of BCG immunotherapy. Lancet 2: 820-821.

Jenkins MJ, Kilpatrick GS (1971). Pulmonary tuberculosis due to BCG. Br Med J 3: 229-230.

Lamm DL (1985) Bacillus Calmette-Guérin immunotherapy for bladder cancer. J Urol 134: 40.

Lamm DL, Stogdill VD, Stogdill BJ, Crispen RG (1986). Complications of Bacillus Calmette-Guérin immunotherapy in 1278 patients with bladder cancer. J Urol 135: 272-274.

Masih N, Majeska j, Yoshida T (1979). Studies on experimental pulmonary granulomatosis. I: Detection of lymphokines in granulomatous lesions. Ann J Pathol 95: 391-406.

Matsaniotis N (1967). Dangers of immunization in immunologically incompetent individuals. Acta Pediatr Scand (suppl) 172: 146-155.

Matsaniotis N, Economou-Mavrou C (1966). BCG fatalities, new aspects of their aetiology. Ann Pediatr 206: 363-378.

McKahn CF, Hendrickson CG, Spitler LF, Gunnarson A, Banerjee D, Nelson WR (1975). Immunotherapy of melanoma with BCG: two fatalities following intralesional injection. Cancer 35: 514-520.

Morales A (1984). Long term results and complications of intracavitary Bacillus Calmette-Guérin therapy for bladder cancer. J Urol 132: 457.

Pinsky C, Hirshault Y, Oettgen H (1972). Treatment of malignant melanoma by intratumoral injection of BCG. Proc Am Assoc Assoc Cancer Res 13: 21.

Pinsky C, Hirshault Y, Oettgen H (1972). Treatment of malignant melanoma by intratumoral injection of BCG. Proc Am Assoc Assoc Cancer Res 13: 21.

Ritch PS, MC Credie KB, Gutterman JU, Hersh EM (1978). Disseminated BCG disease associated with immunotherapy. Cancer 42: 167-170.

Sicevic S (1972). Generalized BCG tuberculosis with fatal course in two sisters. Acta Pediatr Scand 61: 178-184.

Watanabe T, Tanka K, Hagiwara Y (1969). Generalized tuberculosis after BCG vaccination. Report of an autopsy case. Acta Pathol Jap 19: 395-407.

EORTC Genitourinary Group Monograph 6:
BCG in Superficial Bladder Cancer, pages 335–355
© 1989 Alan R. Liss, Inc.

COMPLICATIONS OF BACILLUS CALMETTE-GUÉRIN IMMUNOTHERAPY: REVIEW OF 2602 PATIENTS AND COMPARISON OF CHEMOTHERAPY COMPLICATIONS

Donald L. Lamm, Morgantown, USA; Adolph Steg and Laurent Boccon-Gibod, Paris, France; Alvaro Morales, Kingston, Canada; Michael G. Hanna Jr, Rockville, USA; Francesco Pagano, Padova, Italy; Olaf Alfthan, Helsinki, Finland; Stanley Brosman, Los Angeles, USA; Hugh A.F. Fisher, Albany, USA; Gerhard Jakse, München, FRG; Geoffrey D. Chisholm, Edinburgh, UK; Ad P.M. van der Meijden and Frans M.J. Debruyne, Nijmegen, The Netherlands

INTRODUCTION

The superiority of BCG immunotherapy for superficial bladder cancer treatment and prophylaxis has greatly increased its use throughout the world. This has resulted in an increase in the number and variety of complications of this treatment. This review expands the previous review of 1278 patients reported in 1986 (Lamm, 1986) with the cooperation of multiple investigators by including 1031 patients from the authors' series reported in this book, an additional 70 patients treated by Morales, and 223 patients in an ongoing Southwest Oncology Group study. The incidence of complications and side effects with the various BCG preparations and treatment protocols are summarized and the toxicity of BCG immunotherapy is compared with that of intravesical chemotherapy. The major complications, including sepsis and fatal systemic BCG infection, are reviewed in detail and treatment and prevention discussed in an effort to improve the management of these patients.

The 1986 review included a detailed assessment of common side effects in 195 personal patients, and reviewed serious complications in 134 patients reported in the literature and 949 reviewed by urological investigators. Cystitis occurred in 91% of the patients, 43% had hematuria, 28% had low grade fever, 24% had malaise, and 8% had nausea. Complications identified included fever more than 39.5°C in 50 patients (3.9%), granulomatous prostatitis in 17 (1.3%),

Bacillus Calmette-Guérin pneumonitis or hepatitis in 12 (0.9%), arthritis or arthralgia in 6 (0.5%), hematuria requiring catheterization or transfusion in 6 (0.5%), epididymo-orchitis in 2 (0.2%), bladder contracture in 2 (0.2%), hypotension in 1 (0.1%), and cytopenia in 1 (0.1%). The incidence of significant complications with Armand Frappier, Tice, Connaught, Pasteur, and Glaxo BCG preparations is listed in Table 1.

TABLE 1. Complications in 1278 patients according to substrain of BCG (Lamm et al., 1986)

	Total No.	%	A-F %	T %	C %	P %	G %
Fever 39°C	50	3.9	4.2	6.2	---	1.6	10
Granulomatous prostatitis	17	1.3	1.8	1.5	---	---	--
Pneumonitis/ Hepatitis	12	0.9	0.5	1.5	0.4	1.6	10
Arthritis/ Arthralgia	6	0.5	0.8	---	0.4	---	--
Major hematuria	6	0.5	0.4	---	---	---	--
Skin rash	5	0.4	0.5	---	0.4	---	--
Skin abscess	5	0.4	0.5	---	0.9	---	--
Ureteral obstruction	4	0.3	0.5	0.3	---	---	--
Orchitis/ Epididymitis	2	0.2	0.2	---	0.4	---	--
Contracted bladder	2	0.2	---	0.6	---	---	--
Renal abscess	1	0.1	---	---	0.4	---	--
Hypotention	1	0.1	---	---	---	1.6	--
Cytopenia	1	0.1	---	0.3	---	---	--
Total hospitalized	25	2.0	1.7	1.8	0.9	3.2	10

Differences in the incidences of complications according to strain partly reflect variations in dose and treatment schedule, as well as differences in reporting. There were 648 Armand Frappier (A-F) treated patients reported by Camacho (60), Catalona (41), Douville and associates (6), Herr (250), Lamm (127), Morales (130) and Shellhammer (34). The 325 Tice (T) strain treated patients were reported on by Babayan (70), Brosman (120), Crispen (51), de Kernion (63), and Lamm (21). The 222 Connaught (C) treated patients were reported on by Adolphs (130), Flamm and Grof (45), and Lamm (47). The 59 patients treated with (French) Pasteur BCG (P) were reported on by Martinez-Pineiro and Muntala (29), and Stober and Peter (30). The 10 Glaxo (G) treated patients were reported on by Robinson and associated, and 14 Moreau treated patients (not listed) were reported on by Netto and Lemos.

Updating this experience with a total of 2602 patients treated with Armand Frappier, Tice, Connaught, Pasteur or RIVM BCG, the relative frequency of complication remains similar to that originally reported. High fever (in excess of 39.5°C) remains the most frequently observed toxic reaction aside from the expected irritative bladder symptoms. In all, 2.9% of the patients had high fever. Granulomatous prostatitis decreased from an incidence of 1.3 to 0.9%. Prostatitis may also be acute in onset and may result in urinary retention, as seen in 2 patients (0.1%). Major hematuria was observed with increased frequency in the expanded review, and is now the third most common side effect with an incidence of 1.0%. Systemic BCG infection manifested by pneumonitis and/or hepatitis remains a relatively common and severe complication and was seen in 0.7% of the patients. The most serious, life-threatening complication of BCG sepsis had an alarming increase in percentage from 0.1 to 0.4, Allergic reactions, manifested by arthritis/arthralgia (0.5%) or skin rash (0.3%) were the next most common side effects. The incidence of these and the remaining side effects, ureteral obstruction (0.3%), epididymitis/orchitis (0.4%), bladder contracture (0.2%), were essentially unchanged. The incidence of complications in 2602 patients is illustrated in Table 2.

TABLE 2. Complications of BCG therapy in 2589 patients

	Total		Armand Frappier	Tice	Con- naught	Pasteur	RIVM
	2602		718	726	353	325	129
	No.	%	%	%	%	%	%
Fever	75	2.9	3.8	4.7	4.7	0.6	2.1
Granulomatous prostatitis	23	0.9	1.8	1.0	0.2	0.6	0.0
Pneumonitis/ Hepatitis	18	0.7	0.4	0.8	0.6	1.2	0.8
Arthralgia	12	0.5	0.7	0.1	0.6	1.8	0.0
Hematuria	24	1.0	0.3	0.6	2.4	1.0	0.4
Rash	8	0.3	0.4	0.0	0.9	0.0	0.0
Ureteral obstruction	8	0.3	0.6	0.4	0.2	0.0	0.0
Epididymitis	10	0.4	0.4	0.0	0.2	1.2	0.8
Contracted bladder	6	0.2	0.0	0.3	0.2	0.6	0.0
Renal abscess	2	0.1	0.0	0.0	0.4	0.0	0.0
Sepsis	10	0.4	0.1	0.4	0.9	0.2	0.0
Cytopenia	2	0.1	0.0	0.3	0.0	0.0	0.0

Note that since definitions of side effects vary from one series to another, and all complications were not consi- dered in each series, some assumptions have been made to estimate the overall incidence of complications.

CYSTITIS

Cystitis, induced by BCG typically consists on biopsy of acute and chronic inflammation with granuloma formation. Usually it does not require treatment. Patients generally are symptomatic for one to two days and find relief with symptomatic medication, such as Phenazopyridine and Propan- theline Bromide or Oxybutynin. Repeated BCG administration typically increases the duration and severity of cystitis. If patients suffer severe or prolonged (more than 48 hours) symptoms, treatment with 300 mg Isoniazid daily, Diphenhy- dramine, and Acetaminophen or Ibuprofen is recommended. Treatment is continued only while symptoms persist but is re-instituted and continued for 3 days prophylactically on the morning prior to subsequent BCG instillations. Constitutional symptoms also can be prevented with Isoniazid prophylaxis. It is anticipated that most complications will be prevented with the use of early Isoniazid prophylaxis in patients with increased symptoms, but, as illustrated later, major complication can occur despite Isoniazid prophylaxis.

FEVER

The most common complication, fever more than 39.5°C, was seen in the updated series in 2.9% of all patients (Table 2). Most of the patients with high fever in our experience reported this to us in retrospect and were not hospitalized. The fever typically resolved in 1 or 2 days with anti-pyretics and fluids. However, patients with a simple uncomplicated febrile response to BCG cannot be distinguished from those who will develop progressive systemic BCG infection or anaphylaxis. Such patients should therefore generally be hospitalized and treated with anti-tuberculous drugs.

GRANULOMATOUS PROSTATITIS

Granulomatous prostatitis was seen in 0.9% of the patients over-all. The majority of these patients were asymptomatic and required no treatment. However, acute prostatitis may occur and may cause urinary retention. Since the induration associated with chronic granulomatous prostatitis cannot be distinguished from carcinoma of the prostate, needle biopsy is often required. In patients who are symptomatic 300 mg Isoniazid and 600 mg Rifampin orally each day are recommended.

ALLERGIC REACTIONS

Arthritis or migratory arthralgia (0.5%) and skin rash (0.3%) are considered to be allergic reactions to BCG. These reactions are too uncommon to have a standard treatment protocol, but in patients who are at high risk of tumor recurrence or progression we have not found it necessary to discontinue treatment but simply administer prophylactic Isoniazid and Antihistamines. Patients with severe allergic reactions may require discontinuation of BCG therapy.

COMPLICATIONS OF PERCUTANEOUS BCG

As previously discussed in this volume, data suggest that patients receiving maintenance intravesical BCG have no significant increased antitumor activity with the addition of percutaneous BCG. Significant toxicity can occur from BCG vaccination given intradermally. However, complications are rare. In a review of 117,533 vaccinations for tuberculosis prevention only 51 local complications (0.04%) occurred (deSousa, 1981). The most common complication was abscess (55%), followed by lymph node enlargement (29%), ulceration (12%), and pedunculated lesions (4%). All patients responded to Isoniazid treatment or simple incision. Combined percutaneous and intravesical administration using the Dutch RIVM strain was investigated in a phase I-II study (van der Meijden, 1988). No major complications were reported in 30 patients after 6 weekly percutaneous administrations on alternating upper legs, using a multipuncture apparatus.

EPIDIDYMITIS/ORCHITIS

Patients with localized symptomatic BCG infection, such as epididymitis or orchitis, which occurred in 0.4% of patients, generally will respond to Isoniazid therapy alone. Severe infection with abscess formation may occur and has required orchidectomy in some investigator's experience.

URETERAL OBSTRUCTION

Ureteral obstruction is a potentially serious complication that was seen in 0.3% of the patients in both reviews. Generally, this obstruction is temporary and self-limited, but prolonged anti-tuberculous treatment and postponement of further BCG therapy may be required. Both of our patients who suffered ureteral obstruction had carcinoma in situ and both had complete resolution of intravesical carcinoma in situ following BCG immunotherapy. One patient with a positive ureteral cytology suffered obstruction that required nephrectomy for presumed residual ureteral transitional cell carcinoma. Surprisingly, final pathological examination revealed inflammation and scarring without tumor. In some patients it may be difficult to distinguish obstruction secondary to BCG from that due to ureteral tumor. Patients with flank pain should have renal sonography, urography, or renal scan to exclude the diagnosis of ureteral obstruction.

CONTRACTED BLADDER

Contracted bladder has occurred in 6 patients (0.2%) treated with intravesical BCG. The majority of patients have been treated on a maintenance schedule, and most have not had prophylactic Isoniazid. The absence of bladder contraction in the experience of investigators who have used prophylactic Isoniazid in patients with severe irritative symptoms suggests that prophylactic Isoniazid may reduce the incidence of bladder contracture.

SYSTEMIC BCG INFECTION

Systemic BCG infection manifested by pneumonitis, or granulomatous hepatitis occurred in 18 patients (0.7%). Generally, these patients present with fever and malaise, and have progressively increasing severity of side effects with successive intravesical BCG instillations. Traumatic catheterizations or treatment following extensive tumor resection or bladder perforation can result in systemic BCG infection. Many patients have no acute symptoms, and may be treated with Isoniazid and Rifampin. Patients who are acutely ill with systemic BCG infection should receive triple-drug therapy with Cycloserine for the initial 3 days. Cytopenia (0.1%), is typically associated with systemic BCG infection and is treated accordingly.

RENAL ABCESS

Renal abscess has been reported in 2 patients (0.1%) and is associated with vesico-ureteral reflux. While reflux per se has not been considered a contra-indication to BCG therapy, these patients are likely to be at increased risk of systemic infection, ureteral obstruction, and renal abscess. Renal BCG abscess may present as renal mass and has been confused with renal cell carcinoma. Most patients with BCG abscess will have malaise and fever which can lead one to suspect the correct diagnosis.

TREATMENT CONSIDERATIONS

BCG abscess formation, systemic BCG infection manifested by pneumonitis, hepatitis, or cytopenia, or other
major BCG infection requires aggressive therapy. While it
is true that the BCG organism is attenuated and generally
retains susceptibility to anti-tuberculous drugs, the very
presence of major infection with this organism indicates
that BCG is not a benign organism in some patients. Moreover, BCG has been reported in one patient to cause activation of dormant, Isoniazid-resistant mycobacterial infection (Aungst, 1975). Some physicians have been reluctant to
initiate treatment with Isoniazid, particularly in patients
with hepatitis, since approximately 10% of people taking
Isoniazid for prophylaxis against tuberculosis develop
transient elevation of serum glutamic oxaloacetic transaminase (Scharer and Smith, 1969). Many physicians are not
aware of the fact that BCG infection, particularly in immunocompromised patients, can be progressive and even fatal.
The complications listed clearly point out the necessity of
anti-tuberculous therapy in such patients. BCG is generally
highly sensitive to anti-tuberculous drugs including Isoniazid, Para-aminosalicylic Acid, Streptomycin, Ethambutol,
and Rifampin, and is also generally sensitive to drugs of
lesser activity against mycobacteria such as Kanamycin and
Gentamycin. Patients with serious systemic infection or
abscess are generally treated with the combination of
Isoniazid 300 mg, Rifampin 600 mg, and, depending on the
gravity of the circumstance, Ethambutol 1200 mg daily.
Insufficient data are available to say with certainty how
long patients should be treated. It has been the first
author's policy to treat for only a 2 week period patients
who have high fever and malaise which responds within 48
hours to treatment with Isoniazid and Rifampin. Patients
with pneumonitis or hepatitis, or those with localized
infection which does not respond to treatment within
several days, are treated initially with the 2 drug
combination. Our limited experience, like that of others
(Aungst, 1975), suggests that complete resolution of
infection will occur with continuation of Isoniazid for 3
months. In patients who take several months to have
complete symptomatic or enzymatic response to treatment,
Isoniazid has been continued for as long as 6 months.

Other investigators have been reluctant to use Isoniazid in patients with increasing BCG side effects because of

the concern that such therapy may decrease the antitumor reponse of BCG. As noted, animal studies have shown that excessive BCG administration reduces antitumor response and can, on rare occasion, even result in enhanced tumor growth (Bast, 1974; Lamm, 1982). Therefore, continued growth of BCG may in fact reduce its clinical efficacy. Animal studies have also specifically addressed the question and have demonstrated that concomitant Isoniazid therapy does not diminish the effect of BCG in tumor models (Sparks, 1976).

BCG SEPSIS

Sepsis following intravesical BCG instillation can be fatal. In Lamm's personal series at West Virginia University, 2 of 190 patients (1%) treated with BCG for bladder cancer developed sepsis. Both of these patients survived, but required intensive care plus vigorous anti-tuberculous therapy. One case will be presented to illustrate features which are common in patients who develop BCG sepsis: A 65-year-old man with grade 3, stage T1 transitional cell carcinoma with concomitant carcinoma in situ had negative cystoscopy and biopsies for 3 years following the initiation of BCG therapy, but urinary cytology was reported to be suspicious for high grade malignancy. Cystoscopy with biopsy was therefore repeated, and 6 hours later his 11th intravesical BCG-Tice treatment was given. Eight hours thereafter he had fever to 38.5°C, suprapubic pain, and rigor. Isoniazid, Ampicillin and Gentamicin were given but he developed marked hypotension, confusion, disseminated intravascular coagulopathy, and jaundice. Rifampin and Cycloserine were added to the antibiotic regimen and with intensive monitoring and fluid replacement he gradually improved and recovered without sequelae. All routine as well as acid-fast cultures were negative.

Sepsis has resulted in 2 deaths among 688 patients (0.3%) given intravesical BCG-Connaught on Southwest Oncology Group protocols 8216 and 8507: A 66-year-old man had grade 2, stage Ta transitional cell carcinoma with concomitant carcinoma in situ unresponsive to Mitomycin-C and Adriamycin. He had a prior history of mild liver disturbances due to alcohol abuse. The fifth weekly BCG-Connaught treatment was given after difficulty with urethral catheterization. The patient developed fever to 39°C but responded to treatment with Isoniazid. The 6th dose of BCG was given on Isoniazid prophylaxis. Within 24 hours the patient developed fever and hemoptysis. Ticarcillin, Gentamicin, and Rifampin were given, but the patient failed to respond possibly due to liver toxicity. The patient became progressively lethargic and had increased liver dysfunction, leukopenia, and disseminated intravascular coagulopathy and expired from fulminant sepsis. Postmortem examination revealed BCG organisms in the lungs and inflammatory infiltrates in the liver and kidney.

A 63-year-old man with grade 2, stage Ta transitional cell carcinoma had moderate cystitis after the fourth weekly BCG-Connaught treatment. Two hours after the fifth treatment he became hypotensive without developing fever. Intravenous hydration and Isoniazid were given and he promptly recovered. The 6th dose of BCG was given without Isoniazid prophylaxis. Four days later he became febrile and hypotensive. Isoniazid was resumed, along with Rifampin and Streptomycin, but he developed progressive sepsis with disseminated intravascular coagulopathy, gastric bleeding, and respiratory failure. He died of multi-organ failure and autopsy revealed granulomas with multi-nucleated giant cells in the liver, bone marrow, spleen, and kidney.

These cases illustrate several important principles that have been confirmed by others (Steg et al., 1988). First, while BCG is an attenuated organism with reduced virulence and retained sensitivity to anti-tuberculous drugs, the massive dose given intravesically is a potentially lethal dose if given intravenously. While doses of BCG as high as 1000 mg intravenously have been tolerated in monkeys (Jurczyk-Procyck et al., 1976), considerable clinical experience in cancer patients treated with intralesional or intravesical BCG confirms that fulminant irreversible sepsis is possible in these patients. Sepsis resulting from absorption through inflamed urothelium or direct intravasation resulting from traumatic catheterization are common features of these cases. Both the fatalities occurred during the 6 week induction phase of BCG therapy, and in each case treatment was continued despite evidence of major toxicity: temperature of 39°C and hypotension. One of these patients developed fatal sepsis despite prophylaxis with Isoniazid. These observations suggest that patients who have major toxicity during the induction phase should not receive additional BCG treatments. While we have successfully treated patients with febrile reactions, even those of 39°C, with Isoniazid coverage for subsequent treatments, current experience shows that fatal sepsis can occur even with such coverage. Unless patients have tumor recurrence, the risk of further BCG treatment would seem to exceed the risk of disease progression. Severe cystitis, high fever or other systemic response to BCG suggests that an increased number of organisms are being absorbed or are multiplying. In such circumstances it may be prudent to withhold further BCG for optimal antitumor effect as well as safety.

Fatal reactions to BCG have occurred with highest incidence following intralesional injection. Most of the fatalities result from progressive systemic BCG infection. In exceptional circumstances intracutaneous BCG inoculation alone can produce progressive systemic BCG infection and even fatality. There have been 35 fatalities reported among more than 1.5 billion vaccinations given for tuberculosis prophylaxis before 1975 (Lotte, 1984). Nearly 90% of these fatalities occurred in infants and almost all of these patients had pre-existing defects in cellular immunity. Fatal reactions were seen more commonly (2-1 ratio) in boys than in girls. Interestingly, none of the reported deaths occurred in patients who received BCG orally. While only 1 death per 50 million patients occurred when BCG was given for tuberculosis prophylaxis, a higher mortality (1 death per 12,500 patients) occurred when BCG was given in the treatment of cancer. Most of these deaths resulted from overwhelming BCG infection, sepsis or anaphylactic shock following the intralesional injection of BCG.

In vitro data suggest that Cycloserine, unlike Isonia-zid, Rifampin, Ethambutol, Para-aminosalicylic Acid, and Streptomycin, inhibits BCG growth within 24 hours (Lee and Crispen, 1973). It is known that Isoniazid may take up to a week to decrease growth of BCG in patients (Sparks, 1976). Our very limited experience supports the hypothesis that Cycloserine may be live saving in patients with BCG sepsis. Since patients with fulminant sepsis may not survive the two to seven days required for many anti-tuberculous drugs to inhibit BCG growth, Cycloserine should be given for the first three days and continued until the condition of the patient has stabilized. In 4 patients with fulminant BCG sepsis, two who received Cycloserine survived and two who did not receive cycloserine died.

RARE COMPLICATIONS

Some reported complications occur so infrequently that an incidence cannot reasonably be estimated. Some have been reported in the literature as case reports, and others have been reported by personal communication to the authors. It should be noted that, while it is suspected that BCG had a role in the complications listed, this has not been confirmed in each case.

IMMUNE-COMPLEX GLOMERULONEPHRITIS

Non-specific immunotherapy with Corynebacterium parvum and, in one case, BCG, has been reported to cause immune complex glomerulo-nephritis (Krutchik et al., 1980). This patient with breast carcinoma received intralesional and multiple scarification BCG treatments plus combination chemotherapy. During treatment with BCG, Mitomycin-C, and megestrol acetate she developed peripheral edema and had elevation of creatinine, proteinuria, and microhematuria. Biopsy revealed mesangial interposition and focal mesangial capillary proliferation suggestive of immune complex nephritis. Immunotherapy was discontinued and Prednisone, 60mg/day was initiated but creatinine remained elevated.

CHOROIDITIS

In a review of 352 patients with multiple malignancies treated with BCG-Pasteur by scarification, intradermal, oral, aerosol, or intravenous routes, one case of choroiditis was observed (Schwarzenberg et al., 1976). This was thought to be allergic in nature and resolved with discontinuation of BCG scarifications. One patient among 610 treated with intravesical BCG-Connaught in Southwest Oncology Group protocols has developed choroiditis. This patient, who had enucleation of one eye secondary to a childhood injury, developed marked reduction in vision and ocular findings suggestive of choroiditis. BCG was discontinued and antibiotics begun, but vision has not yet returned. The most frequent ocular complication in children given BCG vaccination is phlyctenular conjunctivitis, followed by benign papillitis, episcleritis, iridocyclitis, choroiditis, and retinal periphlebitis (Lotte, 1984).

NEPHROGENIC ADENOMA

The rare metaplastic change of the urothelium to nephrogenic adenoma, which is in fact an adenomatous metaplasia, has been seen in association with chronic inflammation of the bladder and transitional cell carcinoma of the bladder. Two cases have been reported following BCG immunotherapy, and the possibility that the condition may be caused by the inflammation induced by BCG has been raised (Stilmant and Siroky, 1986).

CARDIAC TOXICITY

BCG immunotherapy for superficial bladder cancer is given to an elder population that has a relatively high incidence of arteriosclerotic disease. Patients on therapy have died of myocardial infarction, but we have not attributed this to BCG therapy. In the Southwest Oncology comparison of Adriamycin and BCG therapy, no increase in cardiac mortality was seen in either group. High fever associated with BCG treatment can result in cardiac toxicity. In a review of over 2700 patients with a variety of cancers treated with BCG, angina pectoris occurred in two patients. Both of these patients had known arteriosclerotic heart disease and both had fever over 40°C. A reduction in dose of scarification decreased the systemic febrile reactions and angina pectoris did not recur.

SUPPURATIVE LYMPHADENITIS

Adenitis is a recognized side effect of BCG vaccination and immunotherapy, with over 6000 cases documented (Lotte, 1984). Nine cases of adenitis were found in 117,500 children vaccinated with intradermal BCG, and 2 of these (0.002%) required surgical drainage in addition to antituberculous drugs. Mesenteric adenitis with fever and abdominal pain has occurred in 10 children vaccinated for tuberculosis, 8 of whom required surgery. Caseating granuloma of paracaecal lymph nodes has been found and cultures have confirmed BCG organisms (Lotte, 1984).

LUPUS VULGARIS

Lupus vulgaris with red, infiltrated, scabbed ulcers and so called "apple-jelly" nodules under the skin rarely occurs after cutaneous immunization (Lotte, 1984). To our knowledge this has not occurred as a result of intravesical therapy.

MUSCULOSKELETAL LESIONS

On rare occasion, intramuscular abscess can occur at sites distant from the site of inoculation (Lotte, 1984). Direct intramuscular injection of BCG can produce abscess and severe fever and malaise with regularity. More commonly BCG can produce a mild chronic osteitis which causes local pain, tenderness and swelling. Joint involvement occurs in about 20% of these cases. The lesions are most common in the long bones and legs. Hands, feet, ribs, and sternum are also frequently involved, but lesions of the vertebrae are very rare. Multiple lesions occurred in only 5% of the patients. Radiographically, limited lacunar lesions or large cavities with or without periosteal reaction are seen.

ABSCESS AND FISTULAE

Administration of intravesical BCG following bladder extravasation can result in pelvic abscess. Similarly, treatment in the face of urethral stricture or disruption can result in abscess or, as has happened in one case, urethral fistula (Andriole, personal communication).

INDUCTION OR PROMOTION OF TUMOR GROWTH

Controlled animal experiments have demonstrated that excessive BCG administration can, in exceptional circumstances, result in enhanced tumor growth. Since patients with one malignancy are at increased risk for a second, and the course of most malignancies is unpredictable, enhancement is most difficult to prove or refute in man. The Southwest Oncology Group randomized comparison of BCG and Adriamycin therapy in superficial bladder cancer provides a rare opportunity to compare the incidence of second malignancies in patients treated with immunotherapy or chemotherapy. Of the 142 patients randomized to receive BCG, 13.4% had a pre-existing second malignant tumor prior to treatment and 14.1% developed a second tumor of other origin after treatment. Of the 130 patients randomized to Adriamycin, 7.7% had a pre-existing carcinoma and 9.2% developed a second tumor of other origin after treatment. There was no statistically significant difference between groups and no evidence to support a role for intravesical BCG as a stimulus for the development or progressions of second malignancies.

COMPARISON OF BCG AND CHEMOTHERAPY TOXICITY

In some instances it is difficult to determine in individual patients whether apparant toxic reactions are in fact due to the treatment given or the disease itself. This is particularly true with toxicities such as contracted bladder, hematuria, and symptoms of cystitis which can occur as a result of bladder tumor or transurethral resection. Controlled trials provide the opportunity to compare the relative frequency of side effects, and several series are available to compare BCG toxicity with that of Adriamycin, Mitomycin, and Thiotepa. The relative incidence of complications may more correctly reflect the true frequency of toxicity related to the treatment itself.

BCG VERSUS ADRIAMYCIN TOXICITY

The Southwest Oncology Group randomized comparison of 120 mg intravesical plus percutaneous BCG-Connaught weekly for 6 weeks, at 3 months, 6 months, and every 6 months thereafter with 50 mg of Adriamycin given weekly for 4 weeks and then monthly provides extensive toxicity data on 230 patients. Table 3 lists the frequency of side effects seen in each group.

As illustrated, the most common side effect seen with intravesical therapy including BCG and chemotherapy, as exemplified in this study by Adriamycin, is irritative bladder symptoms (drug induced cystitis). With BCG-Connaught 52% of the patients had vesical irritation manifested by dysuria. Similarly, 40% of the patients treated with Adriamycin had dysuria. Additional irritative symptoms commonly seen with each bladder treatment include urinary frequency (40% BCG, 28% Adriamycin), and urgency (18% BCG, 12% Adriamycin). The diagnosis of treatment-related cystitis was made in 29% of the BCG group and 20% of the Adriamycin group. Treatment induced temporary urinary incontinence in 6% of the patients in the BCG group and 1% of the patients in the Adriamycin group.

TABLE 3. Toxicity of BCG versus Adriamycin in superficial bladder cancer (SWOG-data)

	BCG-Connaught (112)		Adriamycin (118)	
	No.	%	No.	%
Bladder symptoms:				
Dysuria	58	52	47	40
Frequency	45	40	33	28
Urgency	20	18	14	12
Cystitis	33	29	24	20
Incontinence	7	6	1	1
Hematuria:	44	39	33	28
Urinary infection:	20	18	17	14
Systemic symptoms:				
Fever	43	38	11	9
Chills	38	34	7	6
Nausea	18	16	10	8
Anorexia	12	11	6	5
Diarrhea	7	6	2	2
Arthralgia	8	7	5	4
Hematologic:				
Leukopenia	7	6	6	5
Thrombocytopenia	1	1	1	1
Cardiac morbidity:	3	3	6	5
Pulmonary infection:	3	3	5	4
Hepatic dysfunction:	3	3	1	1
Systemic infection:	3	3	1	1
Ureteral obstruction:	1	1	0	0
Mucositis:	0	0	3	4
Flank pain:	1	1	1	1

Hematuria following transurethral resection for bladder tumor may relate to the surgery, the tumor, or the

treatment. Treatment may induce hematuria by causing cystitis or destruction of residual malignancy. Hematuria may
therefore be associated with response to treatment and may
be improperly considered to be a complication of therapy.
In the SWOG study hematuria was frequent in both treatment
groups: 39% of the BCG group and 28% of the Adriamycin
group.

Patients with bladder tumor who undergo resection with
subsequent catheter drainage are at increased risk of
bacterial urinary infection. While BCG treatment has been
associated with increased resistance to bacterial infection, no protection from infection was apparent with BCG or
Adriamycin. Eighteen percent of BCG treated and 14% of
Adriamycin treated patients had urinary infection. Interestingly, in vitro studies of bacterial adherence have
demonstrated a 2 to 4 fold increase in adherence of bacteria to transitional cell carcinoma line T-24 after BCG
treatment, and BCG treated bladder tumor patients have been
reported to have a 5-fold increase in the incidence of
acquired urinary tract infection (Bruce et al., 1983).

Systemic symptoms, particularly fever (38%) and chills
(34%) were seen much more frequently in the BCG group than
the Adriamycin group (9% and 6 % respectively). Gastro-
intestinal symptoms of nausea (16%), anorexia (11%), and
diarrhea (6%) were seen twice as frequently with BCG. The
immunostimulation resulting from BCG therapy may result in
exacerbation of arthritis. Surprisingly, arthralgia was seen
in both groups: 7% of those treated with BCG and 4% of
those treated with Adriamycin.

Systemic BCG infection may result in myelosuppression.
The primary systemic toxicity of Adriamycin is cardiac and
myelosuppression is less common. In this series leukopenia
was seen in 6% and 5% of BCG and Adriamycin treated
patients, respectively, and 1% of each group had thrombo-
cytopenia. Cardiac morbidity was seen in 3% of BCG and 5%
of Adriamycin treated patients, and may or may not have
been related to treatment.

Additional uncommon events which may or may not be
related to either treatment include pulmonary infection (3%
BCG, 4% Adriamycin), systemic infection, hepatic dysfunction, (3% BCG, 1% Adriamycin each), and mucositis (0% BCG,
3% Adriamycin). Ureteral obstruction occurred in one BCG

treated patient and one patient in each group had flank pain following treatment.

From these data it is apparant that BCG is slightly more toxic than Adriamycin, but this difference is not statistically significant. Of all patients, only 9 discontinued treatment due to toxicity. Of these, 5 were in the BCG group and 4 were in the Adriamycin group.

BCG, THIOTEPA AND ADRIAMYCIN TOXICITY

Martinez-Pineiro (see this volume) compared toxicity of 150 mg BCG-Pasteur given weekly for 6 weeks and then monthly with 50 mg Thiotepa and 50 mg Adriamycin given on the same treatment schedule. The most frequent toxicity with each treatment was symptoms of bladder irritability, which was seen more commonly in the BCG group (28/67, 42%), than the Thiotepa (8/56, 14%) or Adriamycin (7/53, 13%) groups. In addition, the diagnosis of cystitis was made in 16% of the BCG treated patients. Fever was the next most frequent side-effect (7%), but fever was limited to BCG treated patients. Leukopenia (5%) was seen only in the Thiotepa group. These data again suggest that local toxicity is seen more frequently with BCG than with commonly used intravesical chemotherapeutic agents.

BCG VERSUS MITOMYCIN-C TOXICITY

Two studies provide data comparing the toxicity of BCG with Mitomycin-C (MMC) in prospectively controlled, randomized multicenter trials. In the first study, conducted by the EORTC Genito-Urinary Group, BCG-RIVM was compared with MMC and in the second MMC, conducted by the Dutch Southeast Co-operative Urological Group, was compared with BCG-RIVM and BCG-Tice, providing the only controlled comparison of two BCG preparations.

In the initial study (EORTC 30845) thorough toxicity analysis is available on 78 BCG-RIVM patients and 87 MMC patients (Debruyne et al., 1988). Drug induced cystitis was seen in 17% of the patients treated with BCG-RIVM, and 14% of the patients given MMC. It is remarkable that, despite the accepted increased local toxicity of BCG, this multi-center randomized trial demonstrated no statistically significant difference in the incidence of cystitis with BCG or MMC. Bacterial cystitis similarly occurred in 7% and 6% of the patients respectively. Allergic reactions occurred in 1.3% of the BCG treated patients and in 6.4% of the MMC treated patients. Bringing the total incidence of side effects to 40% and 39% respectively. No major systemic complications were seen with either treatment.

In the second study (Dutch Southeast Co-operative Urological Group) preliminary results are available on the toxicity of 44 patients treated with Mitomycin-C, 51 patients treated with BCG-RIVM and 49 patients treated with BCG-Tice. Drug induced cystitis was seen in 18.2% with MMC, 17.6% with BCG-RIVM, and 28.6% with BCG-Tice. Bacterial cystitis was seen in 22.7% with MMC, 41.2% with BCG-RIVM, and 34.7% with BCG-Tice. Other BCG side effects, including fever, malaise, hematuria, and myalgia, none of which required anti-tuberculous therapy, were seen in 27.5% of the BCG-RIVM treated patients and 28.6% of the BCG-Tice treated patients. Again, as with Thiotepa and Adriamycin, the overall number of side effect was higher in the BCG groups than in patients receiving intravesical chemotherapy with MMC. The previously held view that BCG-RIVM is less toxic than other forms of BCG, based on historical comparisons of reported toxicity with other preparations, has not been confirmed in this first randomized comparison of two BCG preparations. Furthermore, it stresses the need for an exact definition of toxicity and side effects to be used by each investigator and the need for prospective comparison of several BCG preparations.

CONCLUSIONS

Serious, potentially fatal complications of intravesical BCG therapy occur. At least 3 deaths from intravesical therapy with BCG have occurred. While the incidence of fatal reactions is difficult to determine, it may be as high as 0.3%, since 2 deaths occurred in 610 patients given BCG-Connaught in the Southwest Oncology Group study. Since no other series has reported fatal BCG reactions, it is hoped that the true incidence is significantly lower. Despite this serious toxicity, the risk to benefit ratio clearly favors the use of BCG in all but those patients who are at low risk of tumor recurrence or progression, i.e. those with primary grade 1, stage Ta papillary transitional cell carcinoma.

Most of the severe irritative side effects and subsequent systemic complications can be prevented with prophylactic Isoniazid given for 3 days, beginning the morning before treatment. Patients with life-threatening systemic Bacillus Calmette-Guérin infection or anaphylaxis should receive 500 mg Cycloserine twice daily for the initial 3 days in addition to combination anti-tuberculous therapy because the rapid action of this drug may be life-saving. Direct intralesional Bacillus Calmette-Guérin immunotherapy can produce sepsis and death, and should be avoided, but it is important to stress that intravesical Bacillus Calmette-Guérin generally is well tolerated and has produced no complications in more than 95% of the patients treated. Furthermore it is essential that general physicians and urologists are keen to recognize possible BCG induced complications as early as possible in order to start immediately adequate treatment.

REFERENCES

Andriole GL (1988). Personal communication.
Aungst WC, Sokal JE, Blair VJ (1975). Complications of BCG vaccination in neoplastic disease. Ann Internal Med 82: 666.
Bast RC, Zbar D, Borsos T, Rapp HJ (1974). BCG and cancer. NEJM 290: 1413.
Bruce AW, Chan RCY, Pinkerton D, Morales A, Chadwick P (1983). Adherence of gram-negative uropathogens to human uro-epithelial cells. J Urol 130: 293.
Debruyne FMJ, van der Meijden APM, Geboers ADH, Franssen MPH, van Leeuwen MJW, Steerenberg PA, de Jong WH, Ruitenberg JJ (1988). BCG-RIVM versus Mitomycin intravesical therapy in superficial bladder cancer. First results of a randomized prospective trial. Urology (Suppl.) 31: 21.
Jurczyk-Procyk S, Martin M, Dubouch P, Gheorghiu M, Economides E, Khalil A, Rappaport H, Mathe G (1976). Toxicity studies of intravenously administered BCG in baboons. Cancer Immunol Immunother 1: 55.
Krutchik An, Buzdar AU, Akhtar M, Blumenschein GR (1980). Immune-complex glomerulonephritis secondary to non-specific immunotherapy. Cancer 45: 495.
Lamm DL, Reichert DF, Harris SC, Lucio RM (1982). Immunotherapy of murine transitional cell carcinoma. J Urol 128: 1104.
Lamm DL, Stogdill VD, Stogdill BJ, Crispen RG (1986). Com-

plications of Bacillus Calmette-Guérin immunotherapy in 1278 patients with bladder cancer. J Urol 135: 272.

Lee TS, Crispen RG (1973). Rapid quantative measurement of drug susceptibility of mycobacteria. Institute for Tuberculosis Research, Chicago, II. Internal publication.

Lotte A, Wasz-Höckert O, Poisson N, Dumitrescu N, Verron M, Couvet E (1984). BCG complications. Estimates of the risk among vaccinated subjects and statistical analysis of their main characteristics. Adv Tuberc Res 21: 107.

van der Meijden (1988). Non-specific immunotherapy with BCG-RIVM in superficial bladder cancer. Histological, immunological and therapeutic aspects. Thesis, University of Nijmegen.

Scharer L, Smith JP (1969). Serum transaminase elevations and other hepatic abnormalities in patients receiving Isoniazid. Ann Internal Med 71: 1113.

Schwarzenberg L, Sinmler MC, Pico JL (1976). Human toxicology of BCG applied in cancer immunotherapy. Cancer Immunol Immunother 1: 69.

deSousa GRM, Sant'Anna C, Lapa e Siva JR, Mano DB, Manhaes NM (1981). Intradermal BCG vaccination complications analysis of 51 cases. Tubercle 64: 23.

Sparks FC (1976). Hazards and complications of BCG immunotherapy. Med Clin N Amer 60: 499.

Steg A. Leleu C, Debré B, Boccon-Gibod L (1988). Systemic Bacillus Calmette-Guérin (BCG) infection in patients treated by intravesical BCG-therapy for bladder cancer. J Urol. 139: 300A.

Stilmant MM, Siroky MB (1986). Nephrogenic adenoma associated with intravesical Bacillus Calmette-Guérin treatment: a report of 2 cases. J Urol 135: 359.

EORTC Genitourinary Group Monograph 6:
BCG in Superficial Bladder Cancer, pages 357–360
© 1989 Alan R. Liss, Inc.

PERSPECTIVES FOR PROGRESS IN THE TREATMENT OF SUPERFICIAL
BLADDER CANCER. THE NEED FOR MULTI-INSTITUTIONAL STUDIES
AND THE POSSIBLE ROLE OF THE EORTC GENITO-URINARY GROUP

Michele Pavone-Macaluso, Vincenzo Serrette

Institute of Urology (M.P.-M.) and Interdepartment
Centre for Research in Clinical Oncology (V.S.),
University of Palermo, Palermo, Italy

Superficial bladder cancers are considered to have a
relatively good prognosis. This is only partially true,
because they tend to recur in at least 70% of the cases and
each recurrence carries a risk of progression in stage and
grade. Therefore, superficial tumors can lead to invasive
cancer and death.

Carcinoma in situ (CIS) is a somewhat different situation. In that there is a much greater potential for producing invasion and death. Topical chemotherapy (or immunotherapy with BCG) has only partially improved the course of
this disease. It is certainly capable of reducing recurrence rate and of prolonging the disease free interval. It
can probably reduce the tendency towards invasion, can lead
to prolonged or permanent regression of CIS and is likely
to reduce death rate of these patients, at least to some
extent. Various drugs and regimens have been found to be
useful, but unfortunately no significant progress has been
made in recent years. Especially in patients with bad risk
factors (multiplicity, prior recurrences, T1 tumors),
progression to a more invasive growth, occurrence of metastases and death from cancer may occur in about 20% of the
patients, in spite of prophylaxis with all the available
drugs.

In particular, despite increasing knowledge of the
prognostic factors, we are unable to detect from the very
beginning the superficial tumors that will show a favorable
course if properly treated with all the presently available
means, including transurethral surgery and chemotherapy or

immunotherapy if appropriate. Such patients cannot be
distinguished from those who will not respond to the treatment and will show an unfavorable course. The EORTC GU-
Group has been involved in several studies of local chemotherapy which have been summarized in recent reports (Kurth
et al., 1983; Denis et al., 1984; de Pauw et al., 1988).

In spite of these contributions, it seems that we have
now reached a plateau with our present methods of treatment, and that no further progress is likely to occur,
unless new thought is given to these problems and new
possibilities are explored.

WHAT ARE THE POSSIBLE NEW AVENUES TO FOLLOW, IN THE HOPE THAT WE CAN GET BETTER RESULTS?

The research for new drugs

It has been shown that many anticancer drugs, due to
the fact that they act in high concentration, are capable
of producing regression of papillary tumors. Some are not
cross-resistant and a response can be obtained even if a
previous drug has failed. There is therefore, a need for
investigating new drugs and new methods of immunotherapy.
No data are available, so far, about the use of Inter-
leukin-2 (IL-2) and Tumor Necrosis Factor (TNF). This can
be achieved by studies of so called "chemoresection" in
cases with multiple papillary tumors, where a marker lesion
is left after resecting the other ones. Local treatment
with the drug under test is then instituted.

The design for a better modality of treatment

The way the topical treatments are administered is
largely empirical and little is known about optimal concentration, interval between instillations and duration of the
treatment. It is likely that higher concentrations and more
prolonged contact time may improve the results obtained
with a given drug. This possibility may be investigated by
comparing standard versus a novel time/concentration
schedule in patients with CIS.

The association of various drugs

The association of various drugs and, in particular, of a "classic" chemotherapeutic agent (such as Thiotepa, Doxorubicin, and Mitomycin-C) or their newest derivatives (Epirubicin) with an immunomodulating agent, such as BCG or IL-2 or TNF, should be tested. It is surprising that, in spite of the widespread use of drug combinations in the systemic treatment of solid tumors, so little information has been obtained in the field of local intravesical treatment.

There is a need for basic information in order to select the most favorable approach:
a. In cell systems. In a suitable cell line or in short-term culture, it would be essential to find out, in a step-wise fashion:
   - which drugs are synergic, additive or counter-productive.
   - which is the best modality of combined treatment: either both drugs present in the same solution at the same time if chemically compatible, or sequential treatment, with the aim of discovering which drug should be used first, and which is the most effective schedule.
b. In experimental models, such as the FANFT-produced bladder tumors in rats.
c. In man, after the previous basic investigations have suggested a preferential approach to be followed.

The identification of more specific risk factors

The identification of more specific risk factors is warranted, e.g. morphological or biochemical differences which may be associated with different patterns of response, in spite of a similar histological appearance. It would be useful if non-responders could be identified, by means of flow-cytometry, computerized morphological analysis, markers, oncogene products, or growth factors. There would be a need for a more sophisticated (albeit more costly and time-consuming) work-up of all patients to be submitted to any kind to topical treatment; so that retrospective analysis could hopefully identify patients who are likely to show a good response from those - e.g. with CIS - who will benefit from immediate cystectomy.

In order to achieve this programme, it is essential that it is rationalized into progressive steps and that all the energies of a large co-operative group are put together, in oder to obtain large numbers of patients for meaningful comparison.

The EORTC Genito-Urinary Group appears to be ideal under this regard.

REFERENCES

Denis L. Pavone-Macaluso M, de Pauw M, and members of the EORTC GU Group (1984). In Küss R et al. (eds): "Bladder Cancer, part B," New York: Alan R. Liss, pp 429-439.

Kurth KH, Schulman C, Pavone-Macaluso M, Robinson M, de Pauw M, Sylvester R, and members of the EORTC GU Group (1983). Current status of EORTC protocols for superficial bladder cancer. Proc 13th International Congress of Chemotherapy, Vienna, Abstract SE 12.1.7/1-4.

de Pauw M, and the EORTC Genito-urinary Group (1988). Ongoing trials in bladder cancer conducted by the EORTC genito-urinary tract cancer co-operative group. In Smith PH, Pavone-Macaluso M (eds): "Management of advanced cancer of prostate and bladder," New York; Alan R. Liss, pp 215-223.

EORTC Genitourinary Group Monograph 6:
BCG in Superficial Bladder Cancer, pages 361–369
© 1989 Alan R. Liss, Inc.

FUTURE CLINCIAL RESEARCH ON THE USE OF BCG FOR BLADDER CANCER

Alvaro Morales, J. Curtis Nickel

Department of Urology, Queen's University, Kingston, Ontario, Canada

Perhaps the easiest and most enjoyable task of this workshop is to address the question of future research directions from the clinical point of view. It simply involves suggesting some of the projects one would like to do if one were to have unlimited funds and the patient accrual capabilities of the European Organization for Research and Treatment on Cancer (EORTC), the Eastern Co-operative Oncology Group (ECOG) and the Southwestern Oncology Group (SWOG) combined!

The organizers of this workshop are to be congratulated for their vision and timing. The clinical use of BCG for superficial bladder cancer has been firmly established for almost a decade but a great deal of important information is either lacking or not widely known. Two fundamental lessons can be drawn from the various studies included in this volume:

1. Much has been learned as to the mechanisms of action of the vaccine both at the experimental and clinical levels. However, our understanding of how it works is still inadequate.
2. There is a critical need for recognition of the more suitable preparations, to establish guidelines for its appropriate side effects and assessment of therapeutic response. Needless to say, but worth emphasizing, these needs can only be fulfilled by the vigorous research efforts of both basic scientists and clinicians.

Although one is fully aware of the current limitations of financial support for biomedical research, we have to deal with the added difficulty of investigating an agent considered "obsolete" by most reviewers from research granting agencies. In an age of amazing achievements in biotechnology the bacterium so carefully developed by Calmette and Guérin 80 years ago may appear as a hold out from the stone age of tumor immunology and immunotherapy.

Undoubtedly, the most important responsibility of those involved in the clinical aspects of superficial bladder research is to provided the practicing physisian with accurate, reliable information regarding available treatments. I believe that in order to accomplish this, future clincial research should be directed, primarily but not exclusively, to the following areas.

HOW IT WORKS

One must assume here that BCG is effective in super-ficial bladder cancer. This is agreed upon. Dr. Ratliff has referred already to the initiator and effector mechanisms of action of the vaccine. Let us first examine the initiator mechanisms. There is a general consensus that the attachment of BCG to the bladder mucosa following intra-vesical administration is a fundamental, early process which must take place if a therapeutic effect is to be achieved. But, how does this attachment take place? Evidence has been presented (Morales and Nickel, 1986) indicating that the initial interaction between the urothelium and the BCG is mediated through an exopoly-saccharide glycocalyx produced by the live, metabolically active bacteria (Fig. 1). Furthermore, as shown by Ratliff, the mediation of fibronectin in this regard may be of crucial importance (Ratliff et al., 1988). These two observations are, obviously, of relevance but by no means conclusive. Therefore, we have to elucidate further the steps of initial interaction between the vaccine and its host. Would it not be wonderful to identify and isolate the subcellular fraction (or fractions) of the bacillus responsible for the anti-neoplastic effects? This is a topic which clearly deserves a major research effort.

Much is currently known about the effector mechanisms of BCG. Thus, enhancement of macrophages, T- and NK-cell activities have been described following administrations of the vaccine (de Jong et al., 1987; Merguerian et al.,

1987). Other immune modulators such as Interferons and Interleukins are also known to be produced after BCG therapy. Little is understood, however, about the therapeutic relevance of these observations. Is each one of these effects important, perhaps crucial? Do some of these mechanisms act synergistically? How can they be enhanced? Why do they fail to operate in some individuals? Indeed, a large research effort appears to be needed just to answer these important but, by no means, all inclusive topics regarding mechanisms of action of the vaccine.

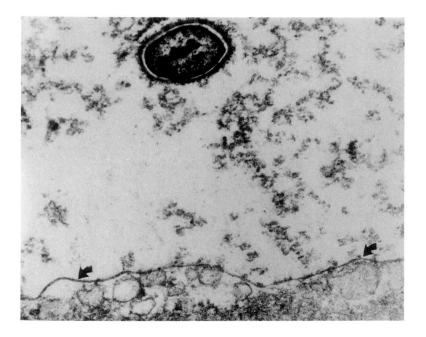

Figure 1. Interaction between the BCG and the urothelium. The arrows demonstrate the urothelial cell wall which is in contact with exopolysaccharide being produced by the bacterium. It is apparent that this represents the primary interaction between the vaccine and its host.

MODE OF ADMINISTRATION

The initial clinical protocol of over a decade ago called for a course of 6 weekly instillations together with intradermal administration. Just recently some modifications to this protocol have been introduced: The abandonment of intradermal administration and various schedules to increase the treatment period to 12 and up to 100 weeks as well as variable intervals between adminstrations. Most investigators agree that a 6 weeks course is sub-optimal but we and others have failed to show that this is the case (Badalament et al., 1987; Morales, 1988). Fortunately this is an area which is receiving much attention and it is expected that firm recommendations may become available in the near future.

A note of caution should be inserted here regarding the abandonment of the intradermal route. This intradermal administration adds inconvenience to the investigator and to the patient. One gets the impression that this has played a major role in its abandonment. Nevertheless, this simple modification has not been researched adequately and deserves further study.

The oral adminstration of BCG as proposed by Netto and Lemos has not received acceptance (Netto and Lemos, 1984). It is fortunate that Dr. Lamm has decided to take a second look at this approach. It is an issue which should be conclusively clarified. Lamm's results will be welcomed by all.

THERAPEUTIC DOSAGE

Early work by us and others showed that the therapeutic dose range of BCG is relatively narrow .... in mice (Morales et al., 1980; Pang and Morales, 1982; Soloway, 1977). However, dose response studies in humans are simply not available. Drs. Pagano and Alfthan (see previous chapters) have found no therapeutic detriment by reducing the dose originally employed (120-150 mg) by half. We have a similar experience with a small group of patients followed for less than 2 years (Morales, 1988). A controlled study addressing this question is of relevance since lower doses may be associated with better tolerance without decreasing the antitumor response.

VACCINE SUPPLIER

All the currently available vaccine is derived from the original strain developed at the Pasteur Institute. The bacterium, however, is not difficult to culture and an number of substrains are being used for cancer research purposes. In urological cancer the following are most commonly used: Frappier (Montreal), Pasteur (Paris), Connaught (Toronto), Tice (Chicago), Trudeau (Lake Saranack), Moreau (Sao Paulo), and RIVM (Bilthoven). However, it should be remembered that many years of independent evolution may have resulted in marked drifting of important biological effects between strains.

It must be reiterated here that one is dealing with a biological product subject to significant variation in activity between batches from the same manufacturer and even inter-manufacturer discrepancies.

This is a crucial aspect at this point of BCG development as an anti-neoplastic agent. While cytotoxic chemotherapeutics from one particular pharmaceutical company is normally consistent and equal in composition and biological activity to the one produced by its competitors, the same is not true in regard to BCG.

It is anticipated that from the current pack of manufacturers, a couple of winners shall emerge. But leadership and confidence are not given or inherited. They are earned by hard work and innovation. In my view those working close with the investigators and clinicians will obtain a definite advantage. The finalists, however, must be the ones with a consistent product of reliable composition, easy to store, mix and administer. In addition, those able to introduce newly developed methods to the manufacturing and delivery systems to increase therapeutic effectiveness and decrease undesirable side effects will be the ones receiving the widest acceptance.

UNDESIRABLE SIDE EFFECTS

In previous chapters of this monograph we have learned that intravesical administration of BCG is not devoid of side effects. Most, if not all, effective anti-neoplastic agents exhibit more or less severe side effects. Fortunately, the majority of BCG-induced complications are minor and self-limiting. They are of concern but, should be assessed against the potential benefits. There are, however, major complications, the most serious being BCG sepsis. It is of interest that this has occured almost exclusively in males with the common denominator being a traumatic urethral catheterization preceding the development of the serious episode. Very vigorous anti-tuberculosis therapy (i.e. Isoniazide, Rifampicin, Streptomycin, Cycloserine) has been recommended together with equally vigorous support measures, on occason requiring intensive care facilities for monitoring and treatment. Fortunately these episodes are exceedingly rare and most probably preventable by experienced individuals using proper delivery systems.

While we are on the topic of anti-tuberculous therapy, the questions of its routine prophylactic use is worth mentioning as a possible subject for further study. It is currently advocated that Isoniazide should be given in the presence of mild systemic (i.e. persistent fever, malaise) or moderate localized symptoms (bladder irritability). Nevertheless, supportive evidence for the routine use of Isoniazide during the course of BCG immunizations is scattered and still unconvincing. Although anti-tuberculous medication may, indeed, not diminish the efficacy of the vaccine, there exists concerns that the initiator events mentioned earlier may be inhibited.

HOST FACTORS

This is a huge area which remains largely unexplored due, in large part, to the difficulties inherent in human research. Intuition, a large body of animal research and some clinical studies suggest that the effectiveness of anti-cancer immune modulation is inversely proportional to the tumor burden. Does this apply to the interactions between BCG and superficial bladder cancer? Are some of the failures related to the extent of the lesions being treated? This does not appear to be a particularly difficult field of investigation, perhaps even one in which a retropective study may shed a great deal of light with a relatively small effort.

One cannot ignore the need for assessing host immuno-competence. A consensus does not exist regarding the relationship between responsiveness to BCG and delayed cutaneous hypersensitivity to PPD. This controversial issue could be easily included in the protocols being developed by the large co-operative groups active in Europe and North America.

COMBINED CYTOTOXIC CHEMOTHERAPY AND BCG

These two modalities are not mutually exclusive. Adolphs reported a better effect of the vaccine when used in combination with Cyclophosphamide, presumably by the latter affecting the suppressor T-cell population (Adolphs and Bastian, 1983). A Finnish study described earlier in this monograph has addressed this phenomenon using Mitomycin. Obviously, several additional cytotoxic agents appear likely candidates for further investigation.

The question of first line of treatment (luckily for the urologist, endoscopic surgery maintains its prominent place!) begs for an answer. Debruyne found no significant difference in effectiveness although Soloway (see previous chapter) has provided evidence suggesting a marginal superiority of BCG over Mitomycin in therapeutic efficacy (Debruyne et al., 1988). Cost considerations give the vaccine a significant advantage. But, is Thiotepa now out of the race? Where does Doxorubicin fit in the therapeutic scheme? Should Epodyl be allowed to fade away gracefully? These questions also remain unsolved.

Above all we should remember that BCG is not the final answer and that the search for new agents (or new applications of old ones) for superficial bladder cancer must be pursued.

Fortunately, comparative trials have been recently activated. Let us hope that they will provide many answers and not further questions.

NEW APPLICATIONS

A very limited experience exists on the use of the vaccine for treatment of superficial tumors in the upper tracts. The well planned and careful approach described earlier by Studer (see previous chapter) provides a path to plan further protocols.

Netto and Lamm have reported their early experience on the use of BCG for minimally invasive disease in a carefully selected population (Lamm, 1987; Netto and Lemos, 1984). The results are encouraging but must be viewed with caution and very guarded optimism. As with the upper tracts, a protocol addressing this issue appears warranted.

A great deal of concern exists for the observation that BCG treatment may eliminate bladder lesions without affecting transitional cell carcinoma of the prostate or lower ureters. While basic research looks for an explanation for such an occurrence, the clinican could explore ways to facilitate contact between the vaccine and the tumor cells. Some suggestions have appeared in the literature (i.e. prostatic resection followed by further BCG administration). Solid research in this area is sorely needed.

FINANCIAL SUPPORT

Finally, one must address the question of financial support for clinical research on BCG. The vaccine has been around for some 80 years and reached its peak of glamour and stardom during the renaissance of non-specific active immunotherapy in the early 1970s. Outside the field of urological oncology it is largely perceived as mostly ineffective at best and dangerous at worst. Changing this erroneous concept in some quarters may be the most difficult task of all!

The message to take home from this workshop is then obvious: Much remains to be learned about BCG. Once all is learned, BCG as we know it today, will be truly a thing of the past to be regarded as a medical curiosity for once its components have been dissected and the therapeutic fractions identified and isolated, they will replace the bacillus that was evolved through the efforts of Calmette and Guérin for purposes they never envisioned.

REFERENCES

Adolphs HD, Bastian HP (1983). Chemoimmune prophylaxis of superficial bladder cancer. Urol 129: 29.
Badalament RA, Herr HW, Wong GY, Gnecco C, Pinsky CM,

Whitmore WF, Fair WR, Oettgen HF (1987). A prospective randomized trial of maintenance vs non-maintenance intravesical BCG therapy for superficial bladder cancer. J Clin Oncol 5: 441.

Debruyne FMJ, van der Meijden APM, Geboers ADH, Franssen MPH, van Leeuwen MJW, Steerenberg PA, de Jong WH, Ruitenberg EJ (1988). BCG (RIVM) versus Mitomycin intravesical therapy in patients with superficial bladder cancer. Urology 31: 21.

de Jong WH, Steerenberg PA, Ruitenberg EJ (1987). BCG and its use for cancer immunotherapy. In "Tumor Immunology - Mechanisms, Diagnosis and Therapy", Amsterdam: Elsevier.

Lamm DL (1987). BCG immunotherapy for superficial bladder cancer. In Ratliff TL, Catalona WJ (eds): "Genito-urinary Cancer," Boston: M. Nijhoff.

Merguerian PA, Donahue L, Cockett ATK (1987). Intraluminal Interleukin-II and BCG for treatment of bladder cancer. J Urol 136: 216.

Morales A, Djeu J, Herberman RB (1980). Immunization by whole cells or cell extracts against an experimental bladder tumor. Invest Urol 17: 310.

Morales A, Nickel JC (1986). Immunotherapy of superficial bladder cancer with BCG. World J Urol 3: 209.

Morales A (1988). Improvements in the use of BCG for superficial bladder cancer. J Urol 139: 310A.

Netto Jr NR, Lemos GC (1984). BCG immunotherapy of bladder cancer. J Urol 132: 675.

Pang ASD, Morales A (1982). Immunoprophylaxis of a murine bladder cancer with high dose BCG immunizations. J Urol 127: 1006.

Ratliff TL, Kavoussi LR, Catalona WJ (1988). Role of fibronectin in intravesical BCG therapy for superficial bladder cancer. J Urol 139: 410.

Soloway MS (1977). Intravesical and systemic chemotherapy of murine bladder cancer. Cancer Res 37: 2918.

Index